Handbook of Patient Care in Cardiac Surgery

Handbook of Patient Care in Cardiac Surgery

Fifth Edition

Gus J. Vlahakes, M.D.
Associate Professor of Surgery, Harvard Medical School; Associate Visiting Surgeon, Cardiac Surgical Unit, Massachusetts General Hospital, Boston

John H. Lemmer, Jr., M.D.
Cardiothoracic Surgeon, Good Samaritan Hospital, Portland, Oregon

Douglas M. Behrendt, M.D.
Professor of Thoracic Surgery, University of Iowa Medical School; Chairman of Cardiothoracic Surgery, University of Iowa Hospitals and Clinics, Iowa City, Iowa

W. Gerald Austen, M.D.
Edward D. Churchill Professor of Surgery, Harvard Medical School; Surgeon-in-Chief, Massachusetts General Hospital, Boston

Little, Brown and Company
Boston   New York   Toronto   London

Copyright © 1994 by Gus J. Vlahakes, John H. Lemmer, Jr., Douglas M. Behrendt, and W. Gerald Austen

Fifth Edition

Previous editions copyright © 1980, 1985 by Douglas M. Behrendt and W. Gerald Austen; © 1972, 1976 by Little, Brown and Company (Inc.)

All rights reserved. No part of this book may be reproduced in any form or by any electronic or mechanical means, including information storage and retrieval systems, without permission in writing from the publisher, except by a reviewer who may quote brief passages in a review.

Library of Congress Cataloging-in-Publication Data

Handbook of patient care in cardiac surgery / Gus J. Vlahakes . . . [et al.]. — 5th ed.
    p.   cm.
  Rev. ed. of: Patient care in cardiac surgery / Douglas M. Behrendt, W. Gerald Austen. 4th ed. c1985.
  Includes bibliographical references and index.
  ISBN 0-316-08779-3
  1. Heart — Surgery. 2. Postoperative care. 3. Therapeutics, Surgical. I. Vlahakes, Gus J. II. Behrendt, Douglas M. Patient care in cardiac surgery.
  [DNLM: 1. Heart Surgery. 2. Patient Care Planning.
WG 169 P298 1994]
RD598.B39   1994
617.4'12 — dc20
DNLM/DLC
for Library of Congress   93-49425
                                                                  CIP

Second Printing

Printed in the United States of America

RRD-VA

Editorial: Nancy Chorpenning
Production Editor: Kellie Cardone
Copyeditor: Cathi Cote
Indexer: Nancy Newman
Production Supervisor: Madeline Belliveau
Cover designer: Hannus Design Associates

Contents

	Preface	vii
1.	Preoperative Evaluation and Management	1
2.	Operative Management	29
3.	Postoperative Management	62
4.	Postoperative Complications Involving the Heart and Lungs	105
5.	Postoperative Complications Involving Other Organ Systems	157
6.	Late Postoperative Management	183
7.	Management of Infants and Children	197
8.	Transplantation	229

Appendixes

1.	Recommendations for Preventing Bacterial Endocarditis	261
2.	Usual Dosages of Drugs Commonly Used in Adults	263
3.	Usual Dosages of Drugs Commonly Used in Infants and Children	270
4.	Desired Serum Concentration of Drugs Commonly Used in the Care of Cardiac Surgery Patients	273
5.	Adjustments in Drug Dose or Dosing Interval for Cardiac Surgery Patients with Renal Impairment	275
6.	Nomogram for Determining Body Surface Area from Height and Weight	280

Index 281

Preface

Handbook of Patient Care in Cardiac Surgery, or *Patient Care in Cardiac Surgery*, as it was known in prior editions, began at Massachusetts General Hospital when Drs. Behrendt and Austen decided to publish the manual written and updated by the MGH cardiac surgical chief residents. The book initially reflected "the MGH way" of rendering postoperative cardiac care. As the field of cardiac surgery has grown and as our cases have become more complex, the book has grown in size and broadened in scope. This is the first edition in which Drs. Gus Vlahakes and John Lemmer have participated as the primary authors, as the tradition is passed from Drs. Behrendt and Austen.

The primary objectives of *Handbook of Patient Care in Cardiac Surgery*, Fifth Edition, are two-fold: First, it is intended as a reference to data referred to frequently during the course of patient care, with tables, charts, and appendixes included for rapid access; second, it is a learning vehicle, allowing a newcomer to sit down and read a chapter on some discrete aspect of patient care and quickly and easily gain an overview of the subject, including selected current references for further study. The book does *not* endeavor to teach contemporary treatment of cardiac disease, nor is it intended to teach cardiac surgical technique beyond the selected aspects necessary for postoperative care.

This book is written for surgical house staff and cardiothoracic trainees involved in the postoperative care of cardiac surgical patients. The nursing perspective is critically important and is incorporated throughout the text. We hope this book will be useful to everyone involved in the postoperative care of cardiac surgical patients.

G. J. V.
J. H. L., Jr.
D. M. B.
W. G. A.

Handbook of
Patient Care in
Cardiac Surgery

Notice
The indications and dosages of all drugs in this book have been recommended in the medical literature and conform to the practices of the general medical community. The medications described do not necessarily have specific approval by the Food and Drug Administration for use in the diseases and dosages for which they are recommended. The package insert for each drug should be consulted for use and dosage as approved by the FDA. Because standards for usage change, it is advisable to keep abreast of revised recommendations, particularly those concerning new drugs.

Preoperative Evaluation and Management

General Considerations

Because of the availability of accurate, quantitative diagnosis, patients being considered for cardiac surgery usually have a detailed evaluation of their pathophysiology, pathologic anatomy, and abnormal hemodynamics. A thorough and precise diagnosis is an essential first step in the surgical treatment of heart disease. Often, this evaluation is done by the referring cardiologist; however, it is the surgeon's responsibility to ensure that the patient's evaluation is complete and that all information needed to plan the appropriate operative treatment has been obtained. In recent years, there has been an increasing trend to rely on noninvasive modalities, such as color Doppler echocardiography; however, although these may help determine the diagnosis, there are many instances in which invasive diagnostic methods are still needed.

Since the last edition of this book in 1985, there have been changes in the indications for surgery for various cardiac lesions. To illustrate, traditionally, prosthetic valve replacement was indicated based, in part, on the patient's symptoms, such as angina, syncope, or shortness of breath. With the availability of valve reconstruction techniques and with the recognition that long-standing valve lesions may predispose to deterioration of heart rhythm and ventricular function, a trend toward earlier intervention for valvular heart disease has developed.

In an analogous way, there has been a tremendous evolution in the indications for coronary artery bypass surgery. The advent of percutaneous angioplasty has dramatically changed the surgical indications, as well as the nature of the patient population requiring operation. Surgeons should expect to see patients who are older, who have more extensive and diffuse distal coronary artery disease, and who may have poor ventricular function as the result of long-standing disease. With the advancing age of these patients, other associated medical problems such as diabetes, chronic renal failure, peripheral vascular disease, and obstructive lung disease pose increasing challenges for postoperative management. These changes in the practice of coronary artery surgery have increased the demands on the team for pre- and postoperative care.

A very important component in the care of each cardiac surgical patient is the orientation and teaching provided the patient by the cardiac surgical nursing staff. This usually begins at the time of admission and occurs in conjuction with medical/surgical evaluation. To obtain maximal cooperation from the patient and to aid in the prevention of postoperative psychosis, the nursing staff should orient the patient (and also a child's parents) to the intensive care unit, monitoring equipment, nursing routines, oxygen masks, and the function of tubes, catheters, and invasive monitoring lines that will be used in the postoperative period. The possibility of and function of prolonged endotracheal intubation and tracheostomy should be discussed, particularly in patients with known, preexisting lung disease. Instructions should be given in proper deep breathing, incentive spirometry, coughing, and leg exercises. Figure 1-1 is a checklist that can be used by the nursing staff as a guideline for preoperative teaching. Teaching aids such as dolls, puppets, and cartoons have proved useful in preparing children for operation.

Preoperative Evaluation and Management

In contrast to those patients referred to other surgical subspecialties, many patients will come for cardiac surgical treatment after an extensive evaluation by a cardiologist. In addition to concerns about proper diagnostic evaluation, it is the responsibility of the surgeon and his or her team to ensure that all preoperative issues are considered. Many of the surgically related aspects may not have been addressed during a cardiology workup. As part of the immediate preoperative evaluation, the collating of patient-related data into a usable database is extremely important. In some institutions, patient histories and data may be placed in a computer-based database, but this may not be applicable to all institutions. Therefore, the use

Does this patient know and understand?	Yes	No	Needs teaching	Sig RN
1. No smoking	☐	☐	☐	☐
2. Daily weights, sodium-restricted diet, and strict fluid limit	☐	☐	☐	☐
3. Role of chest therapist	☐	☐	☐	☐
4. How to turn, cough, deep breathe, and exercise legs	☐	☐	☐	☐
5. Pulmonary function tests	☐	☐	☐	☐
6. Cardiac catheterization (if necessary)	☐	☐	☐	☐
7. Routine chest x-rays, blood work, ECGs, pre- and postoperatively	☐	☐	☐	☐
8. Preoperative prep incl. medications and effect, skin shave, enema, Foley catheter, CVP line	☐	☐	☐	☐
9. Responsibility for personal effects	☐	☐	☐	☐
10. Preanesthesia room	☐	☐	☐	☐
11. Personnel and environment of the surgical intensive care unit, visiting regulations for family, duration of stay	☐	☐	☐	☐
12. Routine equipment encountered postoperatively incl. IVs, blood transfusions, endotracheal tube, respirator, monitor, chest tubes, etc.	☐	☐	☐	☐
13. Transfer to convalescent ward	☐	☐	☐	☐
14. Progression of activity	☐	☐	☐	☐
15. Normal feelings after surgery	☐	☐	☐	☐

Fig. 1-1. Checklist for cardiac surgery preoperative teaching.
Key: Sig RN: Nurse(s) sign or initial to signify that each item on the checklist has been completed. (Courtesy of the Department of Nursing, Massachusetts General Hospital.)

of a data worksheet in the preoperative evaluation and preparation of patients is essential (Fig. 1-2). This brief excerpt of the patient's database should contain pertinent information needed for critical intraoperative decisions and postoperative management. This may be especially difficult for the admitting physicians in an era when insurance carriers are insisting on outpatient evaluation and even same day admissions for open heart surgery; yet it is imperative lest some important piece of data "fall through the cracks."

At the time of admission to the surgical service, the admitting physician must have access to a complete report of the patient's cardiac catheterization. Medical records at the admitting hospital, such as records of a recent admission for preoperative evaluation, must be available for review. Of particular importance are operative reports from previous cardiac, thoracic, or vascular operations. If there has been a recent admission or if the patient has had any recent, specialized laboratory studies, these data should be provided in the preoperative database.

HISTORY AND PHYSICAL EXAMINATION

The database should include a recent list of all of the patient's medications. Any recent changes in medications, such as an increasing diuretic requirement or the need for the addition of antiarrhythmic therapy, should be noted. If any drug dosages have been adjusted according to blood levels, that information should be available, as it will guide possible postoperative use of these medications. Medication allergies, either documented or suspected, should be prominently displayed in the database.

There are certain aspects of the admission physical examination that are important in cardiac surgery and deserve special attention. First, since patients having cardiac surgery will be subjected to extracorporeal circulation, a thorough peripheral vascular examination is essential. This should include surveillance for carotid bruits as well as a detailed recording of peripheral pulses. The peripheral vascular examination has assumed increasing importance in recent years because of the advancing age of the patient population and the increase in the general severity of diffuse atherosclerosis that is being seen by cardiac surgeons. In patients undergoing coronary revascularization surgery, the quantity and quality of the saphenous veins should be assessed. Proper examination is performed with the patient standing. The vein can usually be located on the medial aspect of the ankle. Varicosities and skin changes of chronic venous insufficiency are noted. If there are concerns about absent or diseased lower extremity veins, ultrasound mapping of the greater and lesser saphenous systems should be performed; if this modality is not available, then contrast venography is indicated. In obese patients, it is useful to mark the course of the saphenous veins with an indelible marker at the time of venous mapping [1]. Attention should be paid to the patient's skin, particularly in areas where surgical sites may be located. The presence of acne on the presternal skin or in the inguinal area will increase the risk of wound infection and may require special attention or a delay in surgery, if indicated.

Examination of the patient's dentition should be included in the

```
PREOPERATIVE CARDIAC SURGICAL SUMMARY

NAME_____AGE_____SEX_____ MGH#_____
CARDIOLOGIST_____SURGEON_____TENTATIVE OR DATE_____
DIAGNOSIS_____
HISTORY_____
_____
_____
_____

ETT/Thallium_____
GBPS_____
Echo_____

OTHER MEDICAL PROBLEMS_____
_____
_____

ALLERGIES_____
RECENT MEDICATIONS_____
_____

Other_____
_____

SIGNIFICANT PHYSICAL FINDINGS      BP RIGHT ARM_____      BY LEFT ARM_____    P_____
```

PULSES:		CAROTIDS	BRACH	RADIAL	ULNAR	FEM	POP	POST TIB	DORS PED
	RIGHT								
	LEFT								
	BRUITS								

```
CARDIAC EXAM_____
_____
CHEST AND LUNGS_____
RIGHT SAPHENOUS VEIN_____    LEFT SAPHENOUS VEIN_____
TEETH_____    SKIN_____
RECENT TEMP COURSE_____
RECTAL_____
NEUROLOGICAL DEFICITS_____

CHEST X-RAY DATE_____REPORT:_____
EKG DATE_____REPORT:_____
```

Fig. 1-2. Database worksheet for recording important preoperative patient information.
Key: BT = bleeding time; ABG = arterial blood gases; PFT = pulmonary function studies.

1. Preoperative Evaluation and Management

RECENT LAB	HCT	WBC	PT	PTT	PLATELETS	Na	K+	Cl	CO2	BUN	Cr	BS

	Ca	PO4	Amy	Bili	Alk Phos	CPK	SGOT	LDH	Chol	Tri	HDL	LDL	Digoxin

BT_____ABG's_____PFT's_____

Bacteriology	U/A	Urine	Sputum	Blood	Misc.

Cardiac Cath Data Date:_____   Ventriculogram: EF_____
Aortic Valve_____ _____
Mitral Valve_____
PA_____   LA_____   Coronary Arteries:
RV_____   LV_____   RCA_____
PA_____   AO_____   LM_____
PCW_____ CO_____   LAD_____
                                Diag_____
                                Ramus_____
                                Cfx_____

Issues:
1) <u>Diagnosis</u>_____ OR Date:_____
2) _____
3) _____
4) _____
5) _____
6) _____
7) _____
8) _____
9) _____
10) _____
_____
_____

Other:

preoperative evaluation. Necessary dental work should be completed before surgery, particularly when valve replacement or implantation of any prosthetic material is contemplated [2]. Because dental work can lead to significant bacteremia [3], antibiotic prophylaxis should be used. Amoxicillin is generally included in the regimen because the principal organisms involved in oral-related endocarditis are diphtheroids and alpha streptococci (see Chap. 6 for further discussion).

Routine adult cardiac surgery admission orders are shown in Table 1-1. Laboratory evaluation on admission should include a chest x-ray, ECG, complete blood count, blood typing for subsequent transfusion, and urinalysis. Unless performed during a recent medical evaluation, liver function studies should be obtained; these are particularly important in patients who have right ventricular failure or a history of hepatic dysfunction. Coagulation studies should include prothrombin time, partial thromboplastin time, and platelet count. Platelet function need not be assessed as a routine preoperative study.

Diagnostic Studies

CARDIAC CATHETERIZATION

Cardiac catheterization with cineangiography remains the gold standard in the preoperative evaluation of most types of cardiac disease. It is essential that the original 35-mm film record of the cardiac catheterization be available at the time of operation, particularly for coronary artery surgery. When patients are referred to the cardiac surgical service from an outside hospital, it is important that the original films be sent. If the films appear to be copies, these should be reviewed to ensure that the quality of the reproduction is adequate to show the pertinent anatomy. When patients are referred from centers where cardiac catheterization but not cardiac surgery is performed, it is important to ensure that an adequate study has been done. In general, patients who are more than 35 years old and are having a surgical procedure other than coronary artery surgery should have coronary arteriography as a part of routine cardiac catheterization. This study may be included in the assessment of younger patients if there is anything in the patient's history to suggest risk of atherosclerosis, such as strong family history or known hyperlipidemia. In patients with evidence of peripheral vascular disease, it is important to note whether or not cardiac catheterization was possible or difficult using the femoral approach.

ECHOCARDIOGRAPHY

In recent years, the technology of echocardiography with color Doppler flow analysis has expanded tremendously, and this diagnostic modality has enjoyed increasing importance in evaluating patients for cardiac surgery. Echocardiography provides details about intracardiac anatomy as well as ventricular function. Transesophageal echocardiography provides additional valuable information, particularly in the assessment of the mitral valve and aorta. Thus, for patients who are being considered as candidates for mitral value reconstruction or repair of congenital anomalies, echocardiography

Table 1-1. Routine Cardiac Surgery: Adult Admission Orders

Medication orders only	All other orders
	Scheduled operation
	NPO after midnight
Cefazolin 1 g IM on call to OR	Shave and prep chin to ankles bilaterally, including neck, both groins, and pubis
Hold diuretics	Shower with pHisoHex after prep
Hold digoxin	Paint neck, chest, abdomen, groins, and legs with providone-iodine solution
Magnesium citrate 180 cc PO afternoon prior to surgery	Confirm with blood bank that crossmatch sample is adequate and blood is set up
Fleets enema at bedtime before surgery	Addressograph and vital signs record to OR with chart
Lorazepam 0.5-1.0 mg PO q6h and at bedtime prn	If patient develops chest pain or other symptoms during the night prior to OR, notify MD on-call immediately

is an essential part of the preoperative evaluation. It is essential that cardiac surgeons understand the limitations of echocardiography as well as its capabilities. The echocardiogram may not accurately quantitate the degree of valvular regurgitation. It tends to overestimate valve gradients and, in this setting, may not always be a substitute for cardiac catheterization. Furthermore, the quality of an echo study is dependent not only on the quality of echocardiographic equipment, but also on the experience and knowledge of the echocardiographer. Echocardiography is an interactive study; this is particularly the case in congenital heart disease, where each aspect of the echocardiographic study depends on findings earlier in the study.

THALLIUM SCINTIGRAPHY

The development of thallium scintigraphy is an important milestone in the diagnostic evaluation of coronary artery disease. Thallium-201 chloride is a short-lived, radioactive analogue of potassium that is taken up from the blood into the myocardium in an amount proportional to myocardial blood flow. At our institutions, it is usually injected during peak exercise in an exercise stress test, and scintigraphic images of the heart are recorded at 5 minutes and 3 hours after injection. At 5 minutes, regions of the heart where there are defects in thallium uptake represent areas of decreased perfusion. At 3 hours, if these perfusion defects fill in (thallium "redistribution"), this is evidence of ischemia during exercise in muscle that is potentially viable. Persistent perfusion defects at 3 hours indicate a fixed scar. Thus, in patients in whom there is severely depressed ventricular function with regional akinesia, thallium scintigraphy can help to determine whether a given region of the heart contains viable muscle and will benefit from bypass. In instances where left ventricular filling pressures rise with stress or exercise, increased lung uptake of thallium may indicate ischemia-induced ventricular dysfunction.

Ideally, thallium scintigraphy should be performed at rest and during exercise-induced stress. However, there are some patients who cannot exercise because of peripheral vascular disease or orthopedic problems. In these instances, potentially ischemic myocardial distributions may be revealed by the use of dipyridamole [6] or adenosine [7] with thallium scintigraphy. These agents produce maximal coronary vasodilation, maximizing perfusion and thallium uptake in normal areas of the heart. Areas of the heart perfused through significantly diseased arteries will take up less tracer early after thallium injection and will demonstrate late redistribution, thus identifying regions of the heart with ischemic potential.

PULMONARY FUNCTION TESTING

Although not routinely performed, pulmonary function studies provide a noninvasive means of assessing a patient's pulmonary status and thus may be useful in the preoperative assessment of a patient's risk for surgery if there is severe lung disease. Knowledge of the patient's baseline lung function may help guide therapy in the postoperative period. In any patient in whom there is an extensive smoking history, a history of severe chronic obstructive lung disease or asthma, or symptoms or physical findings to suggest significant chronic lung disease, pulmonary function studies should be considered before elective cardiac surgery. In patients with any component of obstructive lung disease, the response to bronchodilators should be determined. As part of pulmonary function studies, if any significant abnormalities are noted in lung function, a determination of room air blood gases should be made. In patients with more severe chronic obstructive lung disease, it is important to determine whether these patients have chronic hypercarbia and depend on hypoxic drive for respiration. This may be essential information in the ventilatory weaning and management of these patients after cardiac surgery.

ELECTROPHYSIOLOGIC TESTING

In recent years, there have been major advances in the evaluation and treatment of patients with electrophysiologic disorders of the heart. Many patients now come to surgery for primary treatment of either supraventricular tachycardias or ventricular arrhythmias such as recurrent ventricular tachycardia or fibrillation. In patients with ventricular arrhythmias, the decision whether or not to include preoperative electrophysiologic testing remains a complex issue [8]. In patients with concomitant coronary disease in whom rest ischemia is noted on thallium scintigraphy, preoperative electrophysiologic testing may not be indicated because many of these patients will experience amelioration of their arrhythmias after revascularization. Electrophysiologic testing may be indicated, however, in patients with a fixed ventricular scar, to determine if concomitant ventricular surgery is needed to treat the origin of the arrhythmia or to determine if concomitant automatic defibrillator implantation is indicated. In general, if patients have presented with recurrent ventricular tachycardia or out-of-hospital ventricular fibrillation arrest without documented associated myocardial infarction, electrophysiologic testing is indicated.

Special Preoperative Problems

DEPRESSED LEFT VENTRICULAR FUNCTION

Because of advances made in cardiac surgery during the past decade, patients previously thought to be inoperable because of poor left ventricular function are now being considered for cardiac surgery. In particular, patients with advanced coronary artery disease who have intractable rest pain or life-threatening coronary artery anatomy face a dismal prognosis without revascularization. Although it is attractive to think of angioplasty as a good alternative for the high-risk surgical candidate, the severe, diffuse, multivessel nature of these patients' coronary disease often precludes percutaneous angioplasty. Thus, cardiac surgeons increasingly are being called on to manage these challenging patients. To the extent possible, clinical congestive heart failure should be controlled before surgery by careful adjustment of orally administered diuretics or afterload reduction agents. Information regarding the preoperative diuretic requirement may also be useful for postoperative management, as these patients will frequently have ongoing need for chronic diuretic therapy.

In situations where revascularization may not be complete and where operative ischemic time is predicted to be long, we have found it useful in patients with poor left ventricular function to initiate elective, preoperative intraaortic balloon counterpulsation. This is in recognition of the higher-than-usual need for balloon counterpulsation support after surgery. This may be particularly useful in instances where some peripheral vascular disease or vessel tortuosity is present and where fluoroscopic guidance for balloon pump insertion in the cardiac catheterization laboratory is helpful. In this setting, patients are taken to the cardiac catheterization laboratory during transfer to the operating room and an intraaortic balloon pump is inserted over a guidewire using percutaneous techniques, usually in the side opposite from that where saphenous vein harvesting is anticipated. Alternatively, balloon insertion can be done in the operating room before the induction of anesthesia.

Traditionally, balloon counterpulsation has been applied acutely to patients with extreme degrees of ventricular failure, namely patients who present with cardiogenic shock due to coronary artery disease and its complications. Previously, an aggressive surgical approach was employed in the treatment of many patients with cardiogenic shock [9]. The advent of thrombolytic therapy, however, is changing the approach to these patients, and the frequency with which the surgeon must deal with life-threatening cardiogenic shock may be decreasing. With the use of thrombolytic therapy, average infarct size has been reduced, and the incidence of mechanical complications of infarction, such as acute mitral regurgitation and postinfarction ventricular septal defects, has decreased.

LEFT MAIN CORONARY ARTERY DISEASE WITH UNSTABLE ANGINA

Patients with significant disease of the left main coronary artery will frequently present with unstable angina and are at risk for sudden death. These patients are notorious for developing arrhythmias or instability during cardiac catheterization, during the induction of anesthesia for cardiac surgery, and even during the normal handling of the heart before cardiopulmonary bypass. Tight left main coronary stenosis is associated with an increased perioperative mortality rate [10]. Maintenance of medical therapy including the use of nitrates, beta blockers to control heart rate, and heparin are all essential to maintain the patients' stability while they await operation. Any evidence of ischemia on such a regimen mandates immediate stabilization with balloon counterpulsation and early operation. Although these patients can certainly be managed by immediate surgery when they become unstable, their intraoperative course will be smoother and safer if they are initially stabilized by preoperative counterpulsation.

CRITICAL AORTIC STENOSIS

Like patients with left main coronary disease, patients with critical aortic stenosis have the propensity to become suddenly unstable or to die suddenly until the time they undergo valve replacement.

Unlike patients with coronary artery disease, there are no options for support with balloon counterpulsation and no really effective medical therapy that alters the pathophysiology of this lesion. Because of the imbalance between myocardial oxygen supply and demand, the maintenance of systemic pressure is important for myocardial perfusion before the time of surgery. Thus, these patients should not be treated excessively with diuretics because they produce volume depletion and hypotension that would initiate a downward spiral of the patients' hemodynamic status. Likewise, vasodilator therapy should be avoided. Balloon counterpulsation does little to stabilize these patients and, in instances where aortic stenosis is accompanied by some regurgitation, it may actually worsen the hemodynamic status. Thus, patients with critical aortic stenosis should undergo surgery as soon as possible and — if increasing heart failure is noted — on an emergency basis. In selected instances where surgery is not immediately possible because of factors such as concomitant pneumonia or evolving acute renal failure, some patients without regurgitation may be temporarily stabilized by percutaneous aortic valvuloplasty [11].

ACUTE VALVE REGURGITATION AND MALFUNCTIONING PROSTHETIC VALVES

Patients presenting with severe, acute, mitral regurgitation have generally acquired this lesion from a ruptured papillary muscle due to a myocardial infarction or as a complication of bacterial endocarditis. If the lesion is severe enough to produce cardiogenic shock, as may be the case with postinfarction papillary muscle rupture, these patients may be stabilized temporarily by balloon pump counterpulsation and then operated on emergently. Because ongoing cardiogenic shock may have cumulative deleterious effects on critical organ systems, there should be no delay in instituting this sequence of therapy.

In the setting of endocarditis cardiogenic shock is less common. These patients may be initially stabilized with antibiotic therapy, diuresis, and inotropic or afterload reduction medications. Ideally, they should have a period of antibiotic therapy before valve replacement to sterilize the native valve, but valve replacement can be successfully carried out even if this is not possible.

Patients with acute aortic regurgitation usually have this lesion either as a complication of aortic dissection or endocarditis. It results in wide pulse pressure with a low diastolic pressure. A natural cardiac reflex to minimize the effects of aortic regurgitation is tachycardia, which decreases the amount of time that the heart spends in diastole, during which time the regurgitation occurs. Thus, when these patients develop tachycardia, drugs such as beta-blocking agents should be assiduously avoided. Mechanical support by counterpulsation is not an option in this setting, as it requires a competent aortic valve. Surgical replacement or repair of the aortic valve is the essential treatment and it should be undertaken as soon as possible.

Acutely malfunctioning prosthetic valves produce relative surgical emergencies [12]. One situation is thrombosis of a mechanical prosthesis because of inadequate systemic anticoagulation, most commonly in the mitral position. This usually creates a clinical picture of mitral stenosis (± regurgitation) and severe failure. Immediate surgery is mandated. Patients may be heparinized before surgery, but thrombolytic therapy, considered an option by some, is associated with an 18% risk of systemic clot embolization [13] and is not used at our centers. Thrombosis of valves in the aortic position is less common because of the higher shear rate of blood flow past the prosthetic orifice. Acute prosthetic regurgitation may also occur with bioprosthetic tissue valves where calcification has resulted in leaflet stiffening and sudden fracture or with mechanical valves where a disc occluder has escaped from the prosthesis due to strut or disc fracture.

RECENT MYOCARDIAL INFARCTION

Patients who are stable and asymptomatic after an acute myocardial infarction and who require coronary bypass surgery generally should wait at least 1 to 2 weeks before operation. This recommendation may be modified if life-threatening anatomy, such as critical left-main stenosis, is present. Recent evidence suggests that symptomatic patients with recent infarction can undergo operation at any time with little or no increase in risk [14,15]. Each individual patient's treatment must be tailored to the clincial situation; for example, a patient with a large, acute transmural infarction with dyskinesis may benefit from additional time to heal, particularly if a subsequent aneurysmectomy is being considered.

POSTINFARCTION VENTRICULAR SEPTAL DEFECT

Postinfarction ventricular septal defect has become a less frequent occurrence since the advent of thrombolytic therapy and other measures that decrease the severity and size of myocardial infarctions. This is one of the lesions that produces acute cardiogenic shock and remains associated with very high morbidity and mortality. The treatment principles of postinfarction ventricular septal defect with shock have been articulated by many investigators in this field [16]. Stabilization by balloon counterpulsation, immediate cardiac catheterization, and immediate surgery is the preferred treatment sequence. Although some investigators have suggested that these patients could be dealt with in an elective manner, this option is limited to a select group of patients with small shunts who do not develop frank cardiogenic shock [17]. Early operation is essential when cardiogenic shock is present to prevent end-organ complications.

The diagnosis may be strongly suggested by the sudden appearance of a systolic murmur in a patient with an infarct and is confirmed by echocardiography. The patient in shock should undergo placement of monitoring catheters (radial artery, central venous, pulmonary artery) and should have support with intraaortic balloon counterpulsation. The unstable patient should undergo emergency repair of the septal defect. Cardiac catheterization should be done so that associated coronary stenoses can be identified for bypass.

THE FAILED ANGIOPLASTY

The treatment strategy for coronary artery disease changed dramatically with the introduction and growth of percutaneous coronary angioplasty. Although this has revolutionized the treatment of coronary artery disease, particularly single- and double-vessel disease, it has created a small number of patients who require urgent bypass surgery either because of immediate closure of a dilated coronary artery or because of a technical misadventure such as coronary arterial dissection or perforation [18]. Traditionally angioplasty has been performed only when there was an unoccupied operating room and a surgical team available. Because of the burgeoning volume of angioplasty candidates, this practice has been abandoned at many institutions. Certainly angioplasties should be performed only in hospitals where on-site surgical backup is available [19].

In general, patients with a failed angioplasty require urgent surgery if vessel closure or technical misadventure results in regional ischemia that cannot be controlled by immediate, repeat angioplasty [20]. While an operating room is being prepared, several measures can be employed. First, hemodynamics and filling pressures should be optimized, and nitrates may be added intravenously. The cardiologist may attempt to recross the closed vessel if a guidewire is still present and place a multiholed "bailout" catheter to provide temporary flow until surgery can be undertaken [21]. If there is any hemodynamic instability or if the degree of ischemia is severe, intraortic balloon pump support may be added. Once attempts to stabilize the patient are made, the patient should be taken to the first available operating room for complete surgical revascularization. Ideally, the entire process should take less than 2 hours from the onset of ischemia to the institution of cardiopulmonary bypass. Because these patients have not been prepared for surgery blood crossmatching should be initiated as early as possible after the need for surgery is ascertained.

HEMATOLOGIC AND COAGULATION
SYSTEM ABNORMALITIES

Cardiac procedures may be carried out despite known coagulation abnormalities such as hemophilia [22], Christmas disease [23], and von Willebrand's disease [24–26]. The hematologist should be involved early in the care of these patients, both to assist in evaluation and to manage any postoperative problems. The blood bank must be informed that specific component therapy will be required in unusual amounts in the perioperative period. Some elective patients, particularly those with hemophilia, may benefit from preoperative plasmapheresis [27].

Patients with erythrocyte abnormalities are usually identified before surgery. Hereditary spherocytosis or elliptocytosis may produce hemolysis; these patients may require a splenectomy before undergoing cardiac surgery [25]. Metabolic abnormalities such as glucose-6-phosphate deficiency may result in hemolysis that is triggered by certain drugs such as aspirin, quinidine, chloramphenicol, sulfonamides, and nitrofurans. Surgery may be conducted in these patients as long as these triggering agents are avoided [25]. Sickle cell trait (hemoglobin S) is present in the African-American population. These patients may undergo surgery but care should be taken to avoid hypoxia, hypothermia, dehydration, and acidosis, as these conditions may precipitate sickling. Preoperative administration of normal blood may also reduce the sickling risk in these patients [28,29].

Congenital heart disease may be accompanied by cyanosis and significant polycythemia. It is known that these patients can have a wide spectrum of abnormalities of coagulation and platelet function [30,31]. Care must be taken in interpreting laboratory tests because an elevated hematocrit can result in proportionately more anticoagulant than usual being present in the blood test tube as compared with plasma volume, thus resulting in misleading results. The amount of anticoagulation in the test tube should be reduced proportionately when blood samples are obtained from polycythemic patients. In older children and adults with congenital heart disease in whom the hematocrit exceeds 60%, preoperative phlebotomy may be useful, replacing removed red cell volume with fresh frozen plasma. By reducing the hematocrit below 55%, coagulation abnormalities may be improved, reducing postoperative bleeding [32–34]. Cardiac dynamics and oxygen transport after surgery may also be improved [35]. Ideally, phlebotomy should be carried out in a staged manner approximately 1 week before surgery, reducing the hematocrit by no more than 10% at each phlebotomy session. This should be performed most carefully in patients in whom pulmonary blood flow is derived from multiple small collaterals or from a surgically placed systemic-to-pulmonary shunt. In these instances, decreasing viscosity by phlebotomy may decrease systemic vascular resistance, resulting ultimately in decreased pulmonary blood flow and increasing cyanosis [36,37].

RENAL FAILURE

With the increasing number of patients with diffuse vascular disease and of older patients with long-standing diabetes, cardiac surgeons are treating more patients with chronic renal failure. The spectrum of patients includes those with only chemical abnormalities of renal function as well as patients who are functionally anephric and require chronic dialysis.

Patients with severe chronic renal failure requiring dialysis can undergo successful cardiac surgery [38–40]. When surgery is not urgent, patients may be prepared by intensive dialysis to optimize fluid and electrolyte balance and to minimize platelet dysfunction. The anesthetic technique and choice of anesthetic medications and adjuncts should be appropriately tailored to include agents that do not require renal excretion. Intraoperative technique must take into consideration the patient's inability to excrete immediately excessive fluid and electrolytes. Intraoperative ultrafiltration is helpful. Potassium cardioplegia is usually not a problem in anephric patients, as they can absorb a substantial amount of potassium in the intracellular space. Nonetheless, if large amounts of cardioplegia are contemplated or if preoperative hyperkalemia is of concern, cardioplegia should be removed from the circulation by appropriate discard drainage during infusion.

DIABETES

Diabetes management in cardiac surgery does not differ significantly from the approach used in general surgery, with a few caveats. In general, non–insulin-requiring diabetics will need only close monitoring of blood glucose levels after surgery. If patients take agents orally, these should be withheld the morning of surgery and restarted postoperatively when oral intake improves.

Diabetics who require insulin may pose a greater challenge, particularly if there is a history of labile blood glucose control or hospital admissions for ketoacidosis or hypoglycemia. We generally manage these patients on the day of surgery by administration of half their usual dose of insulin, coupled with administration of glucose-containing parenteral fluid up until the time of surgery. Cardiopulmonary bypass with hypothermia will decrease the efficacy of administered insulin, and there should be no excessive efforts to reduce blood glucose levels below 200 to 250 mg/dl, as hypoglycemia can occur when body temperature is restored and administered insulin becomes more effective. Insulin-requiring diabetics experience increased difficulties with wound infection and poor healing. This is especially true for leg incisions. Surgical technique must be particularly meticulous to avoid skin edge trauma. Severe diabetes is a relative contraindication to the use of bilateral internal mammary grafts because of the recognized greater incidence of nonhealing of the sternum and mediastinitis [41].

CHRONIC STEROID USE

Patients may be receiving systemic steroid therapy for a wide variety of disorders, ranging from autoimmune disease to obstructive lung disease or asthma to prior organ transplantation. Steroid use predisposes patients to a higher incidence of complications such as infection, poor healing, and ulcers, or it may exacerbate diabetes in the postoperative period.

In elective surgery, the indication for steroid therapy should be evaluated and the dose employed should be the minimum needed for interim management of the condition for which it is prescribed. These patients are generally managed by hydrocortisone supplementation during the early postoperative period. Hydrocortisone (100 mg) is administered intravenously before the operation. After surgery, it is administered intravenously at a dose of 100 mg every 8 hours and tapered over 3 to 4 days, at which times the patient should be able to resume orally administered steroids at the preoperative maintenance dose.

INFECTION

Traditionally, active infection has been a contraindication to cardiac surgery. In general, this principle still stands. However, with the increasing number of less stable patients, certain exceptions must be considered. Patients who have been in-hospital for more than a few days are always at increased risk for infection or at least colonization with hospital-acquired organisms. Low-grade and even moderate fever may be present without any clear focus of infection. When these patients undergo cardiac surgery, they should have all infusion and monitoring lines changed, and indwelling catheters that have been removed should be cultured [43]. In patients who require urgent surgery, preoperative low-grade fever and even a minor pulmonary infiltrate may be accepted. The risk to the patient is certainly increased, particularly if urgent surgery requires implantation of a prosthetic valve. Even patients with refractory valvular endocarditis may require valve replacement to control infection or heart failure, and this is frequently successful. In general, broad-spectrum antibiotic coverage should be initiated, unless the finding of a specific organism dictates more specific therapy. Postoperatively, frequent surveillance cultures must be continued and strict attention must be paid to line maintenance, pulmonary toilet, and urinary catheter care.

ABNORMAL HEPATIC FUNCTION

Hepatic function may be deranged, particularly in patients who have had long-standing right heart failure. In the extreme, these patients may have decreased serum albumin levels and abnormally elevated prothrombin times, even if they are not anticoagulated. Hepatic function will have been tested in virtually every patient either sometime during the preoperative evaluation or on admission to the hospital for surgery. Any history of recent hepatitis, alcohol abuse, or right heart failure should be an indication to examine hepatic function more closely, including markers of synthetic function such as serum albumin levels or prothrombin time. Vitamin K may be administered parenterally before surgery; in addition, these patients should have additional fresh frozen plasma available in the event that postoperative hemostasis is a problem. In patients with portal-to-systemic shunts, there may be a greater risk of postoperative infection, particularly with gram-negative organisms.

CAROTID ARTERY AND PERIPHERAL VASCULAR DISEASE

With the increase in patient age and severity of coronary artery disease, cardiac surgeons are managing more patients who have severe peripheral vascular disease or carotid artery disease. These patients may have claudication and may have had prior vascular surgery. In all cardiac surgery patients admitted to the hospital, the admission physical examination should include palpation of peripheral pulses as well as screening for carotid and abdominal bruits. Any suspicion of carotid artery disease indicates the need for noninvasive carotid studies. In patients with transmitted cardiac murmurs, it may be difficult to differentiate a murmur from a carotid bruit and, if there is any question, noninvasive studies should be ordered. Although it has been thought that asymptomatic carotid bruits do not pose an increased risk of perioperative stroke [44], this issue is controversial [45]. We favor aggressive evaluation of carotid disease including angiography. If significant carotid disease is present in asymptomatic patients (lumen<1.5 mm), we usually perform concomitant carotid endarterectomy. Patients with symptomatic carotid disease or bilateral disease will have endarterectomy performed with lesser degrees of stenosis. In patients whose heart disease is stable, carotid endarterectomy may sometimes be performed in advance of cardiac surgery, even under local anesthesia, to reduce the risk of perioperative stroke at the time of cardiac surgery.

The presence of peripheral vascular disease should be noted for several reasons. Should a patient require perioperative support by intraaortic balloon pump, it is important to know the state of the aorta, iliac arteries, and femoral arteries. In patients with an increased likelihood of needing a postoperative balloon pump (e.g., those with poor left ventricular function) further noninvasive studies should be undertaken if there is any question of vascular disease. Often, if left heart catheterization was performed successfully using the transfemoral route, the cardiologist who performed the study may have some insight as to the severity of any aortoiliac disease. If peripheral vascular disease is severe enough to compromise local flow, vein harvesting techniques must be particularly meticulous. In patients in whom peripheral vascular surgery is anticipated after cardiac surgery, conduit harvesting from the lower extremities should be coordinated with the vascular surgeon. In general, if peripheral perfusion is particularly poor in one leg, the saphenous vein should be harvested from the opposite side.

PREGNANCY

Pregnancy imposes a substantial stress on the cardiovascular system. Cardiac output progressively rises during pregnancy reaching a peak nearly 1.5 times baseline during the twenty-fifth to twenty-seventh weeks. Although cardiac operations during pregnancy are rare, the usual circumstance involves a woman with underlying heart disease and limited cardiovascular reserve who develops worsening congestive heart failure. Cardiac surgery, including open procedures on cardiopulmonary bypass, may be performed on pregnant women without high maternal mortality [47,48]. However, when cardiopulmonary bypass is employed, fetal mortality may approach 30%. With respect to timing, the risk of surgery to the mother is lowest in the early stages of pregnancy before cardiovascular stress is great, but this is also the period of critical fetal development. The potential for fetal malformation and relative risks are discussed if the mother does not accept therapeutic abortion and cardiac surgery cannot be avoided.

CACHEXIA

Cachexia from cardiac disease may be insidious and may have been present for a considerable period of time, at least in minor degrees, especially in elderly patients [49]. Cachexia can substantially increase the risk of surgery in the perioperative period by reducing the patient's physiologic reserve for ventilatory weaning and, in extreme degrees, from its effects on the immune system. Cardiac cachexia usually occurs in the setting of heart failure from longstanding valvular heart disease, particularly diseases of the mitral valve. In a prior era, this was more common because patients often presented for surgical treatment late in the course of their disease.

There are few preoperative options available for improving cardiac cachexia, particularly in patients with underlying severe valvular heart disease who have a limited ability to handle additional fluid. Parameters indicative of the patient's nutritional status should be noted preoperatively, as these may dictate when postoperative feeding should be instituted. Hypoalbuminemia or elevated PT may be due in part to poor nutrition, or to the long-standing right heart failure that some of these patients have. In children, cachexia or its equivalent, "failure to thrive," may occur when there has been long-standing significant left-to-right intracardiac shunting. Aggressive nutritional support, even the use of intravenous hyperalimentation shortly after surgery, must be considered early in these patients.

CYANOTIC CONGENITAL HEART DISEASE: PROSTAGLANDIN TREATMENT

Cyanosis is a presenting sign in some types of congenital heart disease. In these patients, cyanosis results from cardiac mixing and reduced pulmonary blood flow, as is commonly seen in pulmonary valve atresia, tetralogy of Fallot, and single ventricle with pulmonic stenosis. In a prior era, these patients were often operated on emergently for deep cyanosis shortly after birth. Early after birth, pulmonary blood flow is derived primarily from aortic-to-pulmonary flow across the ductus arteriosus. Spontaneous closure of the ductus arteriosus can result in a marked diminution of pulmonary blood flow and in deep cyanosis. Fortunately, it has been found that the ductus arteriosus may be reopened during the first few days of life by prostaglandin E_1 (PGE_1, PROSTIN PEDIATRIC) in a dose of 10 to 100 ng/kg/min. This produces greater stability and permits surgery to be undertaken in a semielective manner after the patient has had time to improve and stabilize [50], rather than as an emergency as in the past.

There are circumstances during fetal life where the ductus arteriosus provides the pathway for systemic flow. Such circumstances include hypoplastic left-heart syndrome, interrupted aortic arch, and preductal aortic coarctation. In these lesions, ductal closure leads to inadequate systemic circulation. In these newborns, PGE_1 can restore the systemic circulation and permit stabilization and treatment of acidosis. Finally, PGE_1 may also be used in transposition of the great arteries where arterial and venous mixing may be enhanced by ductal patency.

PGE_1 is a potent vasodilator and can therefore cause significant systemic hypotension. It can also cause fever, seizures, and apnea requiring intubation and mechanical ventilation. The side effects may be minimized by using the lowest dosage of PGE_1 that is effective in maintaining ductal patency. PGE_1 has been used preoperatively for up to 29 continuous days without significant complications [50].

Finally, in the preoperative management of cyanotic infants, it is important to maintain a degree of polycythemia with a hematocrit of at least 50%. These babies will often sustain loss of their red cell mass through the usual preoperative investigations, particularly cardiac catheterization, and it is essential that the oxygen-carrying capacity be maintained to offset the effects of cyanosis.

Initial Considerations in Preoperative Medication

NITRATES

Many patients with unstable angina may require therapy with intravenous nitroglycerin. Often, this is administered in high doses to achieve stability in patients with critical coronary anatomy and should be maintained at moderate doses throughout surgery and in the early postoperative period.

CALCIUM CHANNEL BLOCKERS

Many patients undergoing cardiac surgery, including nearly all coronary bypass patients, come to surgery on calcium channel blockers. Although some controversy exists as to the timing of withdrawal of these agents before surgery [51], we generally continue them up to the time of operation. They may inhibit platelet function, but this has never been associated with postoperative bleeding, and their withdrawal may increase the risk of precipitating angina or acceleration of the ventricular response in chronic atrial fibrillation.

DIGITALIS PREPARATIONS

Patients may come to surgery on digitalis preparations. These may be used to control the ventricular rate in atrial fibrillation, and they are also given to patients in heart failure. Digoxin is usually used because it is a short-acting preparation. Digitoxin is much longer acting, and it is more difficult to achieve rapid control of digitoxin levels. Thus, if time permits, digoxin should be substituted for digitoxin therapy for ease of management. Cardiopulmonary bypass does not significantly alter tissue levels of digitalis preparations. Therefore, digoxin is usually discontinued 1 day before operation to reduce the risk of ventricular arrhythmias during surgery [52–54]. The exception may be those patients who require high therapeutic levels of digoxin in order to control the ventricular response in atrial fibrillation.

Although some investigators have suggested the prophylactic use of digoxin preoperatively to reduce the incidence of postoperative atrial flutter and atrial fibrillation, the results of these studies have been inconsistent [55–59]. Hence, we do not preoperatively digitalize patients to prevent postoperative arrhythmias.

BETA BLOCKING AGENTS

Many patients come to surgery on varying doses of beta-blocking agents including longer-acting agents such as sustained-release propranolol, atenolol, or nadolol. At one time, it was thought that the presence of a significant beta blockade at the time of surgery increased the risk of postoperative ventricular dysfunction. It is now recognized that this is not the case. In fact, there is some advantage in maintaining patients on beta blockade, as heart rate tends to be much more controlled, particularly during the induction of anesthesia, and there may be less risk of intraoperative supraventricular arrhythmias. One should be aware that patients receiving long-acting beta-blocking agents may require temporary atrial pacing in the postoperative period to increase heart rate.

ANTICOAGULANT THERAPY

Heparin

Patients with unstable angina awaiting surgery are generally heparinized up to the time of surgery. Patients who have been on intravenously administered heparin may require a larger, initial intraoperative dose of heparin (e.g., 4 mg/kg) to achieve adequate anticoagulation for cardiopulmonary bypass [42]. In addition, these patients may have heparin-associated thrombocytopenia requiring postoperative platelet transfusion [60].

Warfarin (Coumadin)

Some patients admitted for open heart surgery may be receiving warfarin for previous mechanical heart valve implantation, chronic atrial fibrillation, or left ventricular aneurysm with thrombus. Although it is possible to operate on patients who are fully anticoagulated with warfarin, as is frequently the case with heart transplantation, bleeding problems can occur necessitating the administration of large quantities of fresh frozen plasma. Therefore, when circumstances permit, it is desirable to discontinue warfarin anticoagulation a few days before the anticipated surgery. On admission to the hospital, patients can be anticoagulated with heparin until the time of surgery while warfarin is withdrawn. This is particularly important in patients with prosthetic heart valves in whom valve thrombosis or systemic embolization may occur when warfarin has been discontinued. In these patients, vitamin K should *never* be administered, as rapid correction of the prothrombin time may precipitate valve thrombosis. Gradual reversal with fresh frozen plasma, however, is safe in patients with very elevated prothrombin times who must be operated on urgently. When patients are anticoagulated with warfarin, substantial depletion of vitamin K-dependent cofactors must occur before the prothrombin time will increase. Therefore, patients in whom warfarin has been discontinued and in whom the prothrombin time has just become normal may still have significant depletion of cofactors. It is important, whenever possible, to have a 24- or 48-hour interval of normal prothrombin time so that hepatic synthesis of vitamin K-dependent cofactors will be optimal for postoperative hemostasis, particularly if the patient is having repeat open heart surgery.

Patients receiving warfarin undergoing heart transplantation should have a large dose of vitamin K administered (Aqua-MEPHYTON, 10–20 mg IV). In the operating room, it may be difficult to achieve correction of coagulation by the administration of fresh frozen plasma due to volume constraints and hemodilution. A useful technique is to administer approximately 6 units of fresh frozen plasma just before the termination of bypass and remove the excess fluid by hemofiltration.

Aspirin

Increasingly, patients admitted for coronary artery surgery are receiving low-dose aspirin therapy to reduce the risk of myocardial infarction [4,61]. Aspirin causes significant irreversible platelet dysfunction that persists until a sufficient number of new platelets are formed (7 days) and can, thus, significantly increase the risk of bleeding after heart surgery. Ideally, patients who are having elective surgery should discontinue aspirin (or any other medications that potentially affect platelet function) for at least 2 weeks. Table 1-2 is a list of over-the-counter medications known to contain aspirin. In patients who require urgent operation, such as those with unstable angina, there may not be enough time for sufficient platelet turnover to occur. In these patients, provisions should be made to have platelet transfusion available. Although the bleeding time may be a useful indication of the degree of platelet dysfunction in patients who have been on low-dose aspirin therapy, a normal template bleeding time does not necessarily indicate that platelet function-related bleeding will not occur.

HIGH-DOSE DIURETIC THERAPY

Patients with heart failure or long-standing valvular heart disease may require maintenance on high-dose diuretic therapy with agents such as furosemide or bumetanide and may have depletion of total-body potassium stores [62]. It is important that these patients have repletion of potassium before surgery, when surgery is elective. When these patients are admitted to the hospital, diuretics should be reduced in dose or omitted while potassium repletion occurs. This will help avoid serious electrolyte imbalances and consequent cardiac arrhythmias [62,63].

ANTIHYPERTENSIVE MEDICATIONS

In contemporary practice, patients admitted for surgery may be receiving a variety of vasodilator and other medications used for treating hypertension or for reducing afterload in patients with heart failure. In particular, long-acting agents such as the angiotensin-converting enzyme inhibitors enalapril or lisinopril, or older agents such as reserpine or guanethidine may result in hypotension and abnormally low peripheral vascular resistance during surgery. Whenever possible, shorter-acting agents should be substituted, or the above medications should be reduced in dose to the minimum required before surgery. It is important for the team to be aware of these medications so that postoperative blood pressure management can be adjusted appropriately. For example, early after bypass, such patients may need alpha-adrenergic agents to maintain blood pressure.

Intraaortic Balloon Pump Support in the Preoperative Patient

Increasing numbers of patients are admitted with unstable angina requiring intervention on an urgent basis. Many of these patients

Table 1-2. Pharmaceutical Products That Contain Aspirin

A.B.C. Compound
Acoda
Alka-Seltzer
Alka-Seltzer Plus Cold Medicine
Anacin
A.P.C. Tablets
Arthritis Strength Bufferin
Arthritis Pain Formula
Ascriptin
Aspergum
Aspirin and Codeine
Azdone Tablets
Bayer Aspirin
Bayer Children's Cold Tablets
BC Powder
Bufferin
Cama Arthritis Pain Reliever
Congespirin
Damason-P
Darvon Compound-65
Dihydrocodeine Compound Tablets
Easprin
Ecotrin
Empirin w/Codeine Tablets
Equagesic Tablets
Excedrin
4-Way Cold Tablets
Fiorinal
Gelpirin Tablets
Hyco-Pap Capsules
Lortab ASA Tablets
Medigesic Plus Capsules
Methocarbamol and Aspirin Tablets
Momentum Muscular Backache Formula
Moncet (APC) w/ Codeine Tablets
Norgesic Forte Tablets
Norwich Extra-Strength
Oxycodone
P-A-C Analgesic Tablets
Percodan Tablets
Percodan-Demi Tablets
Propoxyphene compound Capsules
Propoxyphene Hydrochloride
Robaxisal Tablets
Roxiprin Tablets
St. Joseph Cold Tablets for Children
St. Joseph Aspirin for Children
Sine-Off Sinus Medicine Tablets-Aspirin Formula
SK-65 Compound Capsules
Soma Compound Tablets
Supac
Synalgos-DC Capsules
Talwin Compound
Triaminicin
Tri-Buffered Bufferin
Ursinus Inlay-Tabs
Vanquish Analgesic Caplets

have been stabilized temporarily by the use of the intraaortic balloon pump [64]. Because this device is now inserted percutaneously, surgeons do not necessarily participate in the decision for its implementation in a given patient. However, it may have significant implications for subsequent surgical management of these patients. First, since the balloon is a prosthetic surface, fibrin and platelets may adhere to it. Therefore these patients are maintained on heparin anticoagulation therapy to minimize platelet loss and coagulation system dysfunction. Second, since these patients are, of necessity, bed-bound during balloon pump support, it is important to minimize the waiting time preoperatively. The relative immobility created by balloon pumping may compromise pulmonary toilet and increase the risk of venous thrombosis and pulmonary embolism. Patients who become agitated or disoriented during balloon pump support often require substantial sedation; this may increase the danger of aspiration and respiratory infection and may mandate intubation. Finally, patients with balloon pumps inserted by the percutaneous route have a significant incidence of peripheral vascular complications, often requiring intervention [65]. Perfusion of the respective leg should be monitored clinically by frequent examination of pulses.

Blood Conservation

Infectious disease transmission is now the most significant risk facing patients who receive homologous blood transfusions. Traditionally, cardiac surgery has required the use of blood transfusions including several units of blood that were incorporated in the cardiopulmonary bypass "prime." With the advent of hemodilution techniques, contemporary intraoperative blood conservation, incorporation of postoperative salvage of shed blood, and tolerance of a degree of postoperative anemia, the amount of blood transfusions that cardiac surgery patients receive has steadily declined. Even with these advances, however, many patients still require transfusions of red cells or other blood components.

The practice of autologous blood donations has been applied to many types of elective surgery, including cardiac surgery, and is certainly an option for those patients facing elective surgery with at least 1 month's notice. For the most part, cardiac surgical patients are capable of participating in an autologous donation program [66,67]. There are a few noteworthy exceptions. Patients with severe aortic stenosis or those with significant left-main coronary disease are not candidates because of the risk of impairing coronary perfusion by acute volume depletion. Patients with underlying anemias and small children are also not candidates.

Patients are started on oral iron replacement in the form of ferrous sulfate (300 mg tid), and blood is collected at 2-week intervals. In general, packed cells and plasma are separated, and plasma is frozen. The patient's hematocrit is checked before each donation, and the donation may be deferred to the following week if the hematocrit is less than 35%. The final donation should be at least 1 week before the anticipated surgical date to allow the patient to resynthesize some red cell mass. It is important that patients are instructed to report any change in cardiac symptoms, particularly any increase in anginal symptoms.

The availability of 2 to 3 units of autologous red cells will often determine whether or not homologous blood is required and will usually result in patients leaving the hospital with substantially more reserve as a result of minimizing the degree of postoperative anemia.

We also offer a "directed donor" program through which a single, carefully screened person (usually a family member) can donate 4 to 6 units preoperatively.

References

1. Lemmer JH Jr, et al. Preoperative saphenous vein mapping for coronary bypass. *J Cardiac Surg* 3:237, 1988.

2. Cohn LH, et al. Bacetrial endocarditis following aortic valve replacement: Clinical and pathologic correlations. *Circulation* 33:209, 1966.

3. Rogosa M, et al. Blood sampling and cultural studies in the detection of postoperative baceteremias. *J Am Dent Assoc* 60:209, 1966.

4. Willard JE, Lange RA, Hillis LD. Current concepts: The use of aspirin in ischemic heart disease. *N Engl J Med* 175:175, 1992.

5. Taggart DP, Siddiqui A., Wheatley DJ. Low-dose pre-operative aspirin therapy, postoperative blood loss, and transfusion requirements. *Ann Thorac Surg* 50:425, 1990.

6. Leppo J, Boucher CA, Okada RD. Serial thallium-201 imaging following dipyridamole infusion: Diagnostic utility in detecting coronary stenoses and relationship to regional wall motion. *Circulation* 66:649, 1982.

7. Verani MS, et al. Diagnosis of coronary artery disease by controlled coronary vasodilation with adenosine and thallium-201 scintigraphy in patients unable to exercise. *Circulation* 82:80, 1990.

8. Brooks R, et al. Current treatment of patients surviving out of hospital cardiac arrest. *JAMA* 265:762, 1991.

9. Sanders CA, et al. Mechanical circulatory assistance. Current status and experience with combining circulatory assistance, emergency coronary angiography, and acute myocardial revascularization. *Circulation* 45:1292, 1972.

10. Hannan EL, et al. Adult open heart surgery in New York State. An analysis of risk factors and hospital mortality rates. *JAMA* 264:2768, 1990.

11. Percutaneous balloon aortic valvuloplasty. Acute and 30-day follow-up results in 674 patients from the NHLBI Balloon Valvuloplasty Registry. *Circulation* 84:2383, 1991.

12. Kontos GJ Jr, et al. Thrombotic obstruction of disc valves: Clinical recognition and surgical management. *Ann Thorac Surg* 48:60, 1989.

13. Graver LM, Gelber PM, Tyras DH. The risk and benefits of thrombolytic therapy in acute aortic and mitral prosthetic valve dysfunction: Report of a case and review of the literature. *Ann Thorac Surg* 46:85, 1988.

14. Kennedy JW, et al. Coronary artery bypass graft surgery early after acute myocardial infarction. *Circulation* 79(Suppl I):I-73, 1989.

15. Applebaum R, et al. Coronary artery bypass grafting within thirty days of acute myocardial infarction. Early and late results in 406 patients. *J Thorac Cardiovasc Surg* 102:745, 1991.

16. Daggett WM. Surgical management of ventricular septal defects complicating myocardial infarction. *World J Surg* 2:753, 1978.

17. Baillot R, et al. Postinfarction ventricular septal defect: Delayed closure with prolonged mechanical circulatory support. *Ann Thorac Surg* 35:138, 1983.

18. Detre KM, et al. Incidence and consequences of periprocedural occlusion. The 1985–1986 National Heart, Lung, and Blood Institute Percutaneous Transluminal Coronary Angioplasty Registry. *Circulation* 82:739, 1990.

19. Pepine CJ, et al. ACC/AHA guidelines for cardiac catheterization and cardiac catheterization laboratories. *Circulation* 84:2213, 1991.

20. Block PC. Emergency surgery for percutaneous transluminal angioplasty: He who calls the tune may have to pay the piper. *Ann Thorac Surg* 40:1, 1985.

21. Ferguson TB Jr, et al. Catheter reperfusion to allow optimal coronary bypass grafting following failed transluminal coronary angioplasty. *Ann Thorac Surg* 42:399, 1986.

22. Brockman SK, Aprill SN, Rabiner FS. Aortic valve replacement in hemophilia. Report of a case. *JAMA* 222:660, 1972.

23. Lawson R, et al. Tricuspid atresia with Christmas disease (hemophilia B). *J Thorac Cardiovasc Surg* 69:585, 1975.

24. Aris A, et al. Open heart surgery in von Willebrand's disease. *J Thorac Cardiovasc Surg* 69:183, 1975.

25. deLeval MR, et al. Open heart surgery in patients with inherited hemoglobinopathies, red cell dyscrasias, and coagulopathies. *Arch Surg* 109:618, 1974.

26. Young PH, Bouhasin JD, Barner HB. Aortic valve replacement in von Willebrand's disease. *J Thorac Cardiovasc Surg* 76:218, 1978.

27. Raish RJ, Witte DL, Goldsmith JC. Successful cardiac surgery following plasmapheresis in a patient with hemophilia B. *Transfusion* 25:128, 1985.

28. Szentpetery S, Robertson L, Lower RR. Complete repair of tetralogy associated with sickle cell anemia and G-6-PD deficiency. *J Thorac Cardiovasc Surg* 72:276, 1976.

29. McGovern E, Otridge BW, Neligan MC. Mitral valve replacement in a patient with sickle cell anemia. *J Thorac Cardiovasc Surg* 35:129, 1987.

30. Ware JA, et al. Defective platelet aggregation in patients undergoing surgical repair of cyanotic congenital heart disease. *Ann Thorac Surg* 36:289, 1983.

31. Colon-Otero G, et al. Preoperative evaluation of hemostasis in patients with congenital heart disease. *Mayo Clin Proc* 62:379, 1987.

32. Ekert H, Sheers M. Preoperative and postoperative platelet function in cyanotic congenital heart disease. *J Thorac Cardiovasc Surg* 67:184, 1974.

33. von Kaulla KN, et al. Preoperative correction of coagulation in tetralogy of Fallot. *Arch Surg* 94:107, 1967.

34. Wedemeyer AL, et al. Serial coagulation studies in patients undergoing Mustard procedure. *Ann Thorac Surg* 15:120, 1973.

35. Rosenthal A, et al. Acute hemodynamic effects of red cell volume reduction in polycythemia of cyanotic congenital heart disease. *Circulation* 42:297, 1970.

36. Rosenthal A, Fyler DC. Effect of red cell volume reduction on pulmonary blood flow in polycythemia of cyanotic congenital heart disease. *Am J Cardiol* 33:410, 1974.

37. Wells R. Syndromes of hyperviscosity. *N Engl J Med* 307:1381, 1982.

38. Connors JP, Shaw RC. Considerations in the management of open-heart surgery in uremic patients. *J Thorac Cardiovasc Surg* 75:400, 1978.

39. Manhas DR, Merendino KA. The management of cardiac surgery in patients with chronic renal failure. A report of three cases. *J Thorac Cardiovasc Surg* 63:235, 1972.

40. Zamora JL, et al. Cardiac surgery in patients with end-stage renal disease. *Ann Thorac Surg* 42:113, 1986.

41. Grossi EA, et al. Sternal wound infections and use of internal mammary artery grafts. *J Thorac Cardiovasc Surg* 102:342, 1991.

42. Cloyd GM, D'Ambra MN, Akins CW. Diminished anticoagulant response to heparin in patients undergoing coronary artery bypass grafting. *J Thorac Cardiovasc Surg* 94:535, 1987.

43. Collins RN, et al. Risk of local and systemic infection with polyethylene intravenous catheters. *N Engl J Med* 279:340, 1968.

44. Reed GL III, et al. Stroke following coronary-artery bypass surgery. A case-controlled estimate of the risk from carotid bruits. *N Engl J Med* 319:1246, 1988.

45. Newman DC, Hicks RG. Combined carotid and coronary artery surgery: A review of the literature. *Ann Thorac Surg* 45:574, 1988.

46. Berens ES, et al. Preoperative carotid artery screening in elderly patients undergoing cardiac surgery. *J Vasc Surg* 15:313, 1992.

47. Becker RM. Intracardiac surgery in pregnant women. *Ann Thorac Surg* 36:453, 1983.

48. Bernal JM, Miralles PJ. Cardiac surgery with cardiopulmonary bypass during pregnancy. *Obstet Gynecol Surv* 41:1, 1986.

49. Rich MW, et al. Increased complications and prolonged hospital stay in elderly cardiac surgical patients with low serum albumin. *Am J Cardiol* 63:714, 1989.

50. Freed MD, et al. Prostaglandin E_1 in infants with ductus arteriosus-dependent congenital heart disease. *Circulation* 64:899, 1981.

51. Murphy CE, Wechsler AS. Calcium channel blockers and cardiac surgery. *J Cardiac Surg* 1987;2:299–325.

52. Lown B, Black H, Moore FD. Digitalis, electrolytes, and the surgical patient. *Am J Cardiol* 5:309, 1960.

53. Morrow DH, Townley NT. Anesthesia and digitalis toxicity: An experimental study. *Anesth Analg* (Cleve) 43:510, 1964.

54. Morgan DB, Mearns AJ, Burkinshaw L. The potassium status of patients prior to open-heart surgery. *J Thorac Cardiovasc Surg* 76:673, 1978.

55. Ivey MF, et al. Influence of propranolol on supraventricular tachycardia early after coronary artery revascularization. *J Thorac Cardiovasc Surg* 85:214, 1983.

56. Parker FB Jr, et al. Supraventricular arrhythmias following coronary artery bypass. *J Thorac Cardiovasc Surg* 86:594, 1983.

57. Roffman JA, Fieldman A. Digoxin and propranolol in the prophylaxis of supraventricular tachydysrhythmia after coronary artery bypass surgery. *Ann Thorac Surg* 31:496, 1981.

58. Selzer A, Walter RM. Adequacy of preoperative digitalis therapy in controlling ventricular rate in postoperative atrial fibrillation. *Circulation* 34:119, 1966.

59. Tyras DH, et al. Supraventricular tachyarrhythmias after myocardial revascularization: A randomized trial of prophylactic digitalization. *J Thorac Cardiovasc Surg* 77:310, 1979.

60. Makhoul RG, et al. Management of patients with heparin-associated thrombocytopenia and thrombosis requiring cardiac surgery. *Ann Thorac Surg* 43:617, 1987.

61. Final report on the aspirin component of the ongoing Physicians' Health Study. Steering Committee of the Physicians' Health Study Research Group. *N Engl J Med* 321:129, 1989.

62. Remencheck AP, et al. Depletion of body potassium by diuretics. *Circulation* 33:796, 1966.

63. Flear CTG, et al. Exchangeable body potassium and sodium in patients in congestive heart failure. *Clin Chim Acta* 13:1, 1966.

64. Creswell LL, et al. Intraaortic balloon counterpulsation: Patterns of usage and outcomes in cardiac surgical patients. *Ann Thorac Surg* 54:11, 1992.

65. Martin RS III, et al. Complications of percutaneous intra-aortic balloon insertion. *J Thorac Cardiovasc Surg* 85:186, 1983.
66. Love TR, et al. Transfusion of predonated autologous blood in elective cardiac surgery. *Ann Thorac Surg* 43:508, 1987.
67. Owings DV, et al. Autologous blood donations prior to elective cardiac surgery. Safety and effect on subsequent blood use. *JAMA* 262:1963, 1989.

Operative Management

Basic Monitoring

An arterial monitoring line is usually inserted into the radial artery by percutaneous technique, although open exposure (cutdown) of the artery is occasionally required. An Allen's test should be performed before cannulation to demonstrate adequate ulnar artery collateral flow to the hand (Fig. 2-1); if the test is positive (i.e., inadequate collateral to the hand), that radial artery should not be used. If neither radial artery can be used, the brachial, femoral, or dorsalis pedis arteries may be cannulated. Usually the radial artery is adequate for postoperative monitoring after cardiopulmonary bypass. On occasion, however, the femoral artery may be more reliable than smaller arteries for pressure measurements because significant postoperative vasoconstriction can produce spuriously low pressure readings in the more peripheral areas of the circulation [1]. In patients with marginal cardiac function, insertion of a femoral arterial line before cardiopulmonary bypass can provide easy access for percutaneous insertion of an intraaortic balloon pump, if needed, in addition to reliable arterial pressure recordings.

Complications of arterial lines should be rare if proper techniques of insertion and maintenance are used. The incidence of thrombotic complications is increased by low cardiac output, hypotension, administration of vasoconstrictor agents, and long duration of use [2–4]. These factors are obviously related to the individual patient and the underlying disease. However, other factors contributing to thrombosis — multiple attempts at cannulation and large catheter size [3] — are related to catheter insertion technique. This emphasizes the need for experienced operators to perform catheter insertion under a careful and standardized protocol.

The risk of infection of arterial catheters is increased by the use of cutdown rather than percutaneous technique, long duration of use, and inflammation at the catheter site. Infection may be less frequent if the fluid in the system is normal saline rather than dextrose and if disposable transducer components are employed [5]. Particular attention should be paid to stopcocks in the pressure monitoring lines; these are contaminated by bacteria in as many as 16% of patients [6]. Femoral arterial catheters may be at somewhat greater risk for infection, but this is controversial [7,8].

Flow-directed pulmonary artery catheters, such as the Swan-Ganz catheter, permit continuous measurement of central venous and pulmonary artery pressures, estimation of cardiac output, determination of mixed venous oxygen saturation, and insertion of pacing wires. We use these in most adult patients undergoing open heart procedures.

Pulmonary artery catheters rarely become infected if removed within 72 hours of insertion [9]. The internal jugular vein provides safe and direct access for insertion (Fig. 2-2). The vein is first located by puncture with a 20-gauge "exploring" needle; in this manner, an inadvertent puncture of the carotid artery can be managed by holding

30 2. Operative Management

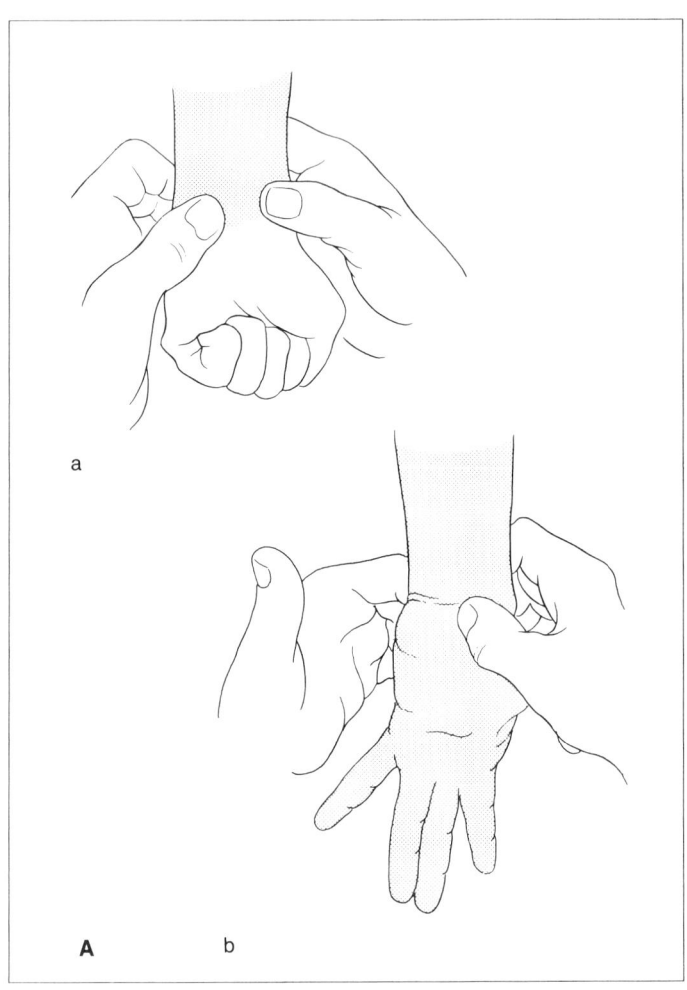

Fig. 2-1. Arterial line insertion. A. An *Allen's test* is used to confirm that the collateral circulation to the hand is intact. The patient is instructed to make a fist which results in blanching of the palmar skin. Both ulnar and radial arteries are then manually occluded (a). The patient is instructed to open the hand and, while the radial artery is kept occluded, pressure is removed from the ulnar artery (b). If the perfusion returns to the fingers, adequate collateral circulation via the ulnar artery is intact and a radial arterial line may be safely inserted.

gentle pressure until there is no risk of hematoma formation. If the larger Swan-Ganz introducer is mistakenly inserted into the artery, the operation should be postponed unless it is urgent or emergent, in which case this complication may require open repair of the carotid artery before institution of heparinization and bypass [10].

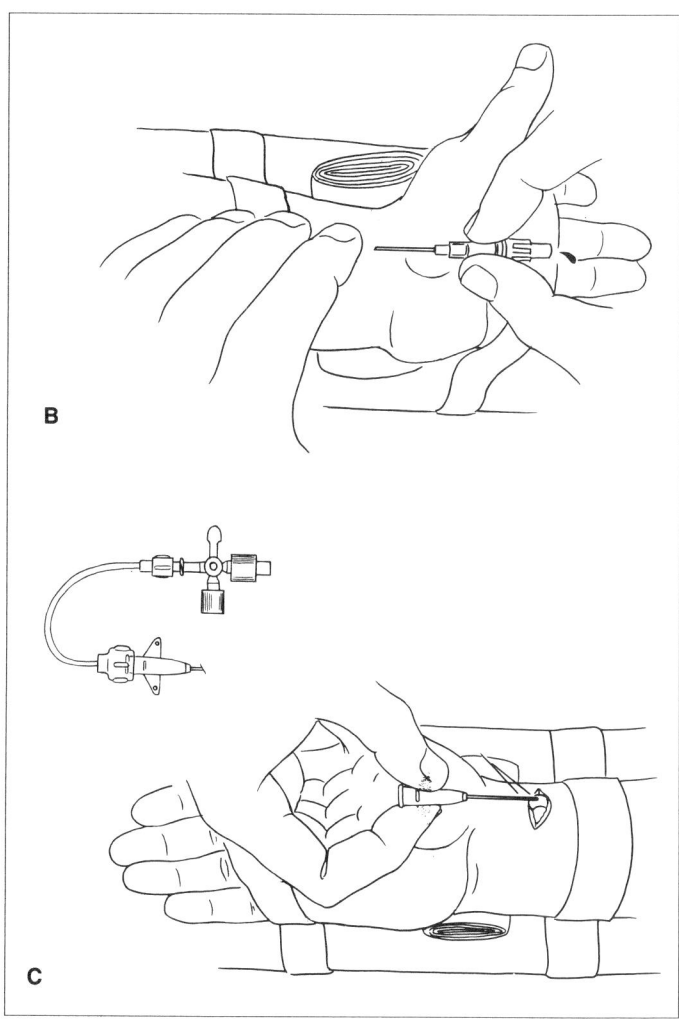

B. A radial line may be inserted using an 18- or 20-gauge intravenous cannula of the catheter-over-needle design. The artery is palpated with one hand to localize it and the cannula is inserted. Generally, the artery is transfixed with the cannula, the needle is then very slowly withdrawn until brisk flow of arterial blood is noted, at which point the cannula is advanced into the artery. **C.** If the cannula cannot be successfully inserted using percutaneous technique, an alternative method is to use a cutdown to expose the artery. A suture sling is placed underneath the radial artery to elevate it, and the cannula is inserted either by a small arteriotomy or by the catheter-over-needle technique, such as used for percutaneous insertion. Whichever technique is used, a short piece of tubing with male and female connectors and Luer-lock hubs are used so that manipulation of a stopcock does not result in kinking of the arterial cannula.

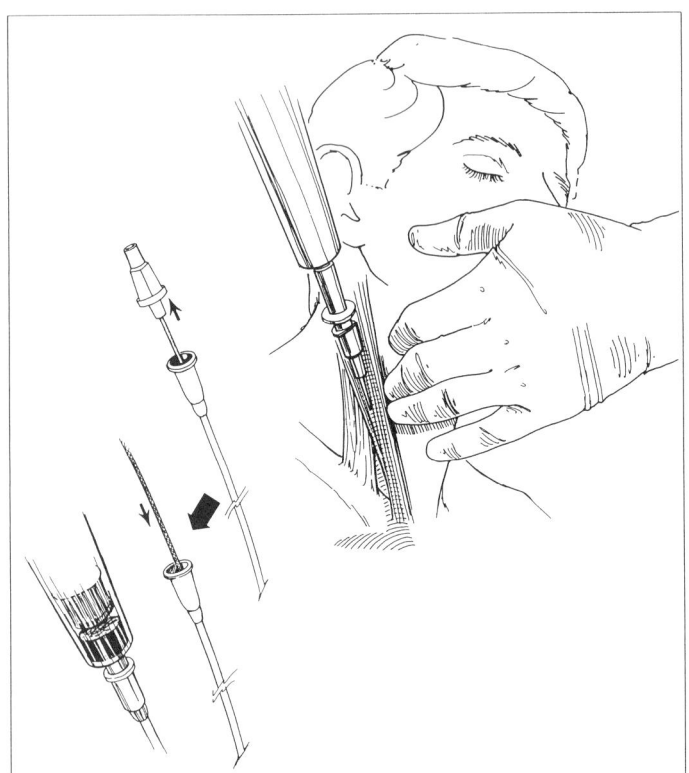

Fig. 2-2. Technique for internal jugular access. The patient is situated in Trendelenburg position with the head turned to the side opposite line insertion. After a sterile prep and draping, the left hand is used to localize the carotid artery. A cannula with needle is then directed between the two heads of the sternocleidomastoid muscle to find the vein. After blood return is confirmed from the needle, the cannula is grasped to immobilize it, the needle is withdrawn, and a guidewire is then inserted into the internal jugular vein. The guidewire may be passed into the central venous position, which may sometimes be confirmed by observing that PVCs have occurred when the guidewire reaches the right ventricle. The central venous catheter (or Swan-Ganz introducer sheath) may then be introduced over the guidewire. The wire is withdrawn and central venous position is confirmed by noting that blood may be aspirated. If central venous pressures are low, air embolism is a potential risk and care must be taken not to allow ingress of air when the syringe is removed from the catheter hub.

The subclavian vein is an alternative site for Swan-Ganz catheter insertion [11]; the risk of pneumothorax and hemorrhage is higher [12,13] but subclavian insertion may be associated with fewer infectious complications [7]. We avoid using the left-sided central veins as access routes in reoperations and other selected cases in which the innominate vein is at increased risk of injury during the surgical procedure.

The technique for catheter insertion is outlined in Figure 2-3. Continuous ECG monitoring is mandatory during the insertion of pulmonary artery catheters; arrhythmias or conduction disturbances may complicate this procedure in as many as 78% of patients [11]. These complications may be reduced by passing the catheter through the right ventricle in an expeditious manner and by avoiding redundant loops of catheter within the cardiac chambers. Prophylactic lidocaine may be administered before insertion in patients who are at particular risk for arrhythmias [14]. Rupture of the pulmonary arteries may occur in up to approximately 0.2% of Swan-Ganz catheter insertions [15,16]. This potentially life-threatening complication is most common in patients with pulmonary hypertension or in those receiving anticoagulants. Manipulation of the heart during cardiac operations, changes in chamber size during bypass, and increasing catheter stiffness due to topical and systemic hypothermia may contribute to this problem [17]. The risk of pulmonary artery rupture can be minimized by limiting the number of balloon inflations in patients at increased risk for this complication and by not leaving the catheters in the wedged position. Rarely is it necessary to intervene surgically for a pulmonary artery rupture; the hemorrhage is usually limited by the low pressure of the pulmonary circulation.

In patients with left bundle branch block, passage of a pulmonary artery catheter can cause failure of conduction down the right bundle branch, resulting in complete heart block. In these situations, we insert a separate pacing wire before pulmonary artery catheter placement, or we use a pulmonary artery catheter that includes a separate port for pacing wire passage.

Additional central venous lines may be inserted via the basilic or cephalic veins. There is a high rate of catheter malposition when these vessels are the route of access [18]. Catheters may also be inserted intraoperatively into the innominate vein or directly into the right atrium. In rare circumstances where mechanical valves have been placed in the tricuspid position, a Swan-Ganz catheter may be inserted into the pulmonary artery during surgery via a pursestring suture in the right ventricular outflow tract.

Esophageal and rectal temperatures are monitored continuously. Urinary catheters are inserted after induction of anesthesia. Nasogastric or orogastric catheters are inserted either after induction of anesthesia or at the end of the operation. Gastric drainage is required to avoid the potentially severe problems of acute gastric dilatation and vomiting. Gastric decompression is essential in patients who require more than a few hours of mechanical ventilation postoperatively, because air swallowing is particularly troublesome in this setting. Transcutaneous oxygen saturation monitors are usually attached to the patient's finger. Although these may be useful in detecting sudden changes in arterial oxygen saturation, they are highly dependent on tissue perfusion and may be unreliable in low-flow states [19].

PACING AND ARRHYTHMIAS

Unexpected sinus bradycardia occurring during induction of anesthesia or in the earliest stages of the operation can be treated pharmacologically. Alternatively, pacing via a pacing port Swan-Ganz

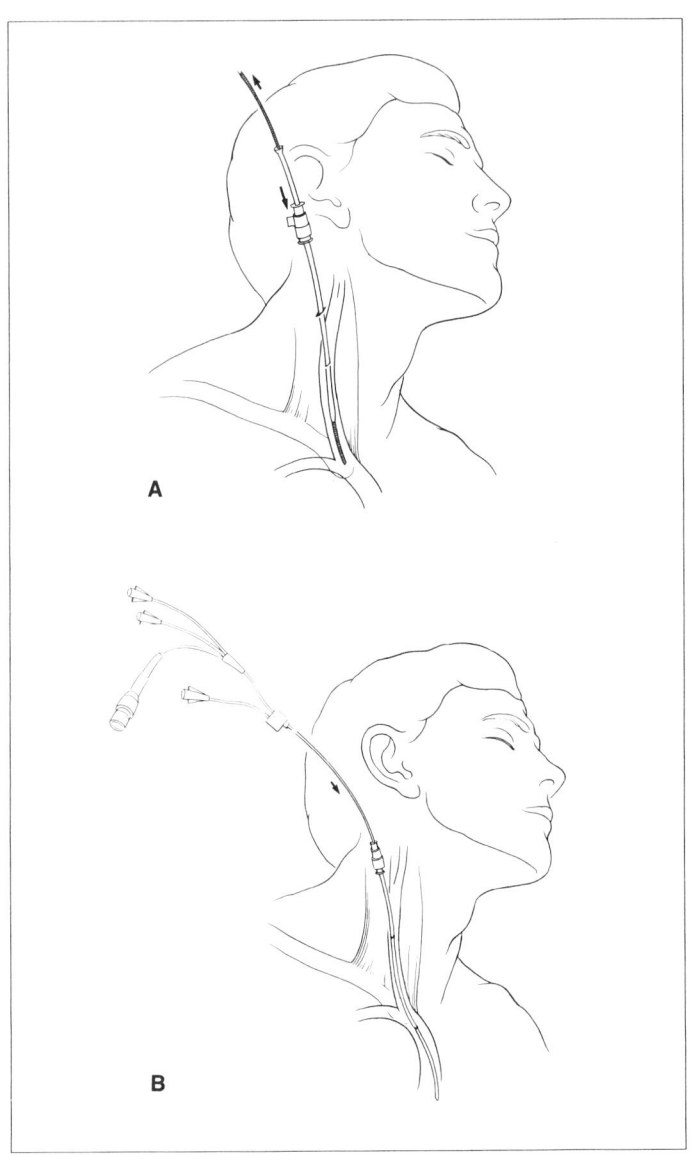

Fig. 2-3. Swan-Ganz catheter insertion. A. Using the technique described in Fig. 2-2, an introducer sheath is placed in the internal jugular vein. Such a sheath usually contains a port for intravenous infusion and will usually contain an O ring seal at the end of the sheath to prevent ingress of air when the Swan-Ganz catheter is not present. B. All ports of the Swan-Ganz catheter are filled with heparinized saline and the distal port is connected to a physiologic monitor. The Swan-Ganz catheter is inserted into the introducer sheath and advanced into the superior vena cava (SVC).

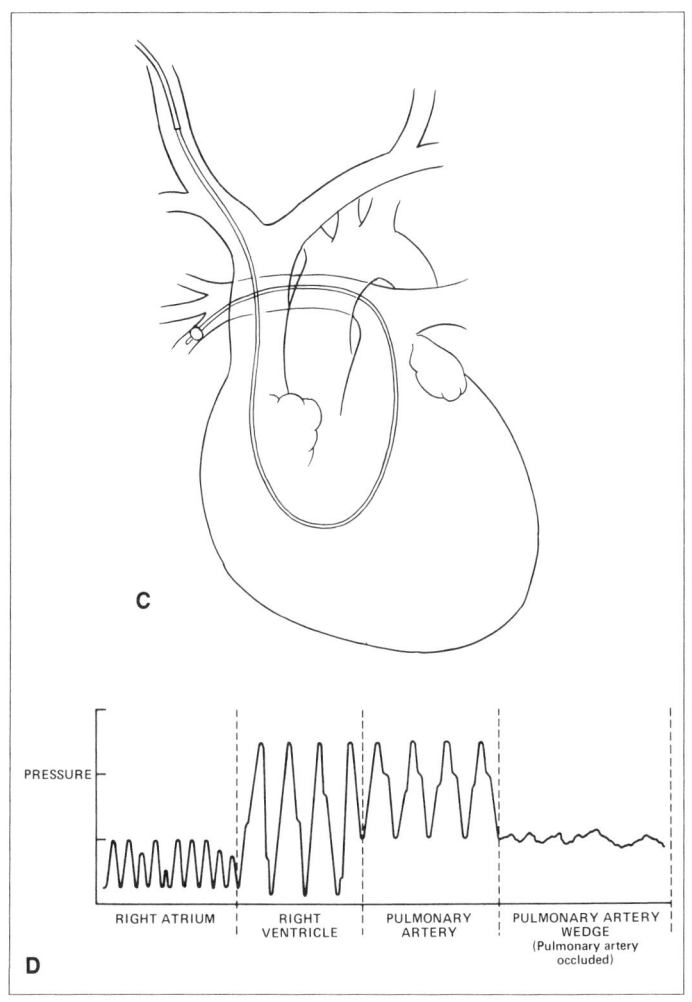

C. Once present in the SVC, the balloon is inflated and the catheter is advanced while the pressure monitor is continuously observed. The catheter is passed from the SVC to the right atrium and into the right ventricle. Subsequently, the catheter may be passed into the pulmonary artery and into the pulmonary capillary wedge position. Transit from right atrium to right ventricle and from right ventricle to pulmonary artery can sometimes be facilitated by having the patient take a deep inspiration which will temporarily bring additional venous return into the heart. D. An example of the hemodynamic tracings obtained during insertion of a Swan-Ganz catheter. The difference between right atrial and right ventricular pressures is often obvious. However, when right ventricular filling pressures are elevated, it may be difficult to distinguish right ventricular from pulmonary artery pressure. A useful guide to note is that during diastole, right ventricular pressures will *increase*, while during diastole, pulmonary artery pressures will *decrease*.

catheter or transesophageal pacing can be useful [20,21]. Note that bradycardia may result from other conditions such as hypoxia during induction of anesthesia.

Patients with previously placed permanent pacemakers should be evaluated carefully before operation. Electrocautery and defibrillation may affect the performance of the pacemaker in a variety of undesirable ways, such as reversion to a backup mode or damage to the sensing and pulse generator circuits. Although modern pacemaker electronics permits safe and uneventful operation in most cases, certain precautions should be employed. These include placing the cautery ground plate as far from the pacemaker as possible, using the lowest possible cautery intensity, and keeping the appropriate pacemaker programmer in the operating room throughout the procedure [22]. Use of bipolar cautery may reduce electromagnetic interference [23]. Rate-dependent demand pacemakers can be inhibited easily by chest wall stimulation or by a temporary pacemaker set at a rate exceeding the permanent device [24].

Anesthesia

Narcotics are an important component of the anesthetic management of the cardiac surgery patient because they have minimal effects on cardiac function and limited interaction with other agents. Morphine is the oldest opiate used in cardiac anesthesia and is still widely popular. Newer agents that produce less vasodilatation include fentanyl and sufentanil; the latter, in particular, may provide more rapid induction and emergence from anesthesia [25] than older agents such as morphine.

Narcotics alone are not always adequate to prevent hemodynamic responses to operative stimuli, particularly in children [26]. For this reason, inhalation agents are often added. Halothane is a frequently used inhalation agent that has a direct negative inotropic effect on the heart without affecting diastolic function [27]. Because halothane is a potent vasodilator, the net effect on cardiac output may be beneficial. Enflurane is another common inhalation agent that has been thought to have less negative inotropic effect than halothane. At equi-anesthetic concentrations, however, the myocardial depression produced by halothane and enflurane is roughly equivalent [28]. Isoflurane has even less negative inotropic effect, but its positive chronotropic effect may be undesirable in patients with myocardial ischemia. Nitrous oxide is less commonly used because of its negative effects on cardiac output and blood pressure, its relative anesthetic impotency, and its ability to worsen any potential air embolism.

Intravenously administered sedatives such as thiopental and the benzodiazepines are frequently added. These drugs reduce response to operative stimuli, but may contribute to myocardial depression. Ketamine is commonly used in children because of its rapidly hypnotic and analgesic effects without depression of respiratory or cardiovascular function; however, ketamine may cause unpleasant hallucinations. Muscle relaxants, including pancuronium, vecuronium, and metocurine, are particularly useful during induction of anesthesia by reducing the muscular rigidity associated with agents such as fentanyl that may make ventilation difficult [29,30].

Conduct of the Operation

The patient should be properly positioned to allow access to all fields of interest. For coronary bypass operations, this usually necessitates adequate exposure of the saphenous vein harvest sites. A circumferential leg prep permits harvesting of greater or lesser saphenous veins. In patients with extensive venous disease or prior bypass surgery, the arm vein may be a last resort for conduit. If use of this conduit is a possibility, the selected extremity must be kept free of intravenous lines and be included in the surgical field. Care must be taken to avoid peripheral nerve complications, which may result from hyperabduction of the shoulders or inadequate cushioning of the arms or legs. All arterial and venous lines must be secure and accessible to the anesthesiologist. Any connections must be securely tightened and any stopcocks properly capped to avoid contamination. Preparing the patient's skin with disinfectant soap must be done thoroughly by experienced personnel after all other manipulation of the patient has ceased. During the preparation, it is poor technique to permit members of the team to start intravenous lines, insert nasogastric tubes, attach cautery ground plates, or otherwise risk contamination.

In selected cases, most commonly reoperations, we apply adhesive defibrillator pads ("R2," R2 Medical Systems, Niles, IL) to the lateral chest walls; these permit the transthoracic administration of electrical countershock even before the heart has been adequately exposed [31]. In all cases, internal defibrillator paddles must be readily available to the surgeon and should be tested at the outset to ensure proper function. The pump oxygenator is primed in the operating room no later than during induction of anesthesia. Sudden hemodynamic deterioration may require emergency cannulation and establishment of bypass. The perfusionist is also in attendance throughout this period.

Although the cosmetic benefits of a small incision may be kept in mind, it is important to make a large enough incision to perform the operation without struggling against the skin and soft tissues. Attention to cosmetics is best focused at the end of the procedure, when proper surgical techniques can provide an acceptable scar. At times, an anterolateral thoracotomy incision can be used, particularly for mitral valve operations or atrial septal defects. A bilateral inframammary incision may permit a median sternotomy, albeit with some compromise of exposure [32].

For primary operations, sternotomy is easily accomplished with an electric or air-powered saw. During this maneuver, the anesthesiologist holds the lungs in expiration to minimize likelihood of opening the pleurae.

For reoperations, the surgeon must read the previous operative note(s) and examine the lateral chest films to prepare for any particularly hazardous anatomy [33]. One important maneuver that reduces the danger of sternal reentry is to have the first assistant elevate the sternum while the surgeon divides the bone with an oscillating saw (Fig. 2-4). Another useful maneuver is to leave the posterior portion of the sternal wires in place while the oscillating saw is applied. In this fashion, precious millimeters of additional space may be available for safe passage of the saw blade. When there have been multiple previous operations, cardiomegaly, elevated right atrial pressures, or other circumstances that cause even greater concern (e.g., ascending aortic aneurysm or false aneurysm), isolation of the femoral artery and vein prior to sternotomy permits rapid cannulation if problems arise. In rare cases, we establish bypass via the femoral route even before attempting sternal division; this is frequently the most prudent approach in reoperations when there is tricuspid regurgitation with significant elevation of right atrial pressure (>20 mm Hg).

HEPARINIZATION

Adequacy of anticoagulation for the purpose of cardiopulmonary bypass is determined by measurement of the activated clotting time (ACT) [34]. The patient's ACT is measured before and after administration of heparin (3 mg/kg). Patients receiving heparin preoperatively tend to require greater doses of heparin to achieve the same degree of anticoagulation for cardiopulmonary bypass [35]; in these patients, the initial dose should be increased to 4 mg/kg. These patients may also have heparin-induced thrombocytopenia that may complicate hemostasis after bypass [36]. Adequate heparin anticoagulation (ACT >400 sec) must be assured before institution of bypass. If the initial heparinizing dose does not achieve adequate prolongation of the ACT, an additional 1 to 2 mg/kg are administered. If this still does not adequately prolong the ACT, antithrombin-III deficiency must be suspected and treated. Fresh frozen

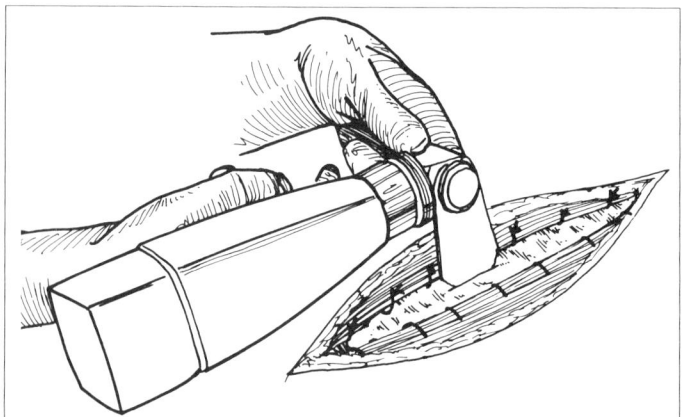

Fig. 2-4. In reoperations for cardiac surgery, the redo sternotomy is generally performed with an oscillating saw. The major concern is adherence of cardiac structures to the posterior table of the sternum. One approach to prevent injury to the aorta or right ventricle is shown: After cutting old sternal wires, they are left in place and used as a guide to the depth of penetration by the oscillating saw, thus decreasing the risk of injuring the aorta or right ventricle.

plasma should be administered (approximately 5 ml/kg) and the ACT should be rechecked before institution of bypass [37]. In all patients, ACT is monitored every 15 minutes, and additional heparin is given as needed to maintain an ACT of more than 400 seconds.

TECHNIQUES OF PERFUSION

The ascending aorta is usually preferred for arterial cannulation. More recently, attention has been directed toward preventing atherosclerotic embolization during ascending aortic cannulation [38]. When selecting a cannulation site, the aorta should be palpated to exclude large plaques (Fig. 2-5). In some centers, intraoperative ultrasound evaluation of the aorta is used to exclude areas of severe atherosclerosis as potential cannulation sites [39]. The ascending aorta may be cannulated safely with one of a variety of commercially available cannulas. Irrespective of the cannula chosen, it is important to ensure that the cannula is not directed into the innominate artery (see also discussion of intraoperative stroke in Chap. 5). Femoral or external iliac access is required for a variety of aortic arch procedures as well as for patients with severe ascending aortic disease that may make direct aortic cannulation hazardous. After cannulation and the institution of bypass, a sudden increase in the pressure in the arterial perfusion line associated with a decrease in the radial artery pressure should raise the suspicion of iatrogenic aortic dissection (Fig. 2-6). In this event, it is mandatory to discontinue bypass immediately and recannulate in another site.

Venous cannulation is most commonly performed via the right atrium with one or two large-bore catheters. One catheter may be inserted via the femoral vein in particular situations; when this is necessary, the right femoral vein usually provides the easiest access to the atrium. Occasionally the right internal jugular or innominate vein can be used for venous drainage. In operations in which the right side of the heart is opened, cannulation of the individual venae cavae and use of caval tourniquets are required.

OXYGENATOR

There are two fundamental oxygenator technologies commonly used today: bubble and membrane or hollow fiber oxygenators. Unlike bubble oxygenators, the latter devices do not allow direct contact between blood and gas; preventing direct blood-gas interaction results in less denaturation of protein and less cell-membrane damage [40–44]. Bubble oxygenators, however, are not associated with significant differences in clinical outcome, organ function, or even certain hematologic indices [41–45].

PROFOUND HYPOTHERMIA AND CIRCULATORY ARREST

Many operations in small infants and certain adult open heart operations, especially those involving the aortic arch, are performed using profound core cooling and circulatory arrest [46]. This provides a completely bloodless field and access to all major intrathoracic vessels. In infants, surface cooling is sometimes performed before use of the bypass circuit in order to avoid large heat shifts from the un-

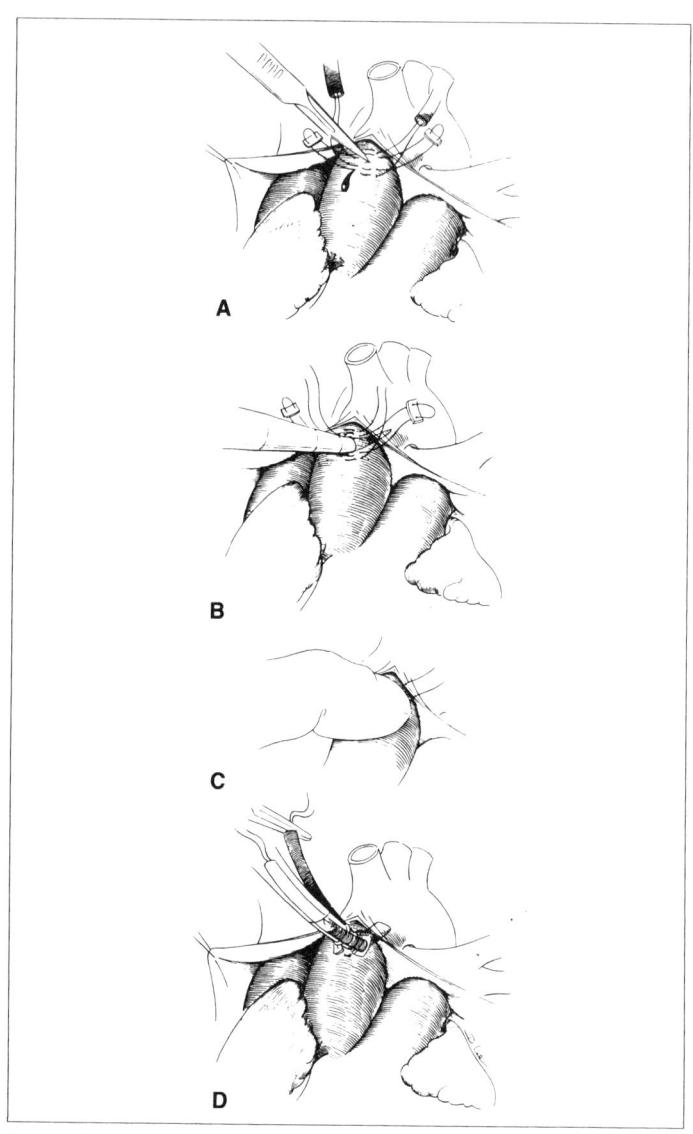

Fig. 2-5. The aorta is palpated to ensure that the site selected for cannulation does not contain palpable plaque. A. Two concentric pursestring sutures are placed around the selected site. An aortotomy is made with a No. 11 or 15 scalpel blade. B. Particularly if some aortic atherosclerosis is present, it may be necessary to dilate the aortotomy site with a tapered dilator. C. After making the aortotomy, temporary control is achieved with gentle digital pressure. D. The aortic cannula is introduced making sure that the tip is facing downstream, aortic pursestring sutures are tightened, and the pursestring suture tourniquets are secured to the cannula using heavy silk ligatures.

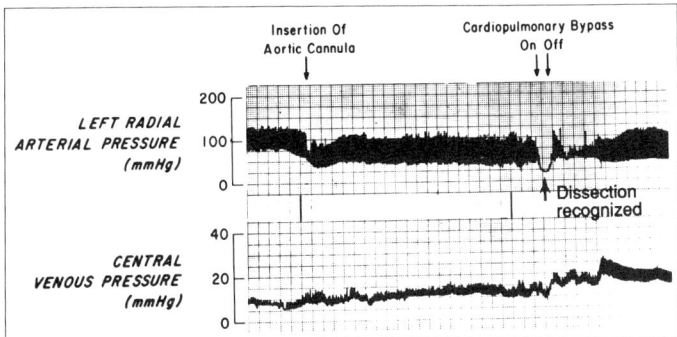

Fig. 2-6. Hemodynamic tracings from a patient where iatrogenic aortic dissection occurred with the aortic cannula being placed initially in a false channel. With the institution of cardiopulmonary bypass, perfusion was initiated in the false channel resulting in loss of perfusion to the left subclavian artery. The dissection was quickly recognized, bypass was terminated, and with the cardiac output directed into the true lumen, the left radial arterial pressure was restored. The patient was recannulated using the femoral artery, bypass was instituted, and during the procedure the iatrogenic dissection site at the ascending aortic cannulation was repaired.

cooled periphery. Core cooling to less than 20°C is performed. Hemodilution is an essential part of the profound hypothermia technique to avoid red cell sludging in the capillaries, which can lead to a "no reflow" phenomenon. Rewarming is performed gradually. Hemostasis may be difficult to achieve at the end of such procedures [47].

MYOCARDIAL PROTECTION

Myocardial protection is a broad concept that includes a number of measures performed to limit injury to the heart muscle. We believe one essential component of myocardial protection is ventricular decompression. The left ventricle may become distended during bypass, most notably during ventricular fibrillation, and this is associated with impaired recovery of ventricular function [48,49]. Prevention of this complication requires knowledge of one or more techniques of venting this chamber. We prefer insertion of a vent into the left ventricle via the right superior pulmonary vein. Other options include venting the aortic root or the pulmonary artery [50] or insertion of a vent via the left ventricular apex.

Formulation of Cardioplegia

For many years, cardiac operations were performed with excellent results with intermittent aortic cross-clamping or with fibrillation arrest; some surgeons continue to prefer these techniques [51]. Today, it is more common to use a cardioplegia solution to arrest and protect the heart [52]. A variety of cardioplegia additives have been proposed to enhance myocardial protection, including calcium channel blockers, metabolic substrates, free-radical scavengers, oxygen, and red blood cells. Traditionally, however, most cardiac surgeons would agree on at least three criteria for an acceptable cardioplegia solution: (1) it must be cold, (2) it must contain potassium in adequate but not excessively toxic concentration, and (3) it must be slightly hyperosmolar [53–55]. More recently interest has emerged in the use of continuous warm blood cardioplegia [56]. However, its superiority over other methods has not been firmly established.

Cardioplegia may be reliably administered by three different methods: (1) infusion into the aortic root, (2) direct cannulation of the coronary arteries, or (3) retrograde perfusion of the coronary sinus. Any of these routes may be satisfactory in some cases, whereas a particular technique may be optimal in others; therefore, the surgeon should be familiar with all of these methods. It is our current preference to use cold (4–6°C), antegrade, dilute oxygenated blood cardioplegia for most operations in adults. Several authors employ retrograde delivery in certain circumstances, such as reoperations.

It is important to administer cardioplegia shortly after induction of cardiac ischemia (aortic cross-clamping) to avoid myocardial injury [57]. Furthermore, the surgeon must be aware that electrical arrest as observed by standard surface monitors may be an insensitive method that may fail to detect myocardial electrical activity. Such activity during cross-clamping may affect the need for postoperative inotropic support [58].

Myocardial Hypothermia

Hypothermia protects the myocardium by reducing its energy demands and increasing its buffering capacity [59]. It also reduces the oxygen and metabolic requirements of the brain and other organs. The myocardial protection provided by systemic hypothermia is superior to that of cold cardioplegia alone [60], possibly due to better maintenance of myocardial cooling. It is maintained by the heat exchanger in the cardiopulmonary bypass circuit; typically, we cool patients to a rectal temperature of 25°C.

Topical cardiac hypothermia is also used in the form of cold saline or iced slush. The addition of topical hypothermia provides significantly improved myocardial protection, particularly when coronary stenoses prevent even distribution of cardioplegia [61]. Care is required in the use of topical hypothermia because of the risk of phrenic nerve paresis associated with excessively cold temperatures. An insulation pad may be used to protect the phrenic nerve when iced slush is liberally used.

SEPARATION FROM CARDIOPULMONARY BYPASS

Preparation for terminating bypass should begin even before all technical maneuvers are completed. Among the most important considerations is removal of air from the heart. Despite the universal awareness of the importance of avoiding air embolism, there is an almost unavoidable introduction of microbubbles into the circulation beginning with aortic cannulation [62]. The use of arterial line filters may reduce this problem [63]. Even after meticulous efforts to remove air, cardiac microbubbles can be detected by echocardiography in 75% of patients undergoing intracardiac operations and in 10% of coronary bypass patients [64,65]. The effect of these small bubbles on postoperative neurologic status is uncertain.

Although we use the steep Trendelenburg position at the time of aortic cross-clamp removal to minimize the passage of air into the carotid arteries, experimental evidence raises questions as to the efficacy of this maneuver [66]. Additional methods of removing air from the heart include vigorous ballottement of the heart while filling it with blood before cross-clamp removal, ventilation of the lungs, and suction of the aortic root and the left ventricular vent [67].

Most cardiopulmonary bypass circuits incorporate multiple safety systems including photoelectric blood level detectors, air-activated ball valves, and automatic shut-off devices. Nevertheless, significant air embolism is estimated to occur in approximately 1 in 1000 open heart operations [68]. When such a catastrophe occurs, the pump should be stopped and the aorta should be vented with the patient in the Trendelenburg position. Reversal of cerebral flow has been proposed by some surgeons [69]. Others have advocated hypothermia, steroids (dexamethasone, 10 mg IV), barbiturates (thiopental, 10 mg/kg IV), and hyperbaric oxygen [68–70].

RHYTHM

Separation from bypass requires a stable cardiac rhythm. In many cases, the heart must be electrically defibrillated in order to achieve this. A bolus dose of lidocaine (2 mg/kg) immediately before removal of the aortic clamp has been shown to reduce the incidence of ventricular fibrillation during reperfusion [71]. Defibrillation should be accomplished with the lowest energy possible to minimize myocardial injury. Myocardial necrosis can occur from defibrillation, but it results only after multiple applications at high-energy levels [72]. Many fibrillating hearts on bypass can be successfully defibrillated with a single shock of 2.5 joules, but the vast majority will be defibrillated with 10 joules [73,74]. Defibrillation is facilitated by an adequate coronary perfusion pressure, higher systemic vascular resistance, physiologic temperature, and a serum potassium in the high-normal range [73]. When initial defibrillation attempts fail, decreasing left ventricular volume and increasing defibrillation energy are two easy methods of improving the results of countershock. In addition, increasing aortic perfusion pressure may also be helpful in the fibrillating heart. Administration of additional lidocaine (1–2 mg/kg) and use of a lidocaine infusion (1–2 mg/min) for adults may assist in preventing refibrillation.

Most arrhythmias that occur during cardiac operations are due to the operative manipulations and preexisting cardiac abnormalities or myocardial ischemia [75]. Diagnosis of arrhythmias is usually easy with the heart under direct observation. Atrial fibrillation, atrial flutter, supraventricular tachycardia, and junctional rhythm may be difficult to distinguish using the surface ECG, but they are readily discerned by inspection of the heart.

Atrial fibrillation may contribute to less-than-optimal cardiac performance during and after separation from bypass. In most cases, electrical defibrillation of the atria should be attempted. If atrial fibrillation occurring after bypass is terminated by cardioversion, the defibrillator should be synchronized to discharge during the refractory period of the cardiac cycle to avoid causing ventricular fibrillation. Even in patients in whom atrial fibrillation has been present for several months preoperatively, sinus rhythm can sometimes be established for at least a portion of the early postoperative period. When a sinus rhythm is established, atrial pacing may help to maintain this rhythm [76].

Rapid atrial pacing is often successful in terminating atrial flutter. This maneuver is performed by applying bipolar atrial pacing at a rate slightly faster than the spontaneous rate. When the atria appear to have been captured by the pacemaker, the rate is further increased until the flutter waves change polarity (usually from negative to positive in lead II). At that point, the pacer is turned off, and the heart often remains in a sinus rhythm at an appropriate rate [77]. This technique is also quite effective in treating paroxysmal supraventricular tachycardia [78].

Temporary cardiac pacing is frequently helpful in maintaining an adequate heart rate, treating arrhythmias, and augmenting cardiac output. Patients with normal cardiac function as well as those with myocardial impairment benefit from the atrioventricular synchrony that pacemakers can provide [79]. As a routine measure, we place two pacing wires on the right atrium and two on the right ventricle. These wires may also permit greater accuracy in diagnosis of postoperative arrhythmias [80,81].

When the patient has been rewarmed to a rectal temperature of at least 35°C and cardiac rhythm is satisfactory, ventilation is resumed. Now the surgeon must ascertain that good lung expansion occurs with ventilation, that there is no closed pneumothorax, and that ventilation compromises no structures (e.g., places tension on an internal mammary artery graft). Failure to achieve adequate ventilation may require repositioning or clearing the endotracheal tube. Mucous plugs or blood clots may create a ball-valve effect on the end of the endotracheal tube, and this may not be resolved by passage of a suction catheter. Complete endotracheal tube removal and insertion of a new tube on bypass must be considered when ventilation is unsatisfactory. Rarely, bronchoscopy must be performed to establish a clear tracheobronchial tree.

Weaning from bypass then requires an adequate filling volume. With guidance from the surgeon, the perfusionist inhibits venous return to the bypass apparatus and progressively transfers volume into the patient. Adequate filling is determined by observation of ventricular size and motion and by palpation of the pulmonary artery and aorta. Measurement of the left atrial, right atrial, and pulmonary artery pressures is helpful as well. Caution must be used in attempting to infer left ventricular end-diastolic pressure or left ventricular volume from pulmonary artery diastolic or pulmonary capillary wedge pressures; the latter are at best unreliable guides to the former [82]. If ventricular performance was reasonably good preoperatively and an effective operation has been performed, bypass can usually be terminated without further delay.

A useful method of predicting cardiac output after separation from bypass has been described [83]. The mixed venous oxygen saturation ($S\bar{v}O_2^{(1)}$) and arterial blood flow ($\dot{Q}^{(1)}$) are recorded just before weaning from bypass is initiated. $S\bar{v}O_2$ is remeasured just after bypass is terminated ($S\bar{v}O_2^{(2)}$). Cardiac output ($\dot{Q}^{(2)}$) is then predicted from the formula:

$S\bar{v}O_2^{(1)}/\dot{Q}^{(1)} = S\bar{v}O_2^{(2)}/\dot{Q}^{(2)}$

This is in contradistinction to the use of mixed venous oxygen saturation to predict cardiac output in the postoperative period, which is much less reliable [84].

If the patient does not manifest adequate perfusion after achieving adequate cardiac filling pressures, the surgeon must attempt to determine a cause. In the absence of a definable, remediable condition, poor myocardial performance may require a return to cardiopulmonary bypass for an additional period of reperfusion before a second attempt to separate. During this time, the use of inotropic agents and afterload reduction may be initiated and may make a difference in separating the patient from bypass. More refractory problems may require use of the intraaortic balloon pump. Because percutaneous insertion of the intraaortic balloon is more difficult when the patient is on bypass, we insert 20-gauge percutaneous femoral artery catheters at the beginning of the operation, when the femoral pulse is easily palpable, in patients in whom we think the possibility of subsequent mechanical support is high. Through these catheters, guidewires, dilators, and introducer sheaths can be inserted, over which the intraaortic balloon can be passed (Fig. 2-7). In high-risk patients with mild aortoiliac disease or tortuous vessels noted during cardiac catheterization, we often insert an intraaortic balloon pump preoperatively in the catheterization laboratory with the help of fluoroscopic guidance. In patients with severe aortoiliac disease, introduction of the balloon pump via the ascending aorta may be required (Fig. 2-8). This technique mandates that the sternum be reopened for balloon removal. Prior vascular surgery, such as graft replacement of the abdominal aorta or an aortoiliac or aortofemoral bypass, does not preclude percutaneous balloon pump insertion [85].

PACING WIRES AND INTRACARDIAC LINES

Temporary pacing wires are placed on the right atrium and right ventricle (Fig. 2-9) and can be used for diagnostic or therapeutic pacing purposes, as discussed further in Chapter 4. In patients receiving bicaval cannulation for cardiopulmonary bypass, atrial pacing wires can be placed under the pursestring sutures used to secure the atrial cannulation sites.

Transthoracic monitoring lines may be used in adults, although this practice varies from institution to institution. If transvenous access is difficult, insertion of a transthoracic right atrial or pulmonary artery catheter may provide the necessary pressure measurements. Left atrial lines may be useful when the pulmonary capillary wedge pressure does not correlate well with the true left atrial pressure [86]. A left atrial catheter also allows administration of drugs into the systemic circulation while minimizing adverse effects on the pulmonary vessels [87,88]. Drug infusion into these lines must be performed with strict precautions to avoid air embolism (Fig. 2-10). Intraoperatively, these lines may be inserted via a pursestring suture in the right superior pulmonary vein (Fig. 2-11), or, if this route is used for insertion of a left ventricular vent, the resulting opening provides easy access for insertion of a left atrial line. Left atrial catheters add the risk of complications, which may include systemic emboli of air and particulate matter and bleeding and catastrophic

46 2. Operative Management

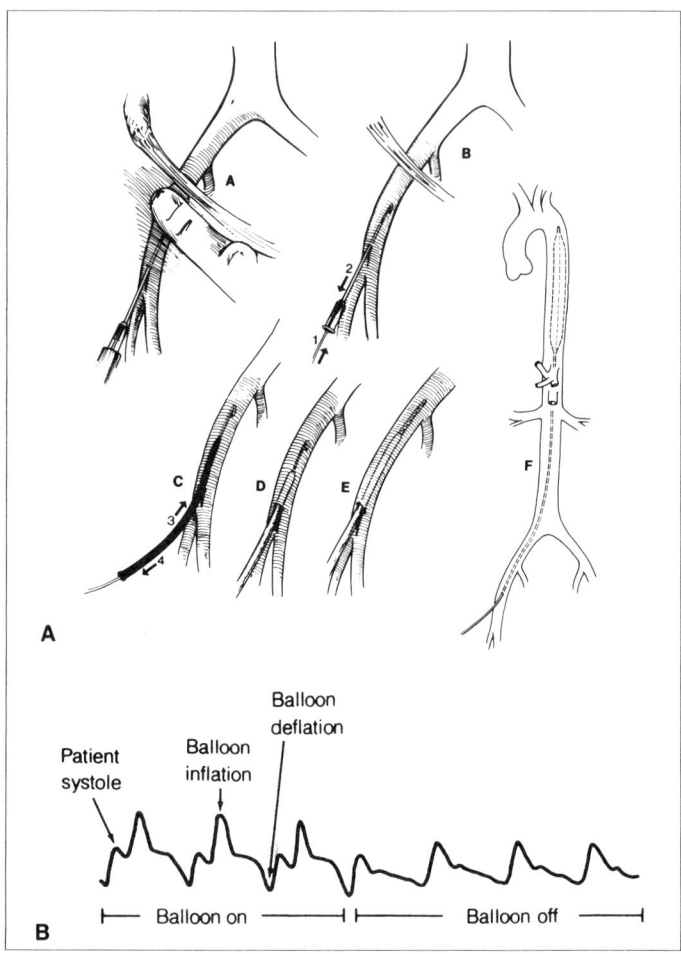

Fig. 2-7. Percutaneous insertion of an intraaortic balloon pump via the femoral artery. A. Insertion technique. If a femoral arterial line is not already present, the femoral artery is localized with a needle and syringe. Ideally, the artery should be entered immediately below the inguinal ligament (A). A guidewire is introduced via the needle (or femoral arterial line, if present) and into the iliofemoral tree (B). The needle is withdrawn over the guidewire, using gentle pressure to prevent bleeding around the insertion site, and dilators are serially introduced over the guidewire to dilate the femoral puncture site (C). An intraaortic balloon pump insertion sheath is then inserted over the final dilator (D, E). The dilator is removed and the balloon is inserted into the sheath. The balloon is then directed into the descending aorta (F). Passage of the balloon can be facilitated if a long guidewire is used (150 cm) to help negotiate the balloon through the iliofemoral arterial system. B. Proper balloon timing is shown in this tracing of arterial blood pressure. Balloon inflation occurs during patient diastole and balloon deflation occurs as the patient's heart ejects so as to produce mechanical afterload reduction.

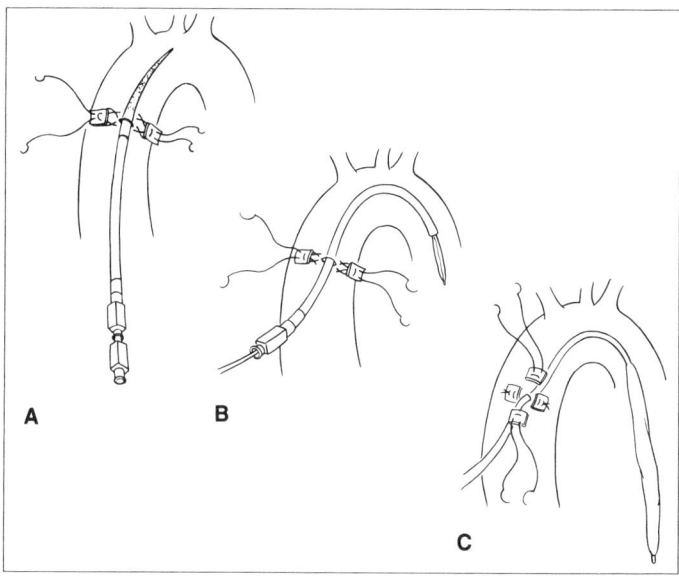

Fig. 2-8. Technique for transthoracic intraaortic balloon placement. Using two concentric pursestring sutures, a guidewire and dilators are introduced into the ascending aorta and passed around the aortic arch into the descending aorta. An insertion sheath is placed over the guidewire and dilators and directed beyond the brachiocephalic vessels (A). The intraaortic balloon pump catheter and balloon are then introduced over the guidewire, via the sheath, into the descending aorta (B). The position must be estimated visually by the surgeon so that the proximal extent of the balloon is beyond the left subclavian artery. (C) The sheath is then withdrawn from the aorta and the pursestring sutures are tightened using short tourniquets. The balloon may be subsequently removed by withdrawing the balloon catheter out the aortotomy, achieving digital control of the aortotomy site, and tightening and tying down the pursestring sutures.

interference with prosthetic disc mitral valves; surgically inserted transthoracic lines do not appear to be more resistant to infection than catheters inserted by percutaneous technique immediately before or after operation [9].

Other lines that are often useful are right atrial lines and lines inserted directly into the pulmonary artery via a pursestring suture in the right ventricular outflow tract (Fig. 2-12). This approach is particularly useful in neonates and infants for measurement of pulmonary artery pressure, pulmonary artery blood sampling, or insertion of thermodilution or oxygen saturation probes. This approach has proved safe, even in relatively hypertensive right ventricles [89].

DECANNULATION

After separation from bypass and administration of the appropriate volume from the bypass circuit, the venous and arterial cannulas

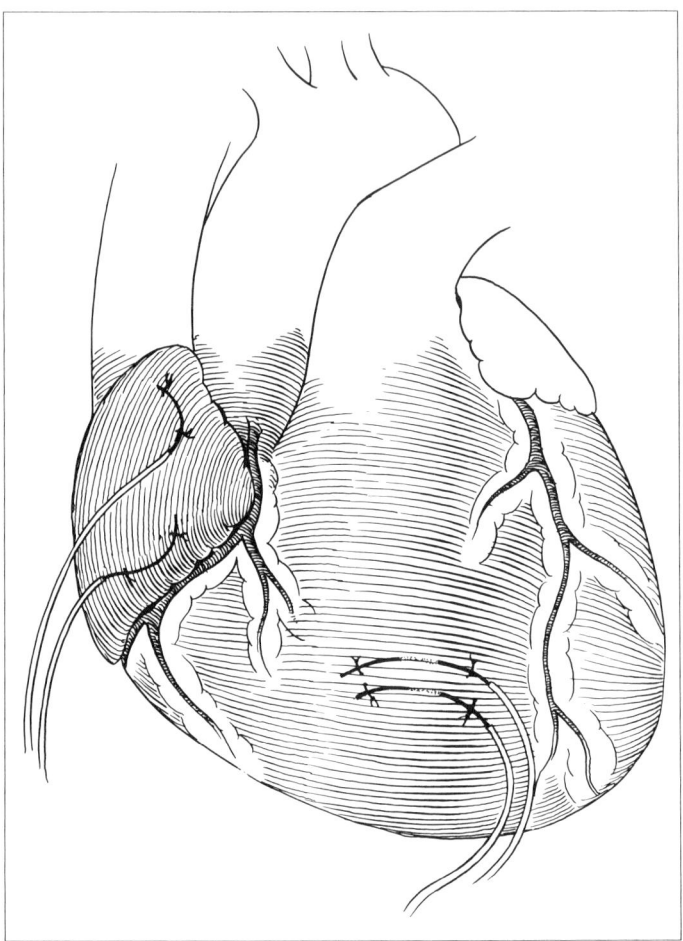

Fig. 2-9. Placement of temporary atrial and ventricular pacing wires at the end of the operation.

are removed, and the surrounding pursestring sutures are secured. Blood remaining in the pump oxygenator circuit is culture-positive for bacteria in over 10% of cases [90]; institutional practices vary as to whether or not this blood is reinfused. Increasingly, it is readministered as part of routine blood conservation measures, without a significant increase in postoperative infection. We usually hemoconcentrate it by recirculation through a hemofilter before reinfusion into the patient, or it can be concentrated by centrifugation.

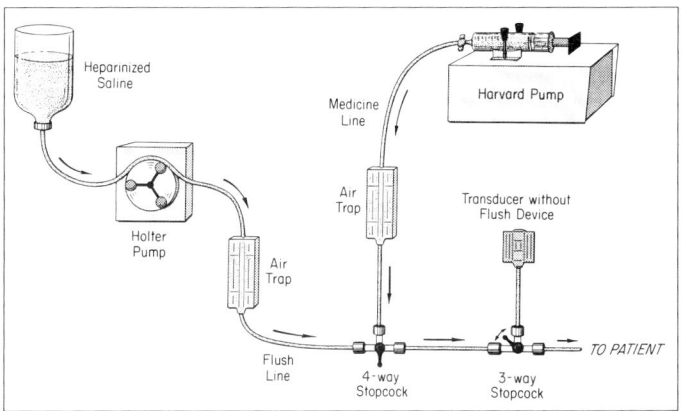

Fig. 2-10. Airtight system for left atrial or central venous catheters to permit simultaneous safe drug infusion and pressure measurement with minimal risk of air embolism.

REVERSAL OF HEPARIN

The dose of protamine required for reversal of heparin is calculated by measurement of the circulating heparin (Hepcon, Englewood, CO) or by administering a fixed dose, followed by confirmation that the ACT has returned to baseline. Even after complete reversal of heparin with confirmation by the heparin analyzer, 30 to 50% of patients may later show evidence of circulating heparin [91,92]. This "heparin rebound" may not be clinically significant and may require no additional protamine unless the patient is bleeding at an unacceptable rate [93].

Protamine typically produces mild hypotension by a direct vasodilation effect [94]; however, it may also cause one of two types of hemodynamic response associated with profound systemic hypotension [95]. The first type is a nonimmunologic reaction related to complement activation and thromboxane release [96]. This causes severe bronchospasm and pulmonary vasoconstriction. Systemic pressure falls as a result of poor pulmonary venous return. Although this response is usually short-lived, support of the circulation sometimes requires reheparinization and return to cardiopulmonary bypass. After several minutes of stabilization, the patient may again be separated from bypass. Because this is not a true allergic response, protamine may be safely readministered, although we prefer to infuse it into the aortic root at a very slow rate. Infusion of low-dose epinephrine or isoproterenol may provide an extra margin of safety to prevent pulmonary vasospasm [97].

The second type of reaction to protamine infusion is a true immune-mediated allergy. Traditionally, it has been thought that a true allergic response to protamine may be seen more commonly in patients receiving neutral protamine Hagedorn (NPH) insulin and in those with seafood allergies [98–100]; more recent evidence casts doubt on these earlier findings [101]. This reaction is mediated by histamine and is associated with low pulmonary artery pressure as

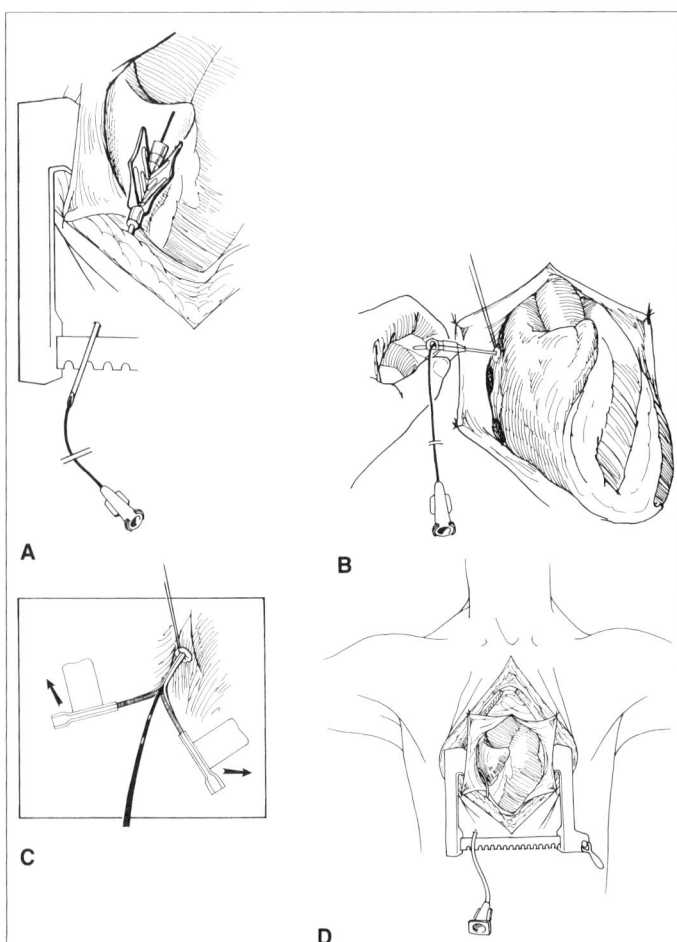

Fig. 2-11. Intraoperative technique for left atrial line insertion. Via a large-bore needle, inserted from inside the epigastric abdominal wall, the left atrial catheter is introduced into the chest (A). Using a split, "break-away" needle, the end of the left atrial catheter is introduced into the left atrium via the proximal right superior pulmonary vein using a pursestring suture to secure hemostasis at the insertion site (B). The "break-away" needle is then extracted and removed (C). Leave a gentle loop of catheter along the right side of the heart to prevent inadvertent extraction of the line when the chest is closed (D).

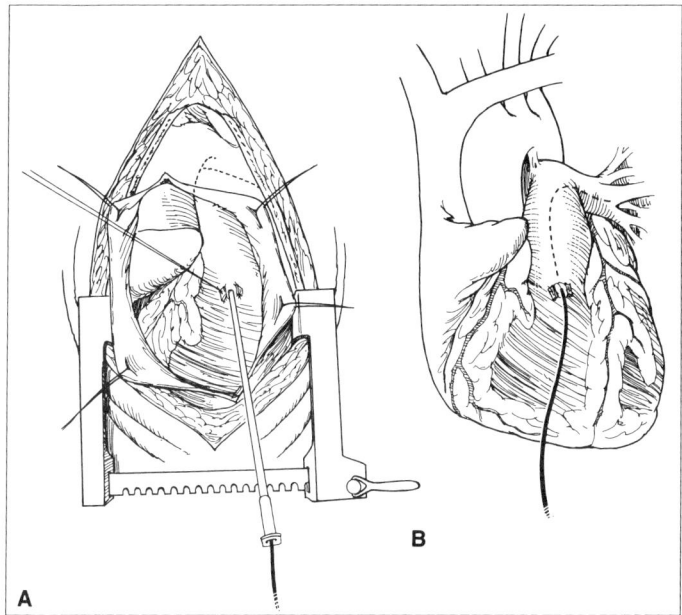

Fig. 2-12. Pulmonary artery monitoring line inserted via pursestring suture in the right ventricular outflow tract. Via a pledget-reinforced mattress suture, a catheter is introduced into the right ventricular outflow tract (A) using an introducer or a cannula-over-needle type of intravenous cannula. The introducer is withdrawn, the mattress suture is tightened, and the catheter is exteriorized through a small stab incision (B).

well as systemic arterial pressure. Resumption of cardiopulmonary bypass may be required. Reversal of heparin should not be attempted again until the patient has received steroids (methylprednisolone, 30 mg/kg IV) and histamine antagonists (chlorpheniramine, 0.15 mg/kg IV, and cimetidine, 5 mg/kg IV). Protamine infusion into the left side of the circulation may reduce histamine release [102], although the hemodynamic advantage of this has not been documented [103]. Rarely, reversal with protamine must be omitted.

PERICARDIAL CLOSURE

Some surgeons believe it is desirable to reapproximate the pericardium in patients in whom reoperation may be possible [33]; in practice, this includes all but the very elderly. Pericardial closure may diminish the formation of adhesions, although this point is debatable. It certainly interposes some tissue between the sternum and the anterior wall of the heart, which may increase the safety of subsequent resternotomy [33]. When pericardium cannot be reopposed, approximation of opposite pleurae may be performed instead. Other surgeons question the value of pericardial closure and express concern as to possible adverse hemodynamic consequences [104]. It is our practice not to close the pericardium if coronary bypass grafting has been performed. In other patients, we close it if it is hemodynamically tolerated. For the patient in whom the native pericardium cannot be approximated or is absent, a variety of pericardial substitutes have been advocated, including bovine pericardium [105,106], silicone rubber [107], and polytetrafluoroethylene [108]. We have been reluctant to use these materials because of their uncertain benefits; very dense adhesions between the prosthesis and the epicardium have been described [106]. Furthermore, serious problems with these materials have been reported, including severe inflammatory reactions [106,109,110], pericardial effusions [107], and calcification.

CLOSURE OF THE CHEST

Large tubes are positioned in the mediastinum before the chest is closed (Fig. 2-13). Conventionally, one tube lies on top of the diaphragm and another behind the sternum. We think that the use of large (32 Fr. or greater) tubes reduces the possibility of tube obstruction due to clots and consequent tamponade. Additionally, the pleural spaces should be drained if they have been entered or if pleural effusions are present.

Closure of the chest must never be performed in a casual fashion. Lack of sternal stability is a principal cause of wound complications [111–113]. The mortality of sternal wound infections dictates a precise and standardized approach to minimize the frequency of this dreaded complication. Excellent results have been obtained by surgeons using a wide variety of materials for sternal reapproximation, including wires, sutures, and metal bands [111,114,115].

SPECIAL PROBLEMS IN CHEST CLOSURE

At times, myocardial edema, acute cardiac dilatation, or other problems may make closure of the sternum impossible. On these occasions, closure of the skin alone [116] or coverage with a silicone rubber sheet [117] may be performed. Struts may be cut from chest tubes to hold the sternal edges apart. In 1 to 4 days, the patient may be returned to the operating room for sternal approximation and complete wound closure when cardiac edema has subsided. This procedure does not increase the risk of mediastinitis or sternal osteomyelitis.

The obese patient and the cachectic patient share a common risk of sternal wound problems, the former because of the increased force applied to the line of closure and the latter because of decreased tissue strength. To a greater degree than patients of normal habitus, these individuals require particular attention to hemostasis, careful approximation of tissues, and avoidance of dead space. It is, at times, helpful to perform the "sternal weave" technique to reinforce the fragile or narrow sternum [112].

Chronic obstructive pulmonary disease is an independent risk factor for the development of mediastinitis [118,119]. The cause of this association is unclear, but it may be related to the greater frequency of nasopharyngeal colonization with pathogens [120,121]. In the absence of any other controllable methods of overcoming

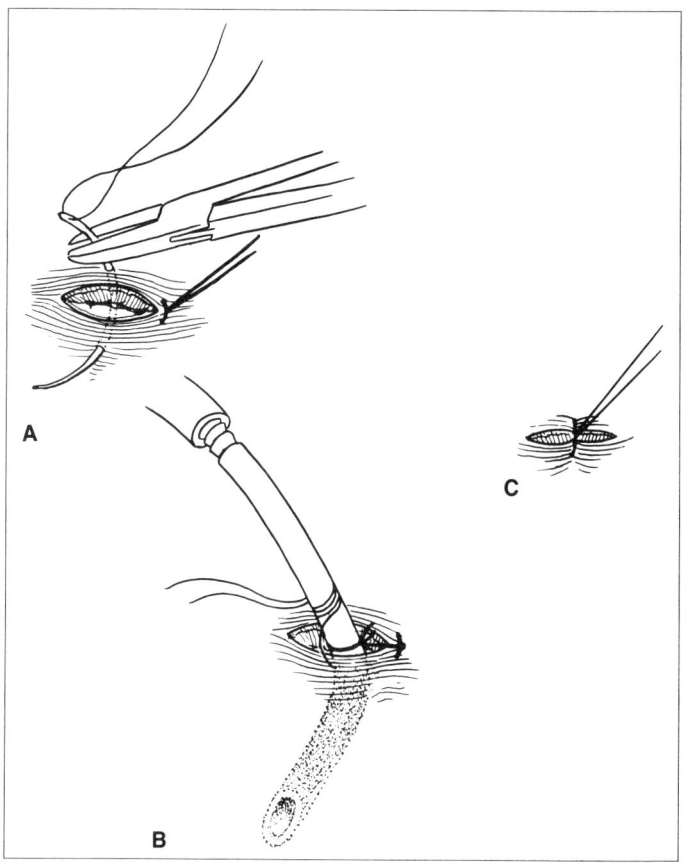

Fig. 2-13. Mediastinal tubes are secured to the skin with heavy silk suture. In addition, a heavy silk suture may be placed for subsequent closure of the chest tube insertion incision (A). The suture is not tied at the time of chest tube insertion, but the excess suture is wrapped around the chest tube (B). After chest tube removal, the suture is tied down to reapproximate the skin edges (C).

this risk factor, meticulous technique remains the best means of prevention.

Closure of the abdominal fascia must not be neglected. Incisional hernia has been reported in 4% of patients undergoing median sternotomy, and up to a third of these may be sufficiently symptomatic to require operative repair. Hernia is most common in males, obese patients, and patients with complicated postoperative courses [122].

TRANSPORT OF THE PATIENT

Movement of the postoperative patient to the recovery area or intensive care unit is potentially hazardous. Narcotic anesthesia may minimize hemodynamic changes during this critical period [123]. Safe transport of the patient from the operating room requires careful attention to all intravascular catheters, infusion devices, and drainage tubes. The patient's ECG, blood pressure, and, ideally, oxygen saturation are monitored continuously with a battery-powered transport monitor. Adequate ventilation and oxygenation must be assured. If the patient is awakening, additional sedation may be necessary to avoid thrashing, which may cause disconnection of a life-supporting piece of equipment. For our pediatric patients, we arrange for the postoperative nurse to come to the operating room to assist in transport. This measure facilitates proper organization and rapid reconnection of essential monitors and drugs on arrival in the intensive care unit.

References

1. Mohr R, Lavee J, Goor DA. Inaccuracy of radial artery pressure measurement after cardiac operations. *J Thorac Cardiovasc Surg* 94:286, 1987.

2. Bedford RF, Wollman H. Complications of percutaneous radial-artery cannulation: An objective prospective study in man. *Anesthesiology* 38:228, 1973.

3. Davis FM, Stewart JM. Radial artery cannulation. A prospective study in patients undergoing cardiothoracic surgery. *Br J Anaesth* 52:41, 1980.

4. Gardner RM, et al. Percutaneous indwelling radial-artery catheters for monitoring cardiovascular function. Prospective study of the risk of thrombosis and infection. *N Engl J Med* 290:1227, 1974.

5. Band JD, Maki DG. Infections caused by arterial catheters used for hemodynamic monitoring. *Am J Med* 67:735, 1979.

6. Shinozaki T, et al. Bacterial contamination of arterial lines: A prospective study. *JAMA* 249:223, 1983.

7. Pinilla JC, et al. Study of the incidence of intravascular catheter infection and associated septicemia in critically ill patients. *Crit Care Med* 11:21, 1983.

8. Singh S, et al. Catheter colonization and bacteremia with pulmonary and arterial catheters. *Crit Care Med* 10:736, 1982.

9. Damen J, et al. Microbiologic risk of invasive hemodynamic monitoring in patients undergoing open-heart operations. *Crit Care Med* 13:548, 1985.

10. McEnany MT, Austen WG. Life-threatening hemorrhage from inadvertent cervical arteriotomy. *Ann Thorac Surg* 24:233, 1977.

11. Elliott CG, Zimmerman GA, Clemmer TP. Complications of pulmonary artery catheterization in the care of critically ill patients. A prospective study. *Chest* 76:647, 1979.

12. Herbst CA Jr. Indications, management, and complications of percutaneous subclavian catheters. *Arch Surg* 113:1421, 1978.

13. Murray IP. Complications of invasive monitoring. *Med Instrum* 15:85, 1981.

14. Shaw TJI. The Swan-Ganz pulmonary artery catheter. *Anaesthesia* 34:651, 1979.

15. Boyd KD, et al. A prospective study of complications of pulmonary artery catheterizations in 500 consecutive patients. *Chest* 84:245, 1983.

16. McDaniel DD, et al. Catheter-induced pulmonary artery hemorrhage: Diagnosis and management in cardiac operations. *J Thorac Cardiovasc Surg* 82:1, 1981.

17. Stone JG, Khambatta HJ, McDaniel DD. Catheter-induced pulmonary artery trauma: Can it always be averted? *J Thorac Cardiovasc Surg* 86:146, 1983.

18. Webre DR, Arens JF. Use of cephalic and basilic veins for introduction of central venous catheters. *Anesthesiology* 38:389, 1973.

19. Kram HB. Noninvasive tissue oxygen monitoring in surgical and critical care medicine. *Surg Clin North Am* 65:1005, 1985.

20. Backofen JE, Schauble JF, Rogers MC. Transesophageal pacing for bradycardia. *Anesthesiology* 61:777, 1984.

21. Buchanan D, et al. Atrial esophageal pacing in patients undergoing coronary artery bypass grafting: Effect of previous cardiac operations and body surface area. *Anesthesiology* 69:595, 1988.

22. Lamas GA, et al. Pacemaker backup-mode reversion and injury during cardiac surgery. *Ann Thorac Surg* 41:155, 1986.

23. Zipes DP. Risk of electrocautery for patients with cardiac pacemaker. *JAMA* 261:2422, 1989.

24. Hakki HI, Goel IP, Mundth ED. Pacemaker inhibition in cardiac surgery. *Ann Thorac Surg* 33:295, 1982.

25. Sanford TJ Jr, et al. A comparison of morphine, fentanyl, and sufentanil anesthesia for cardiac surgery. Induction, emergence, and extubation. *Anesth Analg* 65:259, 1986.

26. Crean P, et al. Fentanyl-oxygen versus fentanyl-N_2O/oxygen anaesthesia in children undergoing cardiac surgery. *Can Anaesth Soc J* 33:36, 1986.

27. Van Tright P, et al. The mechanism of halothane-induced myocardial depression. Altered diastolic mechanics versus impaired contractility. *J Thorac Cardiovasc Surg* 85:832, 1983.

28. Van Tright P, et al. Myocardial depression by anesthetic agents (halothane, enflurane, and nitrous oxide): Quantitation based on end-systolic pressure-dimension relations. *Am J Cardiol* 53:243, 1984.

29. Estafanous FG (ed). *Anesthesia and The Heart Patient.* Boston: Butterworths, 1989.

30. Kaplan JA (ed). *Cardiac Anesthesia.* Vol 2. Orlando: Grune & Stratton, 1987.

31. Bojar RM, et al. Use of self-adhesive external defibrillator pads for complex cardiac surgical procedures. *Ann Thorac Surg* 46:587, 1988.

32. Brutel de la Riviere A, Brom GH, Bron AG. Horizontal submam-

mary skin incision for median sternotomy. *Ann Thorac Surg* 32:101, 1981.

33. Dobell ARC, Jain AK. Catastrophic hemorrhage during redo sternotomy. *Ann Thorac Surg* 37:273, 1984.

34. Bull BS, et al. Heparin therapy during extracorporeal circulation. II. The use of a dose response curve to individualize heparin and protamine dosage. *J Thorac Cardiovasc Surg* 69:685, 1975.

35. Esposito RA, et al. Heparin resistance during cardiopulmonary bypass. The role of heparin pretreatment. *J Thorac Cardiovasc Surg* 85:346, 1983.

36. Glock Y, et al. Cardiovascular surgery and heparin induced thrombocytopenia. *Int Angiol* 7:238, 1988.

37. Cloyd GM, D'Ambra MN, Akins CW. Diminished anticoagulant response to heparin in patients undergoing coronary artery bypass grafting. *J Thorac Cardiovasc Surg* 94:535, 1987.

38. Mills NL, Everson CT. Atherosclerosis of the ascending aorta and coronary bypass. Pathology, clinical correlates, and operative management. *J Thorac Cardiovasc Surg* 102:546, 1991.

39. Waering TH, et al. Management of the severely atherosclerotic ascending aorta during cardiac operations. A strategy for detection and treatment. *J Thorac Cardiovasc Surg* 103:453, 1992.

40. Boers M, et al. Two membrane oxygenators and a bubbler: A clinical comparison. *Ann Thorac Surg* 35:455, 1983.

41. Dancy CM, et al. Pulmonary dysfunction associated with cardiopulmonary bypass: A comparison of bubble and membrane oxygenators. *Circulation* 64(Suppl II):II-54, 1981.

42. Sade RM, et al. A prospective randomized study of membrane versus bubble oxygenators in children. *Ann Thorac Surg* 29:502, 1980.

43. Trumbull HR, et al. A comparison of the effects of membrane and bubble oxygenators on platelet counts and platelet size in elective cardiac operations. *Ann Thorac Surg* 30:52, 1980.

44. van Oeveren W, et al. Deleterious effects of cardiopulmonary bypass. A prospective study of bubble versus membrane oxygenation. *J Thorac Cardiovasc Surg* 89:888, 1985.

45. Tamiya T, et al. Complement activation in cardiopulmonary bypass, with special reference to anaphylatoxin production in membrane and bubble oxygenators. *Ann Thorac Surg* 46:47, 1988.

46. Griepp EB, Griepp RB. Cerebral consequences of hypothermic circulatory arrest in adults. *J Cardiac Surg* 7:134, 1992.

47. Livesay JJ, et al. Resection of aortic arch aneurysms: A comparison of hypothermic techniques in 60 patients. *Ann Thorac Surg* 36:19, 1983.

48. Lucas SK, et al. The harmful effects of ventricular distention during postischemia reperfusion. *Ann Thorac Surg* 32:486, 1981.

49. Olinger GN, Bonchek LI. Ventricular venting during coronary revascularization: Assessment of benefit by intraoperative ventricular function curves. *Ann Thorac Surg* 26:525, 1978.

50. Little AG, et al. Use of the pulmonary artery for left ventricular venting during cardiac operations. *J Thorac Cardiovasc Surg* 87:532, 1984.

51. Akins CW. Noncardioplegic myocardial preservation for coronary revascularization. *J Thorac Cardiovasc Surg* 88:174, 1984.

52. Gay WA Jr, Ebert PA. Functional, metabolic, and morphologic effects of potassium-induced cardioplegia. *Surgery* 74:284, 1973.

53. Buckberg GD. A proposed "solution" to the cardioplegic controversy. *J Thorac Cardiovasc Surg* 77:803, 1979.

54. Gay WA Jr. Potassium-induced cardioplegia: Evolution and present status. *Ann Thorac Surg* 48:441, 1989.

55. Hearse DJ, Stewart DA, Braimbridge MV. The additive protective effects of hypothermia and chemical cardioplegia during ischemic cardiac arrest in the rat. *J Thorac Cardiovasc Surg* 79:39, 1980.

56. Lichtenstein SV, et al. Warm heart surgery: Experience with long cross-clamp times. *Ann Thorac Surg* 52:1009, 1991.

57. Freedman BM, et al. Effects of delay in administration of potassium cardioplegia to the isolated rat heart. *Ann Thorac Surg* 37:309, 1984.

58. Ferguson TB Jr, et al. Monitoring the electrical status of the ventricle during cardioplegic arrest. *Circulation* 68(Suppl II):II-27, 1983.

59. Lange R, The relative importance of alkalinity, temperature, and the washout effect of bicarbonate-buffered, multidose cardioplegic solution. *Circulation* 70(Suppl I):I-75, 1984.

60. Grover FL, et al. Does lower systemic temperature enhance cardioplegic myocardial protection? *J Thorac Cardiovasc Surg* 81:11, 1981.

61. Lazar HL. Rivers S. Importance of topical hypothermia during heterogeneous distribution of cardioplegic solution. *J Thorac Cardiovasc Surg* 98:251, 1989.

62. Padayachee TS, et al. The detection of microemboli in the middle cerebral artery during cardiopulmonary bypass: A transcranial Doppler ultrasound investigation using membrane and bubble oxygenators. *Ann Thorac Surg* 44:298, 1987.

63. Padayachee TS, et al. The effect of arterial filtration on reduction of gaseous microemboli in the middle cerebral artery during cardiopulmonary bypass. *Ann Thorac Surg* 45:647, 1988.

64. Oka Y, et al. Detection of air emboli in the left heart by M-mode transesophageal echocardiography following cardiopulmonary bypass. *Anesthesiology* 63:109, 1985.

65. Topol EJ, et al. Value of intraoperative left ventricular microbubbles detected by transesophageal two-dimensional echocardiography in predicting neurologic outcome after cardiac operations. *Am J Cardiol* 56:773, 1985.

66. Butler BD, et al. Effect of the Trendelenburg position on the distribution of arterial air emboli in dogs. *Ann Thorac Surg* 45:198, 1988.

67. Oka Y, et al. Retained intracardiac air. Transesophageal echocardiography for definition of incidence and monitoring removal by improved techniques. *J Thorac Cardiovasc Surg* 91:329, 1986.

68. Stoney WS, et al. Air embolism and other accidents using pump oxygenators. *Ann Thorac Surg* 29:336, 1980.

69. Mills NL, Ochsner JL. Massive air embolism during cardiopulmonary bypass. Causes, prevention, and management. *J Thorac Cardiovasc Surg* 80:708, 1980.

70. Spampinato N, et al. Massive air embolism during cardiopulmonary bypass: Successful treatment with immediate hypothermia and circulatory support. *Ann Thorac Surg* 32:602, 1981.

71. Fall SM, et al. Prevention of ventricular fibrillation after myocardial revascularization. *Ann Thorac Surg* 43:182, 1987.

72. Kerber RE, et al. Open chest defibrillation during cardiac surgery: Energy and current requirement. *Am J Cardiol* 46:393, 1980.

73. Lake CL, et al. Energy dose and other variables possibly affecting ventricular defibrillation during cardiac surgery. *Anesth Analg* 63:743, 1984.

74. Tacker WA Jr, et al. The electrical dose for direct ventricular fibrillation in man. *J Thorac Cardiovasc Surg* 75:224, 1978.

75. Waldo AL, et al. Diagnosis and treatment of arrhythmias during and following open heart surgery. *Med Clin North Am* 68:1153, 1984.

76. Woodson RD, Starr A. Atrial pacing after mitral valve surgery. *Arch Surg* 97:984, 1968.

77. Cooper TB, MacLean WAH, Waldo AL. Overdrive pacing for supraventricular tachycardia: A review of theoretical implications and therapeutic techniques. *PACE* 1:196, 1978.

78. Waldo AL, et al. Transient entrainment and interruption of the atrioventricular bypass pathway type of paroxysmal atrial tachycardia. A model for understanding and identifying reentrant arrhythmias. *Circulation* 67:73, 1983.

79. Curtis J, et al. Influence of atrioventricular synchrony on hemodynamics in patients with normal and low ejection fractions following open heart surgery. *Am Surg* 52:93, 1986.

80. Malcolm ID, Cherry DA, Morin JE. The use of temporary atrial electrodes to improve diagnostic capabilities with Holter monitoring after cardiac surgery. *Ann Thorac Surg* 41:103, 1986.

81. Waldo AL, Henthorn RW, Plumb VJ. Temporary epicardial wire electrodes in the diagnosis and treatment of arrhythmias after open heart surgery. *Am J Surg* 148:275, 1984.

82. Douglas PS, et al. Unreliability of hemodynamic indexes of left ventricular size during cardiac surgery. *Ann Thorac Surg* 44:31, 1987.

83. Chung RS, et al. Prediction of post-cardiopulmonary bypass cardiac output. *Ann Thorac Surg* 47:297, 1989.

84. Magilligan DJ Jr, et al. Mixed venous oxygen saturation as a

predictor of cardiac output in the postoperative cardiac surgical patient. *Ann Thorac Surg* 44:260, 1987.

85. LaMuraglia GM, et al. The safety of intra-aortic balloon pump catheter insertion through suprainguinal prosthetic vascular bypass grafts. *J Vasc Surg* 13:830, 1991.

86. Raper R, Sibbald WJ. Misled by the wedge? The Swan-Ganz catheter and left ventricular preload. *Chest* 89:427, 1986.

87. D'Ambra MN, et al. Prostaglandin E_1 (PGE_1): A new therapy for refractory right heart failure and pulmonary hypertension after mitral valve replacement. *J Thorac Cardiovasc Surg* 89:567, 1985.

88. D'Ambra MN, Beller JP. Pulmonary circulation: Pharmacologic management. In Grillo HC, et al. (eds), *Current Therapy in Cardiothoracic Surgery*. Toronto: B C Decker, 1989. Pp 278–281.

89. Gold JP, et al. Transthoracic intracardiac monitoring lines in pediatric surgical patients: A ten-year experience. *Ann Thorac Surg* 42:185, 1986.

90. Freeman R, Hjersing N. Bacterial culture of perfusion blood after open-heart surgery. *Thorax* 35:754, 1980.

91. Kesteven PJ, et al. Protamine sulphate and heparin rebound following open-heart surgery. *J Cardiovasc Surg* (Torino) 27:600, 1986.

92. Pifarre R, et al. Management of postoperative heparin rebound following cardiopulmonary bypass. *J Thorac Cardiovasc Surg* 81:378, 1981.

93. Esposito RA, et al. The role of the activated clotting time in heparin administration and neutralization for cardiopulmonary bypass. *J Thorac Cardiovasc Surg* 85:174, 1983.

94. Shapira N, et al. Cardiovascular effects of protamine sulfate in man. *J Thorac Cardiovasc Surg* 84:505, 1982.

95. Horrow JC. Protamine allergy. *J Cardiothorac Anesth* 2:225, 1988.

96. Morel DR, et al. C5a and thromboxane generation associated with pulmonary vaso- and broncho-constriction during protamine administration. *Anesthesiology* 66:597, 1987.

97. Lowenstein E, et al. Catastrophic pulmonary vasoconstriction associated with protamine reversal of heparin. *Anesthesiology* 59:470, 1983.

98. Knape JTA, et al. An anaphylactic reaction to protamine in a patient allergic to fish. *Anesthesiology* 55:324, 1981.

99. Moorthy SS, Pond W, Rowland RG. Severe circulatory shock following protamine (an anaphylactoid reaction). *Anesth Analg* 59:77, 1980.

100. Stewart WJ, et al. Increased risk of severe protamine reactions in NPH insulin-dependent diabetics undergoing cardiac catheterization. *Circulation* 70:788, 1984.

101. Levy JH, et al. Evaluation of patients at risk for protamine reactions. *J Thorac Cardiovasc Surg* 98:200, 1989.

102. Frater RWM, et al. Protamine-induced circulatory changes. *J Thorac Cardiovasc Surg* 87:687, 1984.

103. Katz NM, et al. Hemodynamics of protamine administration. Comparison of right atrial, left atrial, and aortic injection. *J Thorac Cardiovasc Surg* 94:881, 1987.

104. Loop FD. Catastrophic hemorrhage during sternal reentry. *Ann Thorac Surg* 37:271, 1984.

105. Gallo JI, Artinano E, Duran CMG. Clinical experience with glutaraldehyde-preserved heterologous pericardium for the closure of the pericardium after open heart surgery. *Thorac Cardiovasc Surg* 30:306, 1982.

106. Opie JC, Larrieu AJ, Cornell IS. Pericardial substitutes: Delayed reexploration and findings. *Ann Thorac Surg* 43:383, 1987.

107. Laks H, Hammond G, Geha AS. Use of silicone rubber as a pericardial substitute to facilitate reoperation in cardiac surgery. *J Thorac Cardiovasc Surg* 82:88, 1981.

108. Minale C, et al. Closure of the pericardium using expanded polytetrafluoroethylene GORE-TEX Surgical Membrane: Clinical experience. *Thorac Cardiovasc Surg* 35:312, 1987.

109. Mills SA. Complications associated with the use of heterologous bovine pericardium for pericardial closure. *J Thorac Cardiovasc Surg* 92:446, 1986.

110. Skinner JR, et al. Inflammatory epicardial reaction to processed bovine pericardium: Case report. *J Thorac Cardiovasc Surg* 88:789, 1984.

111. Labitzke R, et al. "Sleeve-rope closure" of the median sternotomy after open heart operations. *Thorac Cardiovasc Surg* 31:127, 1983.

112. Robicsek F, Daugherty HK, Cook JW. The prevention and treatment of sternum separation following open-heart surgery. *J Thorac Cardiovasc Surg* 73:267, 1977.

113. Sanfelippo PM, Danielson GK. Complications associated with median sternotomy. *J Thorac Cardiovasc Surg* 63:419, 1972.

114. Breyer RH, et al. A prospective study of sternal wound complications. *Ann Thorac Surg* 37:412, 1984.

115. Mulch J, et al. Closure of longitudinal sternotomy with absorbable sutures. *Thorac Cardiovasc Surg* 34:191, 1986.

116. Milgater E, et al. Delayed sternal closure following cardiac operations. *J Cardiovasc Surg* 27:328, 1986.

117. Josa M, et al. Delayed sternal closure. An improved method of dealing with complications after cardiopulmonary bypass. *J Thorac Cardiovasc Surg* 91:598, 1986.

118. Bor DH, et al. Mediastinitis after cardiovascular surgery. *Rev Infect Dis* 5:885, 1983.

119. Newman LS, et al. Suppurative mediastinitis after open heart surgery. A case control study of risk factors. *Chest* 94:546, 1988.

120. Engelman RM, et al. Mediastinitis following open-heart surgery: Review of two years' experience. *Arch Surg* 107:772, 1973.

121. Frater RWM, Santos GH. Sources of infection in open heart surgery. *NY State J Med* 74:2386, 1974.
122. Davidson BR, Bailey JS. Incisional herniae following median sternotomy incisions: Their incidence and aetiology. *Br J Surg* 73:995, 1986.
123. Insel J, et al. Cardiovascular changes during transport of critically ill and postoperative patients. *Crit Care Med* 14:539, 1986.

Postoperative Management

Postoperative care of the cardiac surgical patient begins at the time of transfer from the operating room to the intensive care unit. This is a hazardous period that requires the strict attention of both the anesthesiologist and the surgeon. ECG and arterial pressure monitoring by a portable, battery-powered unit is essential during the transfer, and basic resuscitation medications (e.g., lidocaine and epinephrine) should be readily available for quick administration en route, if required. Likewise, a spare endotracheal tube and a laryngoscope should be close at hand for emergency reintubation. After arrival in the intensive care unit, transfer of the monitoring leads and transducers to the bedside monitor must be accomplished without delay.

On arrival in the intensive care unit, the monitoring lines are transferred to the bedside monitor and a report is given to the patient's primary nurse and the intensive care unit physician by the anesthesiologist. This includes a brief description of the procedure performed, any problems encountered, details regarding the filling pressure at which the patient's heart appears to function best, and any ongoing drug infusions. Blood samples should be sent *STAT* for arterial blood gas analysis, hematocrit (or hemoglobin) level, and sodium and potassium concentrations. Obtaining these results early will help in the prevention and treatment of serious electrolyte and acid-base abnormalities, which can develop quickly during the early postoperative period. Routine measurement of platelet count and other clotting studies may be performed, but these are unnecessary in the patient who is not bleeding excessively.

The heart is auscultated to provide baseline information such as the presence or absence of murmurs and the loudness of the heart sounds. This baseline examination provides a reference for later examination. For example, the later development of a murmur may indicate detachment of a prosthetic valve or patch, and, similarly, muffled heart sounds later on may suggest cardiac tamponade. The chest is auscultated to determine that there are good breath sounds bilaterally. Any patient who did not have a nasogastric tube inserted during surgery should have one placed shortly after admission to the intensive care unit. A chest x-ray is obtained unless one was performed in the operating room. This provides verification of the position of the endotracheal tube, nasogastric tube, chest tubes, and monitoring cannulas; establishes a baseline measurement of the mediastinal silhouette; and allows one to rule out pneumothorax, hemothorax, or atelectasis. Baseline determinations of the patient's thermodilution cardiac output (or the cardiac index) should be obtained early after arrival in the intensive care unit if a Swan-Ganz catheter is present.

Each patient has a nurse in constant attendance who records the vital signs, fluid input and output, and hemodynamic data at regular intervals on a standardized flow sheet as shown in Figure 3-1. The importance of a permanent staff of nurses trained in cardiac surgical care cannot be overemphasized. Such nurses can accurately record measurements, recognize ECG abnormalities, and initiate treat-

3. Postoperative Management   63

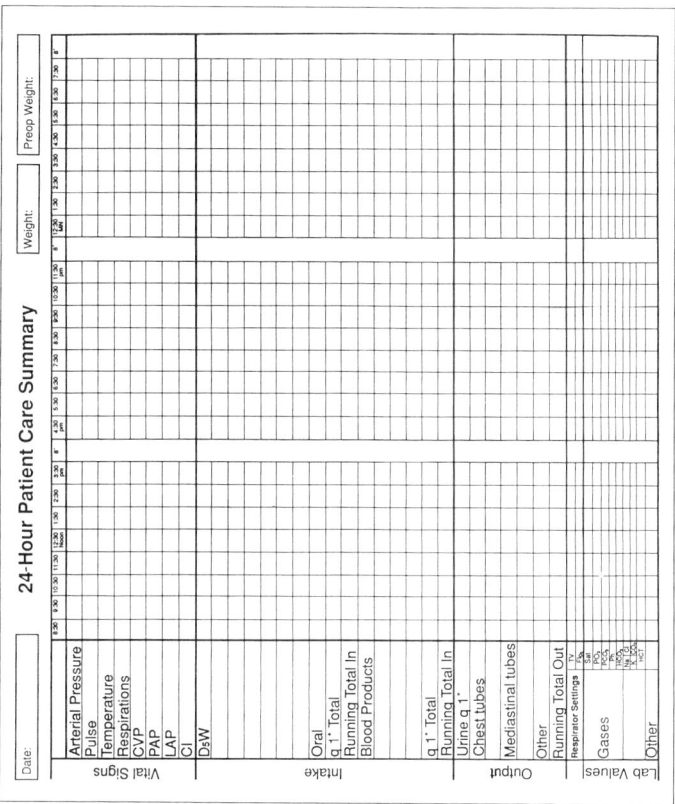

Fig. 3-1. Intensive care unit flow sheet for recording patient data.

ment for problems before they become major ones. Suggestions or concerns raised by an experienced cardiac surgery nurse should not be dismissed lightly by the physicians participating in the care of the postoperative patient.

Once the patient has been admitted to the intensive care unit and all bedside monitors are functioning properly, the postoperative orders are written. We find it convenient to utilize preprinted order sheets (Fig. 3-2) that not only allow for individualization in differing circumstances, but also contain the common orders that are needed for most patients. This increases efficiency and helps prevent the omission of important directives. Likewise, when the patient is ready to be moved out of the intensive care unit, preprinted transfer orders are again employed (Fig. 3-3). It is important to remember to restart orally administered medications that the patient was taking before surgery (such as beta-adrenergic antagonists) when appropriate after the patient has been extubated.

Postoperative Cardiac Surgery ICU Orders

Date & Time	Diagnostic, Therapeutic, and Dietary Orders	✓
	Admit to ICU; Diagnosis: _____ Allergies: _____	
	Continuous ECG, radial artery, pulmonary artery, and left atrial (if present) monitoring	
	Vital signs per ICU standards; Measure I& O; Weigh daily	
	NG tube to low constant suction; Foley to gravity	
	Chest tubes to pleurovacs at -20-cm suction; reinfuse per protocol	
	Lab studies: Hct, Na, K, ABG upon arrival and prn CBC, Lytes, Creat & BUN qAM x 2 days; CK-MB q12 hr x 2 Daily PT?: Yes No	
	CXR within 1 hour of arrival and in AM on POD #1	
	ECG qAM x 2 days	
	Diet: NPO until extubated and NG tube out. Then begin clear liquids and advance to no added salt, low cholesterol diet.	

	Medications, IV, Ventilator Orders	
	IV Fluid: _____ at _____ cc/hr	
	Antibiotics: 1. _____ 2. _____	
	Morphine sulfate _____ mg IV/IM (circle one) q ___ hr prn pain	
	Valium 2–5 mg IV q1–2hr prn agitation	
	When taking PO: Dilaudid 2–4 mg q2–3hr, or, Tylenol #3 1–2 tabs q2–3hr, or, Darvocet-N 1–2 tabs q2–3hr prn pain	

	KCl: for K < 4.0, give 10 mEq in 50 cc D5W over 1 hr
	    for K < 3.0, give 20 mEq in 50 cc D5W over 1 hr
	    Administer through central line. Recheck K after each dose	

	Tylenol 650–1300 mg PO/PR q3–4hr prn T > 101	
	ASA 325 mg PO/PR qd. Begin _____ hours postop, if bleeding less than 50 cc/hr. DO NOT GIVE TO VALVE PATIENTS	
	Antiarrhythmics: 1. _____ 2. _____	

	IV infusions: 1. _____
	              2. _____
	              3. _____	

	Other drugs: 1. _____ 2. _____	
	Ventilator Settings: AC or IMV TV _____ cc; FiO2 ____ %; VR _____ bpm; PEEP ____ cm	

Fig. 3-2. Typical physician's postoperative orders for adults in the intensive care unit following cardiac surgery.

Postoperative Cardiac Surgery Transfer Orders		
Date & Time	Diagnostic, Therapeutic, and Dietary Orders	√
	Transfer to _____ Diagnosis: _____ POD # _____ Allergies: _____	
	Vitals signs per standards; Cardiac telemetry monitor	
	Daily weight; Record I & O	
	Remove Foley on POD # _____	
	Pacemaker orders: _____	
	If chest tubes in: -20-cm suction to pleurovac	
	Lab studies on POD #4 : CBC, Lytes, BUN, Creat; ECG; CXR (PA & Lat) Daily Prothrombin Time?: YES NO	
	Cardiac rehabilitation nurse's instruction per protocol	
	Ambulate as tolerated	
	Diet: _____	
	Fluid restriction: _____cc/day	
	Routine daily wound care	
	Incentive spirometer q2–3 hr when awake	
	Medications, IV, etc. Orders	
	IV fluid: _____	
	Oxygen: _____	
	Dilaudid 2–4 mg PO q3–4hr prn, or, Tylenol #3 1–2 tabs PO q3–4hr prn, or, Darvocet-N 1–2 tabs PO q3-4hr prn	
	If oral pain medication ineffective, give morphine sulfate _____mg IM q3hr prn	
	Benadryl 25 mg PO qhr prn sleep; may repeat x 1	
	Antibiotics: 1. _____ 2. _____	
	Antiarrhythmics: 1. _____ 2. _____	
	Enteric coated ASA - 325 mg PO qd. Do not give to valve patients	
	Colace 100 mg PO bid	
	Milk of magnesia 30 cc PO qhr prn constipation	
	Dulcolax suppository pr 1 qd prn constipation	
	Other medications: 1. _____ 2. _____	

Fig. 3-3. Typical physician's orders for transfer from the intensive care unit to the postoperative cardiac care ward.

Management of the Hemodynamic State

EVALUATION AND MONITORING OF CARDIOVASCULAR FUNCTION

Assessment of the patient's cardiovascular status after cardiac surgery begins with a physical examination. The patient with satisfactory cardiac output and blood pressure typically is alert (if not anesthetized), warm to the touch, and has palpable pedal pulses (in the absence of lower extremity obstructive vascular disease); whereas the patient with inadequate cardiac output and blood pressure typically may be agitated or lethargic, with cool skin and slow capillary refill, and may have no palpable pedal pulses. Infants with inadequate cardiac output often have elevated core temperatures in the face of cold extremities. The patient with cardiac failure, unless hypovolemic, often has jugular venous distention, but more subtle and chronic signs of heart failure such as a third heart sound or pulmonary rales may be difficult to discern in the noisy intensive care unit environment. The physical examination can also be confounded by the effects of hypothermia (causing peripheral vasoconstriction and cool extremities) and anesthetic agents (causing unresponsiveness), which are often present early after surgery. Congestive heart failure in infants is not manifested by peripheral edema or orthopnea as it is in adults. One must search instead for hepatomegaly, facial puffiness, unexplained tachycardia, weight gain, cardiac enlargement, or tachypnea.

Other parameters such as hourly urine output must be taken into account but can be misleading early after open heart surgery [1]. Patients with satisfactory cardiac output and blood pressure usually exhibit a relative diuresis early after surgery due to the effects of hemodilution and of the osmotic agents sometimes administered during cardiopulmonary bypass. Because of these factors, even patients with poor cardiovascular performance early after surgery may continue to produce significant amounts of urine for several hours after operation. Later, when the effects of cardiopulmonary bypass have cleared, urine output becomes a more sensitive measure of cardiac output and blood pressure. In this setting, a low urine output (less than 30–50 ml/hr in adults or 0.5 ml/kg/hr in infants) indicates inadequate hemodynamic performance and requires prompt investigation and treatment.

Invasive measurements provide important complementary information to these noninvasive observations. It must be remembered, however, that all catheters, cannulas, monitors, and tracings may be inaccurate, misread, or mislabeled. *Proper management of the cardiac surgery patient never relies on a single "number" to dictate the direction of therapy, but rather takes into account the results of **all** noninvasive and invasive information that is available.*

Arterial pressure is continuously monitored, usually via a cannula in the patient's radial artery (Fig. 3-4). Although systolic arterial pressure reflects the systolic pressure within the left ventricle (in the absence of obstructive lesions such as aortic stenosis), arterial blood pressure is not a sensitive measure of overall hemodynamic status. The ability of the systemic circulation to vasoconstrict and maintain a relatively normal blood pressure, even in the presence of very poor cardiac function, makes this measure of hemodynamic function often the "last to fall" before total cardiovascular collapse.

Flow-directed (Swan-Ganz) pulmonary artery catheters are utilized routinely for monitoring most adult patients undergoing cardiac surgery at many institutions. These catheters provide continuous measurement of the systolic, diastolic, and mean pressures in the patient's pulmonary artery; allow for thermodilution measurements of the right heart cardiac output; and provide access for blood sampling from the pulmonary artery (mixed venous blood).

The concepts of *preload* and *afterload* are important in the care of cardiac surgical patients. For the ventricle to produce an adequate output, it first must be adequately filled. Technically, the volume

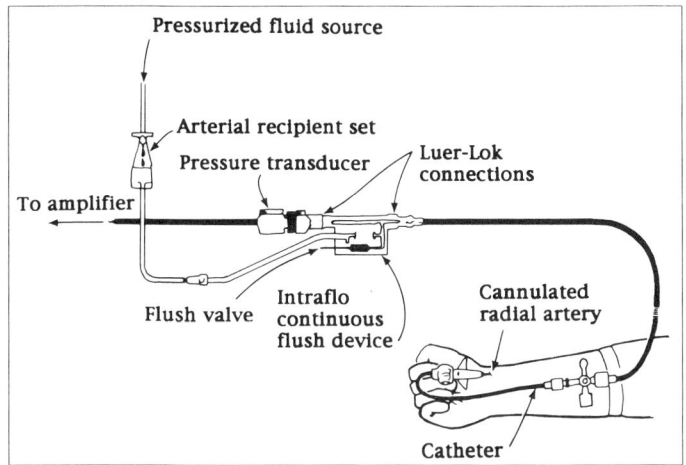

Fig. 3-4. Arterial catheter, transducer, and continuous flush system for arterial lines in adults. A Harvard infusion pump is used for the pressurized fluid source in infants because the infusion volume can be more precisely regulated at 1 to 2 ml/hr through a Y or 4-way stopcock in the arterial line. (From RM Gardner et al. Percutaneous indwelling radial artery catheter for monitoring cardiovascular function. *N Engl J Med* 290:1227, 1974. Reprinted with permission from the *New England Journal of Medicine.*)

of blood within the ventricle at the end of diastole is the best measure of ventricular filling and best reflects the *preload* of the heart, but this is difficult to measure routinely. The left ventricular end-diastolic pressure reflects the ventricular volume (ignoring the effects of compliance). However, to measure the left ventricular end-diastolic pressure, a catheter must be placed within the left ventricle and this has the potential risks of emboli, ventricular irritability, and bleeding through the site of introduction. The mean left atrial pressure is a relatively good measurement of left ventricular filling pressure; left atrial catheters are used for this purpose in selected patients (see Fig. 2-11). Even safer and more convenient, however, is the pulmonary capillary wedge pressure, which is obtained at the end of the pulmonary artery catheter when the vessel is occluded (or "wedged") by temporary inflation of a balloon positioned at the end of the catheter (see Fig. 2-3). The pulmonary capillary wedge pressure closely approximates left ventricular end-diastolic pressure in patients with normal hearts, although it tends to be lower than the end-diastolic pressure in many patients with cardiac disease [2].

Thermodilution cardiac output determination is based on the principle of temperature dilution. The pulmonary artery catheter has at least three lumens: one proximally opening into the right atrium, one at the catheter tip for pressure measurements, and the third for filling the balloon. The catheter and the associated computer derive the cardiac output by analysis of the decrement in temperature in the pulmonary artery produced by a bolus of cold saline injected into the right atrial port; the temperature sensor is at the distal tip of the catheter. Thermodilution measurements of right heart cardiac output (and, on a per-square-meter basis, the cardiac index) provide generally reliable and useful information regarding the hemodynamic state of the patient, since the left ventricular output is usually identical. As a guideline, a cardiac index below 2.0 liter/min/m^2 in infants or below 1.5 liter/min/m^2 in adults indicates an increased probability of death (Fig. 3-5); however, this value can be erroneous due to the improper injection rate or injectate volume of saline or its incorrect temperature. Thermodilution measurement of right heart output is an inaccurate measure of left heart output in the presence of a left-to-right shunt. In such instances (e.g., when the patient has an acute postinfarction ventricular septal defect) the measured thermodilution output is falsely higher than true systemic output of the left ventricle. Tricuspid valve insufficiency also makes the cardiac output determination less accurate by producing artifacts in the thermodilution curve. A significant complication related to the use of the pulmonary artery catheter is pulmonary hemorrhage secondary to overinflation of the balloon, wedging of a catheter that is placed too distally, or prolonged inflation of the balloon [3]. Patients with pulmonary hypertension are especially at risk. Occasionally, ventricular arrhythmias may be produced by the catheter as it traverses the right ventricle during placement.

By measuring the arterial pressure and cardiac output, it is possible to derive the systemic vascular resistance (SVR). This parameter is also referred to as *afterload;* high afterload indicates vasoconstriction whereas low afterload indicates vasodilation. This relationship is as follows:

$$\text{SVR} = \frac{\text{mean aortic pressure } - \text{ right atrial pressure}}{\text{cardiac output}}$$

If the patient does not have a right atrial catheter, central venous pressure may be substituted. The value obtained using this formula provides a useful estimate of the state of vascular constriction; normal adult SVR is 12 to 18 units. SVR may be expressed in dyne-second-centimeter^5 by multiplying the number of units by 80 (normal, 900–1400 dyne-sec-cm^5). It must be realized, however, that the SVR is derived from three other measurements (mean aortic pressure, right atrial pressure, and cardiac output), each of which has potential sources of significant error. Thus the derived vascular resistance should be considered an estimate, but not an accurate determination, of the state of constriction of the circulation.

Likewise, pulmonary vascular resistance (PVR) may be derived as follows:

$$\text{PVR} = \frac{\text{mean pulmonary artery pressure } - \text{ left atrial pressure}}{\text{cardiac output}}$$

The normal PVR is 1 to 3 units or, when multiplied by the conversion factor of 80, 80 to 240 dyne-sec-cm^5.

In some patients, a small catheter may be introduced into the left atrium and brought out through the chest wall to a transducer at the time of surgery for pressure monitoring. These catheters are particularly useful for infants, who are too small for commercially available balloon-tipped pulmonary artery catheters. They allow for

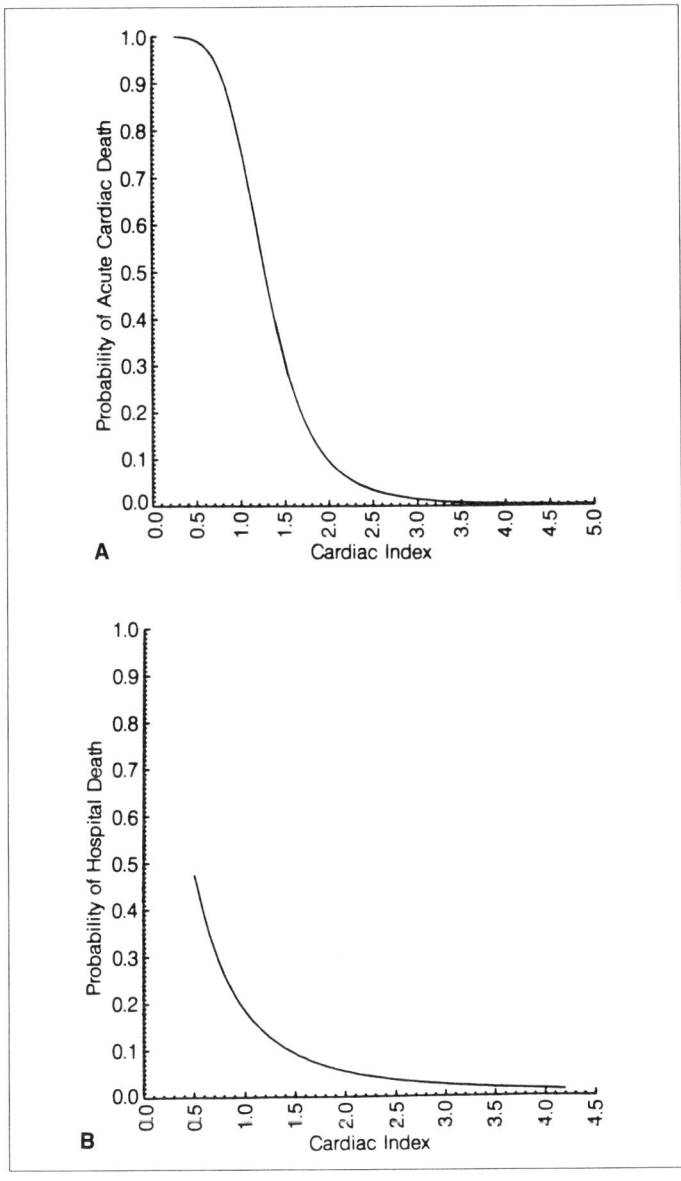

Fig. 3-5. Relationship between postoperative cardiac index (liter/min/m^2) and probability of death for infants (A) and for adults following mitral valve replacement (B). (From NT Kouchoukos et al. Detection and treatment of impaired cardiac performance following cardiac surgery. In JC Davila [ed], *Henry Ford Hospital International Symposium on Cardiac Surgery* [2nd ed]. New York: Elsevier, 1975.)

direct measurement of the left ventricular filling pressure. Because these catheters provide a direct link between the inside of the left heart and the outside of the patient, extreme care must be taken to avoid air or other embolism. The left atrial catheter is sometimes used as a port thorough which inotropic or other cardiovascular active drugs may be infused. This avoids the partial inactivation of the drug as it passes through the lungs, which may occur when such drugs are administered into the right atrium [4]. Left atrial catheters are also used by some surgeons in adults at risk for postoperative low cardiac output. Inspection of the left atrial pressure waveform for the presence of tall "V" waves can serve as a guide to assess mitral valve function. The continuous reading obtained is superior to the pulmonary capillary wedge pressure obtained with a Swan-Ganz catheter, which is measured intermittently and does not always accurately reflect left atrial pressure.

Thermodilution determination of cardiac output is usually made at least every 4 to 6 hours during the first 12 to 24 hours after surgery. If low cardiac output or other problems are present, more frequent determinations are necessary to follow the course of the patient and to determine the effectiveness of therapeutic interventions such as inotropic drug therapy. For most patients who undergo uncomplicated cardiac surgery, intensive hemodynamic monitoring is employed for 12 to 24 hours after operation. If, on the day after surgery, the patient is entirely stable with satisfactory hemodynamic parameters, the pulmonary artery or left atrial catheter (or both) is removed to minimize the risks of catheter sepsis and emboli. The left atrial catheter should not be withdrawn until confirmation of normal coagulation status has been obtained. After removal, the central venous pressure should be watched closely. A rise in the central venous pressure could indicate tamponade secondary to bleeding from the left atrial insertion site. The radial artery cannula may be left in place longer (until the time of transfer from the intensive care unit) to provide access for arterial blood sampling.

MANAGEMENT OF THE CARDIAC OUTPUT

Some degree of ventricular dysfunction invariably follows cardiac surgery utilizing periods of cardiac arrest. Although not usually clinically obvious, even uncomplicated coronary bypass procedures may result in temporary decreases in left ventricular function. This depression reaches a nadir about 4 hours after operation with recovery occurring within 1 to 3 days, depending on the lesion [5–7].

Low cardiac output (defined as a cardiac index of less than 2.0 liter/min/m^2) may result from one or a combination of the following factors: decreased myocardial contractility (of either left, right, or both ventricles), abnormal heart rhythm, inadequate preload, or excessive afterload. The result of low cardiac output is poor systemic perfusion, which causes ischemia of vital organs and, if not successfully treated, the predictable complications of renal, hepatic, neurologic, and further cardiac failure and eventual death. It has been recognized that a cardiac index of less than 1.5 liter/min/m^2 4 hours after surgery or 2.0 liter/min/m^2 on the morning after surgery in adults is associated with an increased incidence of postoperative patient death (see Fig. 3-5) [8]. Despite careful preoperative evaluation, perfect repair of the cardiac lesion, and satisfactory myocardial preservation, low cardiac output still may follow cardiac surgery. Early recognition of the low output state and appropriate management can lead to reversal of the situation and survival of the patient. Management of the low cardiac output state is discussed further in Chapter 4.

Management of the Blood Pressure

POSTOPERATIVE HYPOTENSION

Hypotension in the early period after cardiac surgery may be due to inadequate cardiac output or to lack of vascular tone (i.e., low SVR). The management of low cardiac output is discussed in Chapter 4. Hypotension secondary to low afterload can occur as a cold patient rewarms and vasodilation occurs. Measurement of the SVR (as described previously) allows this diagnosis to be made with assurance. It may be likely in anemic patients because of decreased blood viscosity and is more common in patients who were taking long-acting calcium channel blockers or angiotensin-converting enzyme inhibitors up to the time of surgery, or, it may be the result of sepsis. Hypotension secondary to low afterload frequently responds to volume infusion when the preload is also low. Less often, treatment with an alpha-adrenergic agonist agent such as phenylephrine or norepinephrine (which has both beta- and alpha-agonist actions) is required. Generally, it is desirable to maintain the adult patient's systolic blood pressure at 110 to 120 mm Hg (mean arterial pressure, 60–70 mm Hg). The normal blood pressure of an infant is age-dependent (Table 3-1).

POSTOPERATIVE HYPERTENSION

Hypertension after cardiac surgery is common and the incidence is high in patients undergoing coronary artery bypass procedures. Pain, irritation from the endotracheal tube, emergence from anesthesia, and disorientation all contribute to the adrenergically mediated increase in peripheral vascular resistance and tachycardia that characterizes this state. Early postoperative hypertension is associated with increased myocardial oxygen consumption, bleeding, and disruption of suture lines and may also contribute to neurologic injury. For adults, efforts to lower the blood pressure should be undertaken whenever the mean arterial pressure exceeds 100 to 110 mm Hg. In infants and children, postoperative hypertension is treated at correspondingly lower levels.

A variety of drugs is available for the treatment of temporary postoperative hypertension (Table 3-2). Afterload reduction by continuous infusion of either the short-acting vasodilators — nitroprusside or nitroglycerin — has been the most popular method of treatment for many years. Nitroprusside is a highly effective agent that acts by dilating both the arterial and venous capacitance vessels. Treatment is begun at 0.1 µg/kg/min and the rate of infusion is gradually increased until the desired reduction in blood pressure is achieved. Excessively lowering the blood pressure with nitroprusside in coronary bypass patients may be deleterious for the myocardial oxygen supply-demand relationship; maintenance of the mean blood pressure between 85 and 95 mm Hg is recommended

Table 3-1. Normal values of pulse and blood pressure in the first year of life

Age Group	Pulse rate (beats/min)			Blood pressure	
	Lower limits of normal	Average	Upper limits of normal	Systemic	Diastolic
Premature	80	120	170	60 (50–75)	35 (30–45)
Neonate	80	120	170	75 (60–90)	45 (40–60)
1–12 months	90	120	180	90 (75–100)	60 (50–70)

Source: From JH Moller and WA Neal. *Fetal, Neonatal and Infant Cardiac Disease.* East Norwalk, CT: Appleton & Lange, 1990. P. 170.

Table 3-2. Drugs useful for the treatment of early postoperative hypertension*

Drug	Dosage	Comments
Nitroprusside	0.05–10.00 µg/kg/min	Limit duration of use due to toxicity, especially if renal insufficiency is present.
Nitroglycerin	0.1–5.0 µg/kg/min	Not as effective as nitoprusside but may be better for coronary blood flow.
Nifedipine	10–20 mg sublingual q2–3hr	Use with caution in presence of poor left ventricular function.
Esmolol	Load with 20–40 mg then 1–8 mg/min infusion	Lowers both blood pressure and heart rate; very short duration of effect. Avoid in presence of poor ventricular function.
Labetalol	Load with 5–40 mg over 10 min then 1–3 mg/min infusion	Longer-acting than esmolol. Causes vasodilation in addition to beta blockade. Do not use if ventricular function is poor.

*Adult doses.

[9], particularly when distal disease is severe. Continuous arterial blood pressure monitoring is imperative, and frequent changes in the rate of nitroprusside infusion are usually needed to achieve adequate blood pressure control without causing hypotension. Because of this need for near-constant attention to the blood pressure and the rate of nitroprusside infusion, an automated closed-loop control device (IVAC Titrator) can be used which delivers nitroprusside continuously at a rate that maintains the blood pressure within preset limits [10].

Nitroprusside must be used with care in patients with coronary artery disease. The drug may cause intracoronary steal of blood away from ischemic areas, and tachycardia is common. Experimental evidence suggests that nitroprusside may have detrimental effects of internal mammary artery bypass graft flow [11]. The use of nitroprusside should be limited to 12 hours or less, and to even shorter periods of time in patients with renal insufficiency to avoid thiocyanate accumulation [12,13].

For these reasons, we generally prefer the use of continuous infusion nitroglycerin to nitroprusside, especially for patients with coronary artery disease. Nitroglycerin acts to dilate preferentially the venous capacitance vessels at low doses, affecting the resistance arteries only at higher doses. This probably results in more favorable effects on myocardial metabolism and better internal mammary artery graft flow. Nitroglycerin potentially may cause methemoglobinemia (characterized by high arterial oxygen tension [PaO_2] in the presence of relatively low oxygen saturation) when used at high doses for long periods of time [14]. Also, it is not always effective and may fail to provide adequate control of hypertension in at least 15% of patients [15]. Nitroglycerin infusion in adults is begun at 0.1 µg/kg/min and the rate of infusion is increased by 5 to 10 µg/min every 5 minutes (up to 5.0 µg/kg/min) until the desired reduction in blood pressure is reached. The pediatric dose is 1 to 20 µg/kg/min. Again, continuous measurement of the blood pressure is required to prevent hypotension.

In treating coronary bypass patients with postoperative hypertension, we begin with nitroglycerin and increase the rate of infusion to a maximum of 3 to 5 µg/kg/min. If this does not provide sufficient blood pressure control, nitroprusside is added as a second agent. If high-dose nitroprusside is needed, sublingually administered nifedipine may be used as an additional agent. As the need for drug control is reduced (which usually occurs 6 to 8 hours after surgery), the nitroprusside is withdrawn first and then the nitroglycerin is removed gradually, as indicated by the patient's blood pressure.

Several other types of drugs are useful for the treatment of postoperative hypertension. Calcium channel-blocking drugs (nifedipine, verapamil, diltiazem, isradipine, and nicardipine) lower blood pressure by decreasing afterload (peripheral vasodilation) with variable effects on myocardial contractility [16,17]. These drugs are used extensively to treat patients with heart disease. The five major agents differ somewhat with regard to their relative effects (Table 3-3). Although all five probably impair myocardial contractility to some degree, the beneficial reduction in SVR, in many instances, outweighs the effect on the myocardium and results in a decrease in the left ventricular end-diastolic pressure and improvement of

Table 3-3. Calcium channel blockers frequently used in cardiac surgery patients

Drug	Brand name	Dose	Major Indications	Major side effects	Comment
Diltiazem	Cardizem	Oral: 30–120 mg tid IV: 0.25–0.35 mg/kg bolus then 5–10 mg/hr infusion	Angina, chronic hypertension, arrhythmias. IV for rate control of atrial fibrillation and flutter	Oral: headache, dizziness, ankle swelling IV: high-degree atrioventricular block, asystole	IV dose often first drug used for new-onset atrial fibrillation with rapid ventricular response in postoperative patients. Mild negative inotropic effect.
Nifedipine	Adalat, Procardia	Oral: 10–20 mg tid	Hypertension, angina, coronary artery spasm	Hypotension, negative inotropic effect	Avoid in presence of aortic stenosis.
Verapamil	Calan, Isoptin	Oral: 80–120 mg tid or 240 mg *slow-release* qd IV: 2.5–10.0 mg, repeat in 10 min if required	Hypertension, angina, coronary artery spasm, supraventricular tachycardias. IV for rate control of atrial fibrillation and flutter	Oral: Headaches, dizziness, constipation, hypotension IV: hypotension, atrioventricular block, asystole	Causes elevation of digoxin level.
Isradipine	DynaCirc	Oral: 2.5–10 mg bid-tid	Hypertension, angina	Arthralgia	Does not increase digoxin level.
Nicardipine	Cardene	Oral: 20–40 mg tid	Hypertension, angina	Ankle swelling, dizziness, headache	Does not usually affect digoxin level.

the ejection fraction [18]. For the treatment of postoperative hypertension, nifedipine is convenient and effective. The drug is administered sublingually or intranasally (10 mg initial dose, repeated 1–2 times at 10-minute intervals as needed) and its effect is seen usually within 10 to 15 minutes. The duration of action of nifedipine is 2 to 3 hours. Nicardipine appears to be particularly valuable for the treatment of postoperative hypertension when used as a continuous, titratable infusion [19,20].

Drugs with beta-adrenergic blocking activity have been introduced recently for the treatment of postoperative hypertension and tachycardia. Esmolol is a fast-acting beta-receptor blocking agent that has a very short half-life, allowing for rapid control of the blood pressure with rapid reversal of its effect when discontinued [21,22]. Administration is begun with a loading dose (20–40 mg over 1 minute, followed by a maintenance dose of 1–8 mg/min for adults). The patient's blood pressure and heart rate must be monitored closely to avoid overshooting the desired result. Labetalol, which has both beta- and alpha-receptor blocking properties, is also a useful agent, but must be used with caution or not at all in patients with poor ventricular function [23,24].

In general, however, we refrain from using these drugs with beta-blocking properties in patients with significant left ventricular dysfunction. We find them to be most useful in younger patients with normal contractility, who tend to have hyperdynamic cardiac function during the early postoperative period.

Pulmonary Care

General anesthesia and inhalation anesthetics have been demonstrated to impair pulmonary function significantly. Cardiac surgery utilizing cardiopulmonary bypass results in further postoperative abnormalities of gas exchange. Pulmonary sequestration of activated leukocytes, complement activation, aggregation of platelets in pulmonary capillaries, microemboli (gas or tissue debris), and alveolar hypoperfusion may all be contributing factors to the adverse effects of cardiopulmonary bypass on pulmonary function [25]. Thus, it is not surprising that perioperative pulmonary problems are not unusual in patients undergoing cardiac surgery. In fact, in one study the need for prolonged (greater than 48-hour) postoperative mechanical ventilation was the most common postoperative complication among patients undergoing open heart surgery [26]. Appropriate perioperative management of the pulmonary system is an important aspect of successful care of the cardiac surgery patient.

Identification of patients with compromised pulmonary function before surgery can assist in the management of the patient postoperatively. Note should be made of a history of previous smoking, frequent respiratory infections, episodes of wheezing, chronic sputum production, recent upper respiratory tract infections, and previous cardiac surgery in which damage to a phrenic nerve might have occurred. Preoperative use of the antiarrhythmic drug amiodarone has been associated with a total dose-related, increased incidence of postoperative adult respiratory distress syndrome (ARDS) [27]. For patients with known pulmonary disease or positive risk factors in their history, spirometric studies and room-air arterial blood gas determinations will help detect and quantify abnormalities of ventilation and gas exchange. Patients with known pulmonary dysfunction should be instructed in the use of an incentive spirometer (Fig. 3-6) and should be encouraged to use it every 6 to 8 hours preoperatively (performing 10 maximal sustained inspirations slowly to prevent hyperventilation). Patients with bronchospastic disease should have their medications optimized prior to undergoing operation. Patients who smoke should be encouraged to stop before surgery, although the benefit of doing so is most apparent if the patient quits at least 2 months preoperatively. In fact, quitting for a period of less than 2 months before surgery may actually increase the incidence of postoperative pulmonary morbidity [28].

Young patients, with little or no pulmonary disease, who have undergone an uncomplicated cardiac repair are sometimes extubated in the operating room before transfer to the intensive care unit or soon after arrival in the intensive care unit. Most patients who undergo cardiac surgery are, however, ventilated mechanically for a period of 12 to 24 hours postoperatively, and those with pulmonary or other organ system complications may require assisted ventilation for days or even weeks after operation.

MECHANICAL VENTILATORS

Mechanical ventilators used today provide positive pressure within the airways causing inspiration; expiration follows as a passive pro-

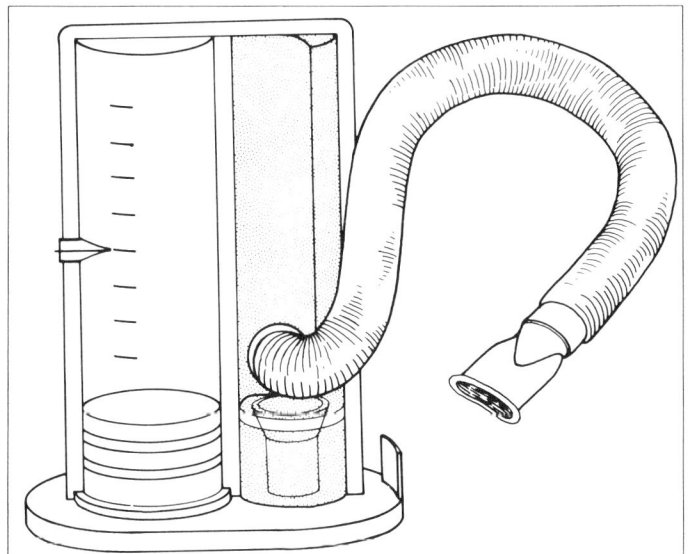

Fig. 3-6. Disposable incentive spirometer. The patient inhales deeply through the mouthpiece. The float on the left rises according to the inspiratory flow rate.

cess. Mechanical ventilators are of two types: flow generator and pressure generator [29]. Flow generator machines cause a predetermined pattern of gas flow in the patient's airway during each inspiration. Lung filling occurs largely unaffected by patient-related factors. Flow generators are the type most commonly used in current practice except for very small infants.

Ventilation of the patient may be entirely controlled (*controlled mechanical ventilation;* Table 3-4) so that the patient has no effect on the actions of the ventilator. This mode is used during surgery when the patient is paralyzed by neuromuscular blocking agents. Conversely, the patient's ventilatory efforts may be augmented (*augmented ventilation*). Augmented ventilation modes, such as *intermittent mandatory ventilation* (Fig. 3-7) are used for awake patients and are especially useful during the process of weaning the patient from mechanical ventilation. The *synchronized intermittent mandatory ventilation* (SIMV) mode detects when patients are taking their own breaths and avoids "stacking" a delivered breath on

Table 3-4. Ventilator setting abbreviations

AV	Augmented ventilation
CMV	Controlled mechanical ventilation
CPAP	Continuous positive airway pressure
IMV	Intermittent mandatory ventilation
IPS	Inspiratory pressure support
MMV	Mandatory minute ventilation
MV	Minute ventilation
PEEP	Positive end-expiratory pressure
SIMV	Synchronized intermittent mandatory ventilation
TV	Tidal volume
VR	Ventilator rate

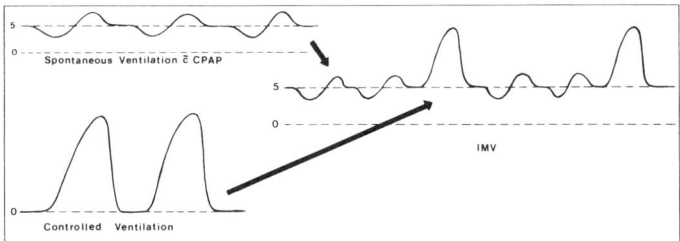

Fig. 3-7. Intermittent mandatory ventilation (IMV). The continuous positive airway pressure (CPAP) system is modified so that the ventilator can inflate the patient's lungs through a one-way valve periodically, thereby augmenting the patient's spontaneous breathing. This provides a useful compromise between spontaneous ventilation with CPAP (*top left*) and conventional, controlled mechanical ventilation (*bottom left*). It is unnecessary to sedate the patient so that (s)he can be "controlled," since (s)he is free to breathe independently of the machine. Weaning is smoothly accomplished by progressively reducing the backup rate of the ventilator until it is not needed. (Adapted from EF Klein, Jr. Weaning from mechanical breathing with intermittent mandatory ventilation. *Arch Surg* 110:345, 1975.)

top of a spontaneous one, thus preventing large tidal volumes and high peak pressures. SIMV senses the drop in pressure as the patient begins to inhale and delivers a breath to the patient in concert with the patient's own efforts; the number of breaths per minute to be assisted in this fashion is preset, and, if the patient does not initiate sufficient breaths per minute, the ventilator will deliver the required number without any effort from the patient. To avoid hypo- or hyperventilation with SIMV mode, the *mandatory minute ventilation* mode can be utilized. This mode monitors the patient's minute ventilation. If the patient is not breathing spontaneously at a sufficient rate to ensure that a preset minute ventilation is reached, the ventilator will deliver breaths so as to make up the difference between the patient's efforts and the preset required minute ventilation. If, however, the patient breathes at a rate and tidal volume equal to, or in excess of, the preset minute ventilation, the ventilator will not deliver breaths to the patient.

In addition to these modes of assisted ventilation, pressure support may be added to the ventilator circuit. *Inspiratory pressure support* provides a constant level of pressure to the airway when the patient initiates a breath. A useful technique for weaning patients from ventilatory support, inspiratory pressure support lessens the work of breathing but does not provide excessive assistance. *Positive end-expiratory pressure* (PEEP) increases the patient's functional residual capacity. This form of pressure support maintains some degree of lung inflation at all times. By decreasing the amount of atelectasis present, arterial oxygenation is increased for the same level of inspired oxygen. PEEP is therefore quite useful for the treatment of respiratory failure characterized by impaired gas exchange; however, this option may have deleterious effects on the patient's cardiac output particularly at higher PEEP levels, which can limit its usefulness in some cardiac surgery patients. This may be particularly true in patients with right heart failure or after the Fontan-Kreutzer procedure. It can be valuable to determine the optimum PEEP for the individual patient. To construct this relationship, cardiac output determinations are made at representative levels of PEEP (e.g., 4, 8, 12, and 16 mm Hg) and the PEEP that provides improvement in oxygenation without lowering the cardiac output significantly is chosen for use. High levels of PEEP may cause rupture of lung bullae (barotrauma) or traction on internal mammary artery bypass grafts, if present. An alternative to PEEP for maintaining lung expansion is the use of a brief inspiratory plateau "hold" (e.g., 0.5 sec) that will have minimal effect on the mean airway pressure.

Early after surgery, the SIMV mode is frequently used even though the patient is not initiating respirations. The SIMV rate and tidal volume are set to provide the minute ventilation that was found during the surgery to provide satisfactory blood gases. For the patient not initiating breaths, this is effectively the same as controlled ventilation. For adults, this is generally a rate of 8 to 12 breaths per minute with a tidal volume of 10 to 15 ml/kg. A PEEP of 5 mm Hg is usually added to help lessen atelectasis. In infants, a rate of 20 to 25 breaths per minute is used at an initial tidal volume of 15 to 20 ml/kg.

USE OF ARTERIAL BLOOD GAS DETERMINATION

Analysis of the arterial blood gases provides valuable information regarding gas exchange and the patient's acid-base status. Significant elevation of the PCO_2 indicates the need for intubation and mechanical ventilation or for a higher minute volume if the patient is already being ventilated. A diminished PO_2 may be caused by a ventilation-perfusion imbalance secondary to atelectasis, pneumonia, or congestive heart failure or by an unrecognized, obligatory right-to-left cardiac shunt. When there is lung disease, increasing the inspired oxygen concentration (FIO_2) will improve the PO_2 significantly. When the PO_2 improves little in the presence of a high FIO_2, there may be a fixed anatomic intracardiac right-to-left shunt or an intrapulmonary shunt. In this situation, proper therapy may include cardiac catheterization or echocardiography to define the defect, transfusion to raise the hematocrit, and percutaneous shunt closure or an operation in some instances.

The base deficit can be determined from the pH and PCO_2, and, from this determination, the amount of sodium bicarbonate necessary to correct any metabolic acidosis can be calculated.

POSTOPERATIVE RESPIRATORY MANAGEMENT

As mentioned previously, most patients are ventilated mechanically overnight after open heart surgery. Adults usually keep the endotracheal tube that was placed at the time of surgery; in infants, however, the tube may be replaced with a new one before transfer to the intensive care unit because the old tube is sometimes partially blocked by blood clots or retained secretions. Tubes for infants must be uncuffed and should fit the trachea loosely, but they should not be allowed to slide up and down as the infant moves. Nasotracheal tube placement in neonates and infants allows for more secure fixation and better oral hygiene and provokes fewer oral secretions; however, with proper technique, an oral tube also may be securely fixed in position (Fig. 3-8). Adequate sedation or even muscle-paralyzing agents are used as required to prevent the child from thrashing about while "tethered to a respirator by the endotracheal tube" [30].

If the patient is hemodynamically stable by the early morning after the day of surgery, narcotic administration is minimized, the ventilator rate is decreased gradually, the patient is encouraged to breathe more and more on his or her own, and respiratory excursions are observed. The alert patient who has an unlabored respiratory effort is placed on a T-piece or a positive-pressure apparatus, breathing through the endotracheal tube but without mechanical assistance, with 50% inspired oxygen concentration for 20 minutes or so, and arterial blood gases are checked. If satisfactory, the endotracheal tube is removed. For borderline patients, simple pulmonary function tests (*weaning parameters* — i.e., vital capacity, tidal volume, and inspiratory force) can be obtained to aid in the decision regarding extubation (Table 3-5). Some patients, particularly older ones, may still be too somnolent for extubation 12 to 18 hours after operation and may require several more hours of ventilatory assistance, during which time narcotics and sedatives should be administered only if absolutely necessary.

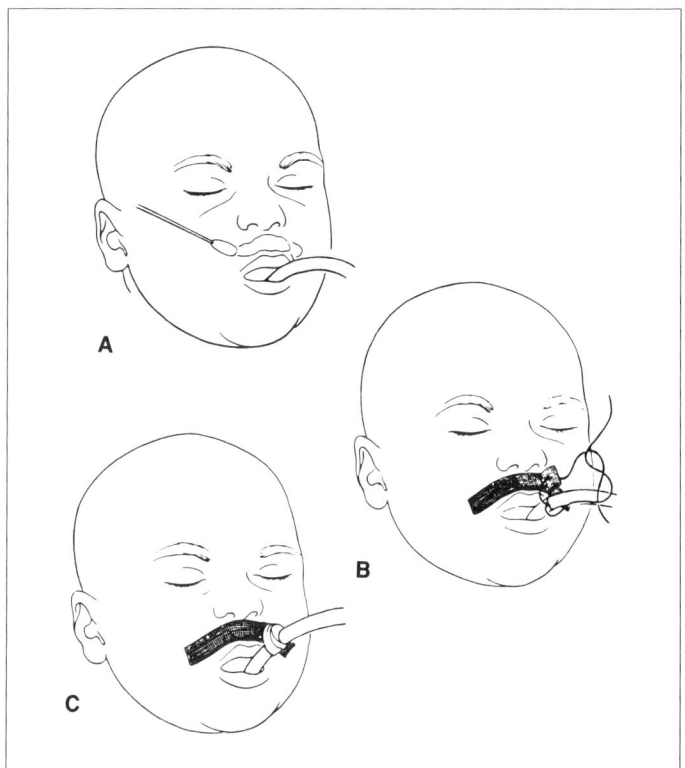

Fig. 3-8. Technique for securing an orotracheal tube in an infant or neonate to minimize the risk of dislodging the tube. (A) Skin overlying the maxilla is first painted with benzoin. (B) A strip of Elastoplast or cloth adhesive tape is applied with a fold in the center. A heavy silk ligature is tightly tied around the tube, indenting the wall slightly; and the ligature is then sutured through the folded tape. (C) Finally, half-inch tape is applied over the suture to provide additional stabilization. By this method, the tube is secured to the maxilla, which moves relatively little, and saliva will not loosen its fixation.

After extubation, humidified oxygen is delivered to the patient by face mask (usually beginning at 50% concentration). The inspired oxygen concentration is decreased gradually over 8 to 24 hours with regular measurements of the arterial blood gases. When the patient is comfortable (with satisfactory blood gases) on 35 to 40% oxygen concentration, the mode of oxygen delivery is changed to nasal prongs. These are generally more comfortable for the patient and more convenient for eating and drinking. The patient is usually on nasal-prong oxygen at the time of transfer from the intensive care unit to the postoperative care ward. Over the next few days, the nasal-prong oxygen delivery rate is reduced gradually and then discontinued.

Table 3-5. Guidelines for weaning and extubating patients on ventilators*

1. *Criteria for initiating weaning for short periods from assisted ventilation to intermittent mandatory ventilation (IMV):*
   Arterial PO_2 more than 90 mm Hg on 40% O_2 in absence of right-to-left shunt.
   Adequate neuromuscular coordination.
   Full consciousness.
   Stable cardiovascular function; i.e., satisfactory cardiac output at reasonably low filling pressure, no pulmonary edema, arrhythmias controlled, substantial inotropic or pressor drug support not required.
   Chest x-ray and auscultatory findings acceptable.

2. *Criteria for weaning the patient progressively to an IMV rate of zero (to T-tube or CPAP):*
   Vital capacity more than 10 ml/kg.
   Arterial PO_2 above 70 mm Hg on PEEP or CPAP of 5 cm H_2O or less (PO_2 may be lower in patients with right-to-left shunts).
   Respiratory rate less than 20–25 breaths/min (higher in infants).
   Respiratory effort appears reasonable.
   Patient denies dyspnea.
   Inspiratory force of at least -20 cm H_2O.

3. *Criteria for extubation following 20- to 30-minute trial of T-tube or unassisted breathing on CPAP of 5 cm H_2O or less:*
   Arterial PO_2 greater than 70 mm Hg on FiO_2 of 40% or less.
   Arterial PCO_2 30–45 mm Hg.
   Vital capacity more than 10–15 ml/kg ideal body weight.
   Respiratory rate less than 25–30 breaths/min (higher in infants, depending on size).
   Patient denies dyspnea.

*Generally, progression from steps 1 to 2 to 3 occurs as the patient meets the stated criteria with progress delayed in borderline situations. Exceptions must be made in the application of these guidelines; for example, in patients with chronic pulmonary disease or congenital heart disease with right-to-left shunts.

Respiratory care during the early postoperative period is simple but important. At the time of surgery, the patient's chest and mediastinal tubes are connected to a commercially available three-chamber system (e.g., Pleurovac) to prevent the intrathoracic accumulation of blood and fluid (Fig. 3-9). Alternatively, a collection system that permits reinfusion of shed blood may be used. For the intubated patient, frequent endotracheal suctioning, full humidification of the inspired gases, and frequent changes of position are the keys to prevention of retained secretions and atelectasis. Chest percussion and vibratory therapy are useful for mobilization of retained secretions. The patient is encouraged to sit up, dangle his or her legs, and begin to use an incentive spirometer the day after operation if the hemodynamic condition is stable. Use of the incentive spirometer is as effective in preventing postoperative atelectasis as is intermittent positive-pressure breathing treatment and is likely more cost-effective [31]. Early ambulation is encouraged as soon as it is tolerated and the level of exercise is increased gradually. The

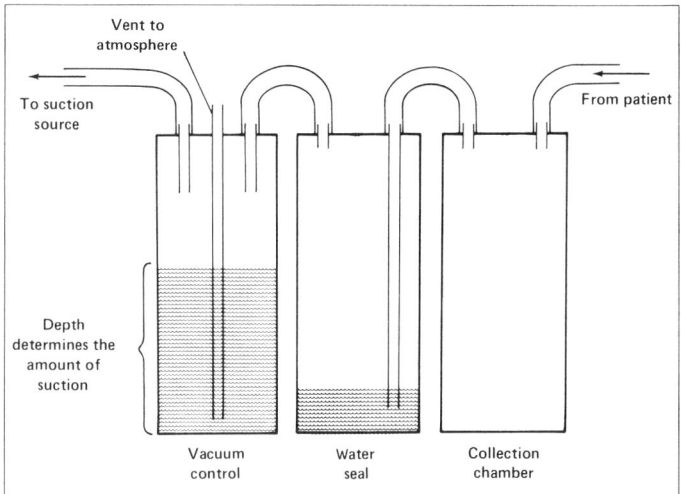

Fig. 3-9. Principles of a chest-tube suction system. The essential components of commercially available suction systems for chest-tube drainage are: (1) A fluid collection chamber (*right*) in which the fluid or blood draining from the chest may be collected sterilely, measured accurately, and (in some systems) detached for connection to an IV line so that the shed blood can be reinfused into the patient. (2) A water seal chamber (*middle*) that functions as a one-way valve to prevent the backward flow of air into the chest and as a monitor for air leakage from the chest. Leaking air appears as bubbles from the underwater portion of the tube. The water level in this chamber is usually set at 2 cm. (3) A vacuum control chamber (*left*) in which the water level is usually set at 20 cm of water, the amount of negative pressure applied to the chest tubes through the other chambers. The connection to atmosphere will relieve any negative pressure in excess of this amount that is applied by the wall suction. The suction source should be adjusted to provide gentle, continuous bubbling in this chamber to assure that the intended vacuum is being maintained. Excessive bubbling will result in a lowered water level and decreased suction.

patient's chest tubes are removed when drainage through them has become negligible (usually on the first or second postoperative day), which usually helps in decreasing the pain of breathing.

Fluids and Electrolytes

POSTOPERATIVE FLUID MANAGEMENT

Patients who undergo cardiac surgery using hemodilution cardiopulmonary bypass perfusion are invariably total body fluid–"overloaded" at the end of the procedure. This gain in predominantly extravascular fluid occurs as the result of the bypass circuit prime fluid volume, hemodilution (with loss of plasma oncotic pressure), and capillary leakage during the period of cardiopulmonary bypass. The degree of interstitial tissue edema is proportional to the length of time on cardiopulmonary bypass and is greatest in very small children [32,33]. Thus, vigorous fluid administration during the early postoperative period is usually not necessary for cardiac surgery patients (as compared, for example, with patients who have undergone major abdominal surgery). Fluid orders should specify a low fluid infusion rate: 50 ml/hr for adults and one-half of maintenance rate for pediatric patients. To minimize the sodium load, 5% dextrose solution is used. Further fluid and electrolyte administration is tailored to the individual patient based on hemodynamic criteria. Typical metabolic patterns experienced by patients early after heart surgery are summarized in Table 3-6.

Despite an increase in total body fluid of up to 20 to 30%, the intravascular volume status of the patient during the early postoperative period is dynamic, and volume administration may be required to maintain adequate filling of the heart, i.e., preload. The effects of hemodilution, redistribution of fluid, vasodilation due to rewarming, and other factors may result in a decreased intravascular volume despite the gain in total body fluid, and volume administration is often required at some point in the early postoperative period to maintain adequate ventricular preload. Monitoring the heart rate, arterial pressure, cardiac output, central venous pressure, pulmonary artery pressure, left atrial pressure (if a left atrial catheter is present), and urine output provides information to allow one to adjust colloid or crystalloid administration to the patient appropriate to the circumstances. When arterial pressure, filling pressures, and urine output are low, a trial of volume infusion should be given. Intravascular depletion would also be expected to cause tachycardia, but this response may be blunted in patients who took beta-adrenergic antagonists preoperatively. Use of a colloidal volume expander such as plasma protein fraction, albumin mixed in a crystalloid solution, or the polysaccharide hetastarch is customary. Although a crystalloid solution (in the form of one-half normal sa-

Table 3-6. Usual metabolic patterns in the immediate postoperative period in patients who have undergone surgery utilizing cardiopulmonary bypass

1. Extracellular fluid volume is increased from preoperative level, often by as much as 20–30%.
2. Intravascular fluid volume may be decreased from preoperative level (especially early after surgery). Thus the patient usually requires fluid administration despite overall total body gain in fluid volume.
3. Sodium excretion falls to low levels (less than 10 mEq/liter of urine). Total body sodium increases, even if its administration is severely restricted. Serum sodium concentration may decrease due to dilution.
4. Potassium is excreted in large amounts, often as high as 100 mEq/liter of urine (in patients with normal renal function). Serum potassium concentration falls, necessitating large daily infusions of potassium chloride.
5. The glomerular filtration rate, represented by the creatinine clearance, increases during the first few postoperative days.
6. Plasma catecholamine and vasopressin levels are elevated.

line) will also be effective, its effects are more transient and a further increase in the extracellular fluid volume will result. Routine use of blood products such as plasma or red blood cells for the purpose of volume expansion should be minimized because of limited supply, higher cost, and risk of transmitted infection. Minimizing their use is usually possible unless the patient is bleeding substantially. For the adult patient with obviously depleted intravascular volume, a bolus of 250 to 500 ml of colloid solution is administered over 20 to 30 minutes with careful monitoring of the patient's hemodynamic parameters. If the filling pressure (central venous, pulmonary artery diastolic, or left atrial) rises above 15 mm Hg, the bolus infusion should be slowed and the situation reassessed. For infants, the usual trial fluid bolus is 5 to 10 ml/kg.

In an effort to reduce interstitial edema, patients with an uncomplicated postoperative course are usually fluid-restricted to approximately 50% of normal requirements beginning the first day after surgery. Intravenous fluid administration is minimized, and, if able, the patient is allowed to take small amounts of fluid by mouth. Mild diuretic therapy is also usually employed in an effort to return the patient to his or her preoperative weight within 5 to 7 days after uncomplicated cardiac procedures.

POTASSIUM

Of the electrolyte abnormalities that may occur after cardiac surgery, hypokalemia is the most common. Patients on long-term preoperative diuretic therapy frequently have decreased total body potassium stores even though their serum potassium levels may be within the normal range. Relatively high intraoperative urine output with concomitant potassium loss is common to most patients with good renal function who undergo cardiopulmonary bypass using hemodilution-perfusion techniques. This effect usually continues for several hours after the operation and will be exacerbated in hyperglycemic patients. The associated potassium loss can be considerable and may result in severe hypokalemia.

Hypokalemic patients suffering myocardial infarctions have an increased incidence of ventricular arrhythmias [34]. Likewise, in open heart surgery patients, hypokalemia results in ventricular irritability with an increased incidence of ventricular arrhythmias. Serious hypokalemia also results in muscular weakness, metabolic alkalosis, ECG changes (T-wave flattening and inversion, U-wave prominence, and ST-segment depression), and increased susceptibility to digoxin toxicity.

Careful attention must be paid to the patient's serum potassium concentration during the early postoperative period. Depletion of serum potassium levels can occur quickly; therefore, frequent potassium level determinations and replacement as required are essential. For infants, potassium chloride may be given through a central line in doses up to 0.5 mEq/kg/hr mixed in 3–5 ml/kg of 5% dextrose. For adults, potassium is administered at a rate of 10 to 20 mEq/hr: This should be mixed in 100 ml of 5% dextrose and given through a central vein catheter to prevent vein irritation. The rate of infusion must be controlled by an infusion pump (such as an IVAC) to prevent inadvertent rapid delivery, and the patient should be monitored continuously by ECG because fatal arrhythmias may result from too-rapid administration. In this manner, the serum potassium level should be maintained between 4.0 and 5.0 mEq/dl. After the first 24 hours, the tendency to excrete potassium will be decreased; however, administration of diuretics will continue to lower the serum concentration and supplemental potassium will need to be given. If potassium-sparing diuretics (such as triamterene [Dyazide], spironolactone [Aldactazide], or amiloride [Moduretic]) are used, a regularly scheduled dose of potassium *should not* be given because dangerous hyperkalemia may result.

Although uncommon, hyperkalemia may occur after cardiac surgery, most frequently in patients with impaired renal function. The combination of preexisting renal insufficiency, large doses of hyperkalemic cardioplegic solution infusion, red cell damage during cardiopulmonary bypass, and (when low cardiac output is present) hypoperfusion of tissues with release of intracellular potassium can quickly result in dangerous hyperkalemia in the early postoperative period. Use of hemofiltration during operation can help lessen this problem. One maneuver useful for the patient with mild hyperkalemia (serum potassium, 5.5 to 6.0 mEq/liter) and relatively normal renal function is to administer a moderate dose of furosemide (40 mg IV) and to replace the resultant urine output with a crystalloid, potassium-free solution. Severe hyperkalemia (above 7.0 mEq/liter) causes weakness, paresthesia, and ECG changes (peaked T waves, atrioventricular block, and widened QRS complex) and may lead to arrhythmic death of the patient. Specific treatment is begun when the serum potassium level exceeds 5.5 mEq/liter. If ECG changes are present, calcium gluconate should be administered (10 ml of 10% solution IV over 3–5 minutes); however, calcium reversal of the cardiac effects of hyperkalemia will be short-lived. Glucose (50 ml of 50% dextrose solution) with insulin (10 units of regular insulin added to the solution) may be administered over 10 minutes to drive serum potassium into the intracellular space. Likewise, alkalinization of the blood with sodium bicarbonate (2–3 ampules added to a liter of 5% glucose infused over 1–2 hours) also moves potassium into the cells and lowers the serum concentration. Definitive removal of excess potassium from the body requires the use of the cation-exchange resin sodium polystyrene sulfonate (Kayexalate, 20–60 g mixed with 70% sorbitol to prevent constipation) given either orally or rectally. Peritoneal dialysis or hemodialysis can be employed to treat hyperkalemia associated with severe renal failure, but the total potassium load removed by this technique is less than that removed with cation-exchange resin [35].

SODIUM

As mentioned previously, open heart surgery using cardiopulmonary bypass causes a significant increase in the patient's total body fluid volume. This is frequently associated with a moderate reduction in the serum sodium concentration but not in the total body sodium content. Loss of the accumulated extra free water over the first few days after surgery (often assisted by the administration of diuretic agents) generally leads to an increase in the sodium level. Treatment of the asymptomatic mild or moderate hyponatremia in the early postoperative period by administration of sodium-containing solutions is usually not indicated: The fundamental problem is water overload and hemodilution, not sodium deficiency; therefore, mild to moderate fluid restriction is in order. When determining the total daily fluid intake of the patient, it is important to include sources of fluid input, such as volumes of saline injected for cardiac output determination (10 ml per injection) and heparin flush volumes for the arterial cannula and pulmonary artery catheter. These volumes can add up to a substantial amount of fluid inputs without being recognized as such, and they may be significant, especially in the smaller patient.

CALCIUM AND MAGNESIUM

Ionized (and total) serum calcium levels decrease during cardiopulmonary bypass and, if untreated, remain below normal during the early postoperative period largely due to hemodilution. There is no known adverse consequence of this temporary derangement when it is mild, and it usually returns to normal during the first 24 hours after operation [36]. Serum-ionized calcium levels may also be decreased by: (1) hyperventilation with alkalosis, (2) rapid heparin administration, (3) intravenous lipid administration, (4) radiographic contrast media, (5) hyper- and hypomagnesemia, and (6) sodium citrate administration [37]. Citrate is present in anticoagulated banked blood, and hypocalcemia is a potential result of blood transfusion. However, this effect is very transient (citrate is cleared quickly) and requires very fast rates of blood infusion (1.5–2.0 ml/kg/min). The routine intravenous administration of calcium with red cell transfusions is not recommended and may actually be harmful [38]. Most postoperative hypocalcemia is the result of dilution, although patients with disorders of vitamin D metabolism may be susceptible to prolonged symptomatic hypocalcemia in the early postoperative period.

Symptoms develop when the ionized calcium level falls below 3.0 mg/dl, the level at which replacement is recommended. Manifestations of hypocalcemia include low cardiac output, hypotension, arrhythmias, and ECG abnormalities (prolongation of QT and ST segments, and T-wave inversion). Noncardiac effects of hypocalcemia include tetany, muscle spasms, seizures, apnea, bronchospasm, laryngospasm, and psychosis. When administered to correct significant hypocalcemia, elemental calcium should be given intravenously. Initially, a bolus of 100 to 200 mg of elemental calcium (10–20 ml of 10% calcium gluconate or 4–8 ml of 10% calcium chloride) is given, followed by infusion of 1 to 2 mg/kg/hr. Administration through a central line is mandatory because calcium solutions are irritating to peripheral veins. In particular, calcium chloride should not be given through a peripheral vein because it can cause tissue necrosis. Care should be taken to avoid hypercalcemia in patients receiving digoxin, as this may precipitate digoxin toxicity.

Hypocalcemia tends to occur most often in newborn infants undergoing operation, likely as a result of inadequate calcium stores and immature parathyroid glands. In the infant, significant hypocalcemia may be manifested by twitching, jitteriness, and seizures. Treatment is by *slow, central venous* catheter injection of 10% calcium gluconate, 10 to 20 mg/kg, or 10% calcium chloride, 5 mg/kg (Table 3-7).

Table 3-7. Drugs that should not usually be administered via peripheral intravenous catheters

Potassium at high concentration (above 20 mEq/liter)
Sodium bicarbonate bolus
Calcium chloride (10% solution)
50% dextrose
Norepinephrine
Epinephrine
Dopamine
Phenylephrine
Vancomycin
  (Preferably given via central line. If administered peripherally, solution should be dilute and intravenous line should be secure to prevent extravasation)

A significant decrease in the patient's serum magnesium level occurs after cardiac surgery utilizing cardiopulmonary bypass [39]. This decrease is out of proportion to that expected to occur simply due to hemodilution, and there is a gradual return to normal over a period of about 10 days. The relationship between hypomagnesemia and cardiac arrhythmias is uncertain and available information is conflicting. Although magnesium infusion may be useful therapy for a variety of supraventricular and ventricular arrhythmias, this effect appears to be nonspecific and there is no certain relationship between hypomagnesemia and postoperative cardiac arrhythmias [40]. In fact, routine intraoperative administration of magnesium during open heart surgery may have adverse effects [41]. Thus, we do not usually measure serum magnesium levels or routinely administer magnesium after open heart surgery.

Acid-Base Balance

ACIDOSIS

Metabolic acidosis after cardiac surgery is most often due to low cardiac output and poor systemic perfusion with release of lactate from tissues secondary to anaerobic metabolism. Impaired excretion of organic acids due to poor renal perfusion is also a contributing factor. Hyperventilation, the respiratory response to metabolic acidosis, develops slowly (over 12–24 hours) and cannot be relied on as compensation [42]. Furthermore, most patients are intubated and on controlled ventilation. In any case, respiratory compensation for metabolic acidosis does not correct the proximate cause of the problem. Acidosis results in reduced myocardial contractility, thereby worsening the low cardiac output state. Furthermore, vasopressor and inotropic agents such as epinephrine are less effective when administered to the acidotic patient.

Evaluation of the acidotic patient begins with measurement of the arterial blood gases (Fig. 3-10). This provides the information necessary to determine the relative contributions of metabolic and respiratory causes of increased hydrogen ion concentration. Respiratory acidosis due to inadequate ventilation is characterized

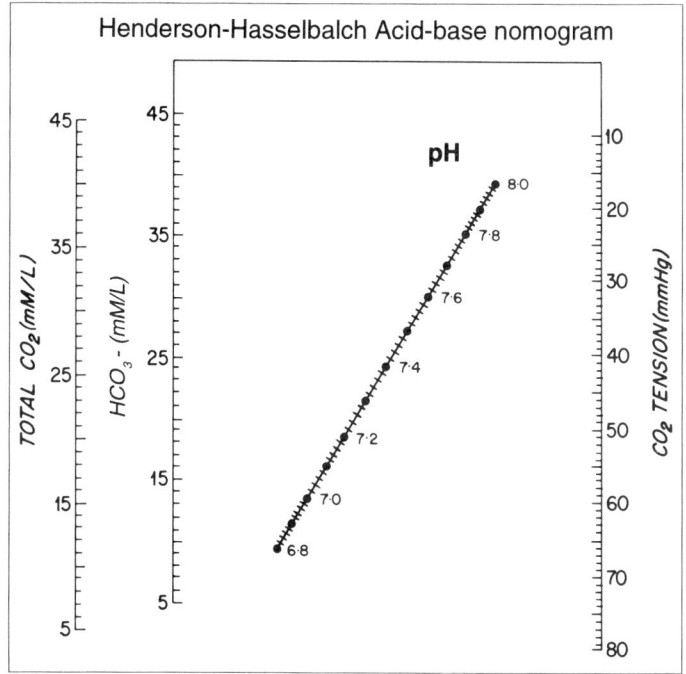

Fig. 3-10. Henderson-Hasselbalch acid-base nomogram relating total CO_2 and bicarbonate HCO_3^-, PCO_2 (*right*) and pH (*center*). (From FC McLean. *Physiol Rev* 18:495, 1938. Reproduced with permission.)

by hypercarbia and a mild increase in the bicarbonate concentration. Such hypercarbia is to be avoided, as elevation of the PCO_2 in postoperative patients has been shown to cause large increases in pulmonary vascular resistance, which may result in impairment of right ventricular function [43]. Respiratory acidosis in the early postoperative patient who is on a mechanical ventilator is usually simple to correct: Increasing the minute ventilation by increasing the ventilator rate or delivered volume will lead toward normalization of the CO_2 tension and arterial pH. A portable chest x-ray will help rule out mechanical causes of compromised ventilation such as pneumothorax or large pleural effusion.

As mentioned above, metabolic acidosis early after open heart surgery is most often due to low cardiac output; this may be confirmed by thermodilution measurement of the patient's cardiac index. If verified, appropriate measures to improve the low output state are in order (evaluation to rule out cardiac tamponade, optimization of filling pressure, inotropic drugs, vasodilators, and mechanical support, as needed).

Metabolic acidosis should be corrected partially by the intravenous administration of sodium bicarbonate in doses sufficient to raise the pH above 7.30. Determination of how much sodium bicarbonate to administer to the acidotic patient is simple if the base excess is known. The *base excess* is the calculated nonrespiratory component of the acidotic state of the patient. Expressed as milliequivalents (mEq) of base per liter of blood, the base excess is derived from the pH, PCO_2, and hematocrit of the sample analyzed, and this value is provided by the arterial blood gas analyzer. It may also be estimated by subtracting 25 from the patient's serum bicarbonate level; when negative, the patient has metabolic acidosis. The number of milliequivalents of bicarbonate that should be administered to the acidotic patient is calculated as follows: Divide the patient's weight (in kg) by 3 to determine the extracellular space volume (since about one-third of the weight is extracellular fluid) and multiply the base excess value by the extracellular space volume to obtain the number of milliequivalents of bicarbonate required to reverse completely the negative base excess. To avoid overcorrection, administer only one-half of this calculated dose and repeat the blood gas determination in 20 to 30 minutes. For example, a 60-kg patient with a base excess of -5 would receive 50 mEq of sodium bicarbonate; since each ampule contains 44.6 mEq, we would begin by giving the patient a single ampule and then recheck the arterial blood gases.

Overcorrection of metabolic acidosis by the administration of bicarbonate must be avoided as the resultant alkalosis is also detrimental to cardiac function and may predispose to arrhythmias, result in increased CO_2 production, and impair oxygen delivery to the tissues by increasing hemoglobin's affinity for oxygen. Rapid correction of extracellular acidosis may actually cause worsening of intracellular acidosis [44,45]. Because of the potential detrimental effects of administered bicarbonate, it is important that any respiratory component to the acidosis be quickly corrected first to lessen the need for bicarbonate. Generally, bicarbonate should be administered only when the patient's pH is less than 7.30. Furthermore, sodium bicarbonate administration provides a large sodium load (44.6 mEq per ampule) and can lead to hypernatremia and volume overload, especially in infants. Tromethamine (THAM) can be substituted for sodium bicarbonate, especially when the serum sodium level is above 155 mEq/liter. It is an effective buffer and does not provide a large sodium load to the patient. However, because the required volumes of infusion are large and it is a respiratory depressant, we rarely use it.

ALKALOSIS

Alkalosis during the early period after cardiac surgery is most often respiratory in etiology secondary to ventilator-induced hyperventilation. Typically, the arterial blood gases will exhibit a low CO_2 tension and a decreased bicarbonate concentration. For the early postoperative patient still on mechanical ventilation, this is easily corrected by decreasing the patient's minute ventilation. Metabolic alkalosis, characterized by an elevated arterial bicarbonate concentration, can be induced by hypokalemia, excessive losses of gastric juice with chloride depletion, hypovolemia (since renal retention of sodium prevails over correction of alkalosis), or the very rapid transfusion of large amounts of blood containing sodium citrate. Some degree of respiratory compensation for metabolic alkalosis can occur in the patient who is not being ventilated mechanically. Severe hypoventilation will not usually develop because this response is limited by the hypoxic respiratory drive. The tendency to retain CO_2 to compensate for significant metabolic alkalosis may hamper efforts to wean the patient with respiratory compromise from mechanical ventilation.

Frequently during the first few days after uncomplicated cardiac surgery, a mild form of metabolic alkalosis may develop. This is related to the use of diuretic agents to rid the patient of accumulated water without sufficient potassium and chloride replacement. Hypokalemia-induced alkalosis will be reversed with the administration of potassium chloride with the goal of raising the serum potassium level above 4.5 mEq/dl. A mildly low serum potassium level (e.g., 3.5 mEq/dl) indicates a severe total body depletion of potassium, and significant amounts of potassium chloride may be needed to restore the total body reserves. In fact, patients on chronic diuretics or who are chronically overventilated may have a profound intracellular potassium deficit with a normal serum potassium level and severe metabolic alkalosis. Large volumes of potassium chloride are required to correct this, and, rarely, administration of dilute hydrochloric acid (0.15 Normal HCl at 0.2 mEq/kg/hr IV for 12 hours via a central line) or ammonium chloride is necessary.

Use of Blood Products in the Perioperative Period

Cardiac surgery utilizing cardiopulmonary bypass results in significant trauma to blood components and in bleeding. The intraoperative use of heparin, platelet dysfunction, and dilution of platelets and serum clotting factors all lead to significant operative blood loss and postoperative anemia. Therefore, an important part of the management of the patient undergoing cardiac surgery involves the rational use of blood products.

Despite the anemia present after cardiac operation, it is not necessary to restore the adult patient to the normal hematocrit of 38 to 48% to maintain optimal postoperative cardiopulmonary function and uncomplicated recovery from surgery. In fact, the hazards of disease transmission (hepatitis and acquired immunodeficiency syndrome [AIDS]), transfusion reaction, and the possible detrimental effect on immunologic defenses are becoming increasingly realized. This realization has intensified efforts to perform cardiac surgery with minimal transfusion of blood products [46–49]. Although the estimated risk of contracting AIDS from a blood transfusion is low (1:40,000 to 1:1,000,000), the risk of developing non-A, non-B hepatitis (hepatitis C) is significantly higher (up to 1:100) [50]. Because of the hazards associated with blood transfusion, efforts to avoid transfusion are important; part of this effort involves allowing the patient to have a below-normal red cell volume after surgery. Although oxygen delivery would be expected to be decreased because of the decreased hemoglobin level, compensatory increases in cardiac output (by increasing stroke volume and heart rate) occur. Even severe anemia is well tolerated in patients with relatively normal left ventricular function [51]. There is no evidence that moderate anemia increases bleeding, adversely affects wound healing, contributes to postoperative infections, or increases the length of the postoperative hospital stay [49,52]. Thus, most patients tolerate a postoperative hematocrit of 25% without difficulty, and, for patients with no cardiopulmonary compromise, this threshold for transfusion of red blood cells can be lowered even further [53]. At our institutions, adult patients with uncomplicated postoperative courses generally are given transfusions of red blood cells only when the hematocrit falls below 21 to 24%.

Infants with cyanotic heart disease are dependent on the increased hematocrit that is usually present. In a patient undergoing a palliative procedure (such as Blalock-Taussig shunt), the hematocrit should be maintained at a level appropriate to the oxygen saturation; that is, an infant with an oxygen saturation in the 90s requires a hematocrit of at least 40%, whereas an infant with an oxygen saturation in the 70s requires a hematocrit in the high-50% range. Elevating the hematocrit above the mid-50% range should be avoided, however, as this increases the blood viscosity too much and could result in thrombosis of a systemic-to-pulmonary shunt.

The primary determinants of the need for blood transfusion during the perioperative period are the patient's preoperative red blood cell volume and the amount of postoperative bleeding. Low preoperative hematocrit values are more likely to be present in patients who are female, elderly, nonsmoking, and of small body size; such patients are likely to require postoperative transfusion [54,55]. Patients with stable cardiac disease and relatively normal red cell volumes who are scheduled to undergo elective surgery may predonate their blood to be returned to them during the perioperative period, thus significantly reducing the need for transfusion of homologous blood. Such autologous donations have been found to be safe for adults and children with severe heart disease, although patients with unstable angina or severe aortic valve stenosis are usually excluded [56–58].

Many other measures are utilized to decrease the need for perioperative red cell transfusion [59]. Preoperative aspirin therapy in coronary bypass patients definitely increases the need for perioperative blood transfusion and may increase incidence of reoperation for bleeding [60]. We, therefore, advise avoidance of aspirin for 7 days preoperatively, if possible, to prevent aspirin-induced platelet dysfunction. After cannulation of the adult patient, but before the institution of cardiopulmonary bypass, 1 to 2 units of heparinized blood may be withdrawn from the patient and stored (if the patient's preoperative hematocrit is relatively normal). This whole blood, containing functional platelets and soluble clotting factors, is then reinfused into the patient after discontinuation of bypass and administration of protamine. Blood lost during surgery after heparinization is returned to the bypass circuit via the cardiotomy sucker. Intraoperative blood loss that occurs before heparinization or after the administration of protamine can be collected by a system (e.g., Cell-Saver) that washes and concentrates the red cells for retransfusion. After discontinuation of cardiopulmonary bypass, the blood contained within the pump circuit can be emptied into the Cell-Saver or hemoconcentrated by recirculation through an ultrafiltration circuit (e.g., Hemocor), thus providing a significant volume of red blood cells for transfusion back to the patient. Blood from mediastinal drainage tubes in the early postoperative period can be collected in a special collection system (e.g., Pleurovac autotransfusion system) and reinfused into the patient.

Pharmacologic agents are also being used in an effort to decrease the need for perioperative red cell transfusion. Recombinant erythropoietin administered to anemic patients or to those predonating their own blood before elective surgery has been shown to reduce the need for autologous transfusion during the perioperative period [61,62]. The protease inhibitor aprotinin, administered during cardiopulmonary bypass, appears to be effective in reducing bleeding, but it is not yet approved for use in the United States [63,64]. Desmopressin acetate (DDAVP), administered intraoperatively to improve platelet function after protamine reversal of the heparin effect, has also been utilized for this purpose; however, its efficacy has not been confirmed and its routine use is not currently recommended [65,66]. Patients scheduled for elective surgery (whether or not they predonate) may be treated preoperatively with ferrous sulfate (325 mg 3 times daily) to build up iron stores.

Despite these efforts to decrease the need for perioperative blood transfusion, many patients do require red blood cell replacement. It is common practice for blood blanks to separate donated blood into its various components (packed red blood cells, platelet concentrates, fresh frozen plasma, and coagulation factor concentrates). Thus, the practice of whole blood transfusion is infrequent, and donated blood is maximally utilized.

The decision to transfuse the cardiac surgery patient with red blood cells is based on a number of factors. The following patient data must be taken into account: hematocrit, age, presence or absence of symptoms, underlying cardiopulmonary status, presence or absence of perioperative complications, and nutritional status. For example, a postoperative hematocrit of 23% may be quite satisfactory for a younger patient who is basically healthy, who has well-preserved left ventricular function, and who is stable and not bleeding excessively after an uncomplicated operation. Conversely, even though the hematocrit is 27%, it may be advisable to replace red blood cells in the older, nutritionally deficient patient who has poor left ventricular function and who is bleeding in the early postoperative period. Thus, these decisions must be individualized. There are no absolute guidelines that are applicable to all patients. Anemic patients may be discharged from the hospital on iron replacement with no apparent adverse effects; the hematocrit usually returns to 80% of the preoperative hematocrit level by 3 weeks after surgery [67]. Because of the potential risks, all blood component transfusions must be justified by the circumstances, and the reasons for the transfusion should be documented in the medical record.

Blood components other than red blood cells are useful in the management of the cardiac surgery patient, especially when coagulopathy and excessive bleeding are present. Routine prophylactic administration of platelets, plasma, or other clotting factors is not, however, beneficial and should not be performed because of the risk of disease transmission [68]. Similarly, blood products should not be used routinely for volume expansion of the hypovolemic patient who is not bleeding excessively. Crystalloid or colloid solutions such as plasma protein fraction or hetastarch provide volume replacement without the risks associated with fresh frozen plasma. Clotting factor components (platelets, fresh frozen plasma, and cryoprecipitate) should be reserved for the patient who is experiencing excessive postoperative bleeding associated with abnormal clotting studies (see Chap. 5).

Pain Control

Morphine is usually the drug of choice to control pain during the early postoperative period. Mechanically ventilated adults are given 2 to 10 mg by slow intravenous bolus at 1 mg/min; the infant bolus dose is 0.1 to 0.5 mg/kg at a rate of 0.1 mg/min. The main hemodynamic effect of morphine is vasodilation, thereby reducing ventricular preload and afterload with favorable effects on myocardial oxygen consumption. If the patient is hypovolemic, however, dangerous hypotension may result. Thus, morphine is given slowly with careful monitoring of the patient's arterial blood pressure and filling pressure(s). Small, frequent intravenous doses are preferable to larger, less frequent intramuscular injections during the early postoperative period because of the variability in absorption when the intramuscular route is used. For infants and children, we often employ a continuous morphine infusion (5–100 μg/kg/hr). After extubation, care must be used to avoid excess narcotic administration, which may result in respiratory depression. Conversely, insufficient pain relief will result in splinting and failure of the patient to cough and clear secretions. For adults, we generally switch to intramuscularly administered morphine (4–10 mg every 4 hours as needed) at the time of transfer from the intensive care unit. Younger adult patients are often given a patient-controlled analgesia pump so they can regulate their own pain medication administration. This technique must be used with caution in older patients lest they become oversedated. As oral intake is resumed, most patients find relief with combination codeine and acetaminophen preparations taken orally. In patients who do not tolerate narcotics, we have found ketorolac (Toradol) 10 mg qid very useful. Some patients note an enhanced analgesic effect when a nosteroidal antiinflammatory agent is added.

Patients occasionally require sedation during the early postoperative period to prevent dangerous agitation and "fighting the ventilator." For this purpose, diazepam (Valium) is used in small intravenous doses (2–5 mg every 2–3 hours for adults; 0.04–0.20 mg/kg every 2–3 hours for children). Chloral hydrate, 30 to 100 mg/kg by mouth or rectal suppository, is a very useful sedative in infants and it does not depress cardiac or respiratory function. Diazepam is not well absorbed from intramuscular injection so the intravenous route is preferred. Occasionally, adequate sedation of infants cannot be achieved with narcotics, and chloral hydrate, diazepam, or midazolam (Versed) with a muscle relaxant such as pancuronium (Pavulon; 0.04–0.10 mg/kg IV) is used. Infants sometimes struggle while intubated, which causes trauma to the trachea and risks inadvertent extubation and dislodgement of intravenous catheters; therefore, they must be adequately sedated or pharmacologically paralyzed.

It must be remembered, however, that *a patient who becomes restless or apprehensive may be hypoxic or in a low output state*. If this is the case, the administration of analgesics or sedatives does not correct the basic problem and may be very hazardous.

Diuretic Therapy

Patients who undergo cardiac surgery are commonly treated with diuretic drugs to increase sodium excretion. Congestive heart failure results in increased total body sodium content with secondary edema, and many patients with heart failure are treated chronically with diuretic drugs. Likewise, cardiac surgery using cardiopulmonary bypass results in total body excesses of sodium and water so that diuretic agents are frequently prescribed on a temporary basis during the postoperative period. The mechanism of action of commonly used diuretic agents is to block part of the tubular reabsorption of sodium resulting in increased sodium excretion. The major groups used clinically today are: (1) loop diuretics (furosemide, ethacrynic acid, or bumetanide), (2) thiazide diuretics (hydrochlorothiazide, chlorthalidone, or metolazone), (3) potassium-sparing diuretics (spironolactone, triamterene, or amiloride), and (4) combination products (hydrochlorothiazide plus either spironolactone, triamterene, or amiloride).

On the first morning after uncomplicated open heart surgery, when cardiac function has returned toward the preoperative level and the patient is fully rewarmed, a dose of a loop diuretic (most often furosemide, 10–40 mg IV for adults, 0.5–1.0 mg/kg IV for infants) is often given to promote diuresis. Patients with cardiac failure, high filling pressures, and pulmonary edema are treated with higher doses of intravenous furosemide with careful monitoring of the ventricular filling pressures and serum potassium levels. In this setting, furosemide has the additional beneficial effect of increasing venous capacitance and decreasing left ventricular end-diastolic pressure and pulmonary edema [69]. Patients on preoperative diuretic therapy may require higher doses after surgery, particularly if they were receiving high doses for a long period of time. After extubation, when the patient is able to take medications orally, it is common practice to administer either furosemide or a combination diuretic (such as triamterene 50 mg plus hydrochlorothiazide 25 mg) for several days. The combination diuretic helps prevent hypokalemia, although the patient's potassium level should be checked regularly during the early postoperative period. Concurrent administration of a daily dose of potassium with a combination diuretic containing a potassium-sparing agent is contraindicated because of the possibility of dangerous hyperkalemia. The patient is weighed daily; when the preoperative weight is approached the diuretic is discontinued. Important diuretic drug interactions include: potassium-sparing diuretics plus angiotensin-converting enzyme inhibitors such as captopril (may cause dangerous hyperkalemia); spironolactone plus digoxin (raises digoxin levels); and triamterene plus indomethacin (may cause renal failure) [70,71].

Diabetes Management

Patients with diabetes mellitus have an increased incidence of coronary artery disease, and, therefore, a significant proportion (10–

15%) of patients undergoing coronary revascularization procedures are diabetic.

Diabetes mellitus is identified in some studies as a risk factor for perioperative mortality in patients undergoing coronary artery bypass procedures [72]. Additionally, diabetic patients have increased lengths of postoperative hospital stay and increased perioperative morbidity, in particular, sternotomy complications and renal insufficiency [73,74]. Diabetic patients (insulin-dependent, on oral agents, or diet-controlled) as well as previously unrecognized "borderline diabetics," frequently become very hyperglycemic during the early postoperative period due to the stress of surgical trauma. Additionally, hyperglycemia is exacerbated by the use of catecholamine support medications. The most frequent consequence of untreated hyperglycemia is osmotic diuresis with intravascular volume depletion. The renal threshold for spilling glucose into the urine with concomitant loss of water and electrolytes is a serum glucose level of approximately 200 mg/dl. Other potential adverse effects of postoperative hyperglycemia include increased risk of infection and impaired wound healing, presumably secondary to impairment of lymphocyte and phagocyte cell function. On rare occasions, hyperglycemic hyperosmolar coma or ketoacidosis results from an uncontrolled blood sugar level; this is most likely to occur with the development of other complications such as infection [75].

Management of diabetic patients in the perioperative period requires administration of both glucose and insulin. On the morning of surgery, the insulin-dependent diabetic should receive one-half of his or her usual morning dose of insulin by subcutaneous injection, in the form of an intermediate-acting preparation. Patients who were not taking insulin before surgery (even though managed by an oral agent or diet) should not receive insulin on the morning of surgery. For both groups, an intravenous infusion of 5% dextrose at 75 to 100 ml/hr is begun in the morning. After arrival in the operating room, and hourly during surgery, the blood glucose level should be measured. Hyperglycemia can be treated intraoperatively with small intravenous boluses of regular insulin (1–5 units) or concomitant infusion of glucose and variable rates of constantly infused insulin [76]. In the intensive care unit after operation, the blood glucose level should be maintained between 100 to 220 mg/dl by continuous infusion of 5% dextrose and the intravenous administration of regular insulin at a rate of 1 to 10 units/hr until enteral intake is resumed. The blood glucose level should be measured every 1 to 2 hours with a portable analyzer (e.g., the Accu-Check blood glucose monitor) and the insulin dose adjusted accordingly. When the patient begins to receive enteral caloric support (either in the form of oral intake or tube feedings), conversion to longer-acting preparations may be accomplished. During this transition phase, insulin is frequently administered on a sliding scale basis. Continued frequent blood glucose measurements (every 4–6 hours) are important during this period of recuperation due to the patient's unpredictable caloric intake.

Hypoglycemia in adult patients is unusual, except for that resulting from excessive exogenous insulin administration. If it does occur, it can be counteracted by the intravenous administration of 50% dextrose. To prevent this occurrence, some glucose should be administered at all times (in the form of intravenously administered 5% dextrose) to the diabetic patient receiving insulin but who is not eating normally. Only when normal caloric intake is achieved should the patient be placed back on his or her preoperative drug regimen (insulin or oral agent). Infants, due to decreased hepatic glycogen stores, are at increased risk for hypoglycemia. Thus, severe perioperative hypoglycemia may occur in newborns (below 30 mg/dl in full-term infants, below 20 mg/dl in the premature), leading to seizures. This usually can be prevented by using an intravenous maintenance solution with adequate glucose (10% dextrose) and frequent determination of the baby's blood glucose level.

Nutritional Support

Nutritional deficiencies can lead to heart failure, and heart failure can result in nutritional deficiencies. The protein-calorie malnutrition associated with chronic congestive heart failure is known as the syndrome of cardiac cachexia. Preoperative malnutrition is a risk factor for postoperative complications and prolonged hospital stay in patients undergoing cardiac surgery. A preoperative albumin level of less than 3.5 g/dl is associated with an increased frequency of postoperative complications in elderly patients [77]. Preoperative nutritional supplementation, however, is rarely feasible due to the urgency of operation. Also, the benefits of such therapy have not been demonstrated conclusively. The realization that preoperative deficiency may exist should lead to early postoperative nutritional assessment and supplementation.

Many infants with congenital heart disease and heart failure are unable to feed normally, and "failure to thrive" frequently enters into the decision to recommend surgical repair for the underlying cardiac lesion. After operation, these patients need early protein and caloric supplementation. Thus, a nasogastric tube is inserted after operation. Initially this is used for gastric drainage, but, as soon as bowel activity returns, tube feedings may be started. The tube should be fine-bore to prevent obstruction of the nares (infants are nose-breathers) and soft to prevent gastric perforation or nasal erosion. Initial feedings in infants consist of a clear fluid such as 5% dextrose at 5 to 10 ml/hr. The residual amount left in the stomach after each hour is determined by aspiration. If low residual amounts are present, tube feedings are advanced both in amount and substance. For newborns, expressed breast milk may be available; this is preferable to commercially available formulas. The infant may need a pacifier to satisfy the urge to suck. Once on full tube feedings and sucking well (usually after just a few days), the infant is allowed oral intake with the tube in place. Supplements are given by tube until full calories are ingested by mouth.

Likewise, adults who have preoperative complications should receive early postoperative alimentation. Patients with postoperative complications that prevent the oral intake of sufficient protein and calories should also be started on early nutritional supplementation to prevent so-called nosocomial cardiac cachexia (Table 3-8) [78]. This can frequently be accomplished via a feeding tube (nasogastric or, preferably, nasoduodenal) to avoid the problems of maintaining venous access, fluid overload, and infection associated with central

Table 3-8. Adult enteral formulas commonly used

	Replete with Fiber	Jevity	Osmolite	Osmolite HN	Ensure	Ensure Plus	Nutrivent	Tolerex
Calories/ml	1.00	1.06	1.06	1.06	1.06	1.50	1.50	1.00
Protein source	Calcium caseinate	Sodium & calcium caseinates, soy isolates	Sodium & calcium caseinates	Sodium & calcium caseinates, soy isolates	Sodium & calcium caseinates, soy isolates	Sodium & calcium caseinates, soy isolates	Calcium caseinate	Free amino acids
Fat source	Canola oil, MCT oil	Safflower, MCT oil, canola oil	Safflower, MCT oil, canola oil	Safflower, MCT oil, canola oil	Corn oil	Corn oil	Canola oil, MCT oil, corn oil	Safflower oil
CHO source	Maltodextrin, corn syrup solids, soy polysaccharides	Hydrolyzed cornstarch, soy polysaccharides	Glucose polymers	Glucose polymers	Corn syrup, sucrose	Hydrolyzed cornstarch, sucrose	Maltodextrin, sucrose	Hydrolyzed starch
Protein (g/liter)	62.5	44.4	37.2	44.4	37.2	62.6	68	20.6
Fat (g/liter)	34	36.8	38.5	36.8	37.2	50	94.8	1.5
CHO (g/liter)	113	151.7	145	141.2	145	199.9	100.8	226.3
Osmolality (mOsm/kg)	300	310	300	300	470	650	450	550
Na^+K^+ (mg/liter)	500/1560	929/1564	635/1013	929/1564	846/1564	1184/1818	750/2240	468/1172
Ca^+PO_4 (mg/liter)	1000/1000	909/756	530/530	758/758	530/530	1056/1056	1200/1200	556/556
Comments	14 g dietary fiber per liter. Lactose free	14 g dietary fiber per liter. Lactose free	Lactose free, low residue, isotonic	Lactose free, low residue, isotonic	Lactose free, low residue	Lactose free, low residue	Lactose free, designed to lower CO_2 production in pulmonary patients	Elemental, low fat

Table 3-8 (continued)

	Vital High Nitrogen	Perative	Amin-Aid	Lipisorb	Suplena	Nepro	Vivonex T.E.N.	AlitraQ
Calories/ml	1.00	1.30	2.00	1.35	2.00	2.00	1.00	1.00
Protein source	Free amino acids (13%), peptides (87%)	Partially hydrolyzed sodium caseinate	Crystalline essential amino acids	Sodium & calcium caseinates	Sodium & calcium caseinates	Calcium, magnesium, & sodium caseinates	Free amino acids	Hydrolyzed soy, whey, & free amino acids
Fat source	MCT oil, safflower oil	Canola oil, MCT oil, corn oil	Soybean oil, lecithin, mono- & diglycerides	MCT oil (85%), soy oil (15%)	90% high-oleic safflower oil, 10% soy oil	High-oleic safflower oil, soy oil	Safflower oil	MCT oil, safflower oil
CHO source	Hydrolyzed cornstarch, sucrose	Hydrolyzed cornstarch	Maltodextrin, sucrose	Maltodextrin, sucrose	Hydrolyzed cornstarch, sucrose	Hydrolyzed cornstarch, sucrose	Hydrolyzed starch	Hydrolyzed cornstarch, sucrose
Protein (g/liter)	41.7	66.6	19.4	57.4	30.0	69.9	38.2	52.5
Fat (g/liter)	10.8	37.4	46.2	56.5	95.6	95.6	2.8	15.5
CHO (g/liter)	185.09	177.2	365.6	160.4	255.2	215.2	206	165
Osmolality	500	425	700	600	600	635	630	575
NA^+K^+ (mg/liter)	566/1400	1040/1730	<345/117	1000/620	783/1116	829/1057	460/782	1000/1200
CA^+PO_4 (mg/liter)	667/667	867/867	—	700/700	1385/728	1373/686	500/500	733/733
Comments	Powder, elemental, BCAA's, trace lactose, meat & whey protein	Low residue designed for metabolic-stressed patients. Lactose free	Essential amino acids for management of renal disease	Designed for fat absorption. Lactose free	High calorie, low protein, low electrolyte	Dialyzed patients. Moderate protein, low electrolyte	Elemental, low fat	Glutamine enriched

Key: MCT = medium-chain triglycerides (fractionated coconut oil); BCAA = branch-chain amino acid.
Source: Table courtesy of Mary Whalen, R.D., Department of Dietetics, Massachusetts General Hospital.

venous hyperalimentation. The gastrointestinal ileus associated with cardiac surgery usually clears within a few days allowing for nutrition via the gastrointestinal tract. Various enteral formulas are commercially available and the type of formula can be tailored to the needs of the patient (see Table 3-8). Tube feedings may be preferable to efforts at oral supplementation in some patients because they are independent of the patient's appetite and allow for continuous delivery (avoiding abdominal distention and wide swings in the blood glucose level). As the patient's general condition improves, he or she can be converted gradually to a full oral diet.

Parenteral nutrition may be required for pediatric or adult patients who are unable to receive nutrition via a feeding tube. This may be delivered via a central or peripheral vein and typically consists of a glucose solution containing electrolytes, vitamins, trace minerals, and amino acids, in addition to a daily infusion of an emulsified lipid solution. During parenteral alimentation, the patient is monitored closely with regard to urine output, urine glucose, serum electrolytes, glucose and blood urea nitrogen, liver enzymes, and blood count.

Patients with normal preoperative nutritional states and uncomplicated postoperative courses typically have depressed appetites and occasional nausea early after surgery, and this is of little consequence. Generally, they are prescribed a low-salt (2 g sodium) diet as their total body sodium is usually elevated, and they are discharged home on a "no-added" salt diet unless indications for continuing significant sodium restriction are present (e.g., heart failure or hypertension). After about a week, the appetite usually returns with discharge from the hospital and the return to "home cooking." Patients with hyperlipemia or obesity who require special dietary management should be placed on these special diets 4 to 6 weeks after surgery.

References

1. Kohanna FH, et al. Cardiac output determination after cardiac operation: Lack of correlation between direct measurements and indirect estimates. *J Thorac Cardiovasc Surg* 82:904, 1981.

2. Flores ED, Lange RA, Hillis RD. Relation of mean pulmonary arterial wedge pressure and left ventricular end-diastolic pressure. *Am J Cardiol* 66:1532, 1990.

3. Fleisher AG, et al. Management of massive hemoptysis secondary to catheter-induced perforation of the pulmonary artery during cardiopulmonary bypass. *Chest* 95:1340, 1989.

4. Hochberg MS, et al. Pulmonary inactivation of vasopressors following cardiac operations. *Ann Thorac Surg* 41:200, 1986.

5. Breisblatt WM, et al. Acute myocardial dysfunction and recovery: A common occurrence after coronary bypass surgery. *J Am Coll Cardiol* 15:1261, 1990.

6. Gray, R, et al. Scintigraphic and hemodynamic demonstration of transient left ventricular dysfunction immediately after uncompli-

cated coronary artery bypass grafting. *J Thorac Cardiovasc Surg* 77:504, 1979.

7. Czer L, et al. Transient hemodynamic dysfunction after myocardial revascularization. *J Thorac Cardiovasc Surg* 86:228, 1983.

8. Kirklin JK, Kirklin JW. Management of the cardiovascular subsystem after cardiac surgery. *Ann Thorac Surg* 32:311, 1980.

9. Fremes SE, et al. Effects of postoperative hypertension and its treatment. *J Thorac Cardiovasc Surg* 86:47, 1983.

10. Cosgrove DM, et al. Automated control of postoperative hypertension: A prospective, randomized multicenter study. *Ann Thorac Surg* 47:678, 1989.

11. Jett GK, et al. Vasoactive drug effects of blood flow in internal mammary artery and saphenous vein grafts. *J Thorac Cardiovasc Surg* 94:2, 1987.

12. Kaplan JA, Guffin AV. Perioperative management of hypertension and tachycardia. *J Cardiothorac Anesth* 4:7, 1990.

13. Patel CB, et al. Use of sodium nitroprusside in post-coronary bypass grafting surgery — a plea for conservatism. *Chest* 89:663, 1986.

14. Bojar RM, et al. Methemoglobinemia from intravenous nitroglycerin: A word of caution. *Ann Thorac Surg* 43:332, 1987.

15. Kaplan JA, Jones EL. Vasodilator therapy during coronary artery surgery. A comparison of nitroglycerin and nitroprusside. *J Thorac Cardiovasc Surg* 77:301, 1979.

16. Brush JE Jr, et al. Comparative effects of verapamil and nitroprusside on left ventricular function in patients with hypertension. *J Am Coll Cardiol* 14:515, 1989.

17. Mullen JC, et al. Postoperative hypertension: A comparison of diltiazem, nifedipine, and nitroprusside. *J Thorac Cardiovasc Surg* 96:122, 1988.

18. Bauer JH, Reams GP. The role of calcium entry blockers in hypertensive emergencies. *Circulation* 75(Suppl V):V-174, 1987.

19. IV Nicardipine Study Group. Efficacy and safety of intravenous nicardipine in the control of postoperative hypertension. *Chest* 99:393, 1991.

20. van Wezel HB, et al. The efficacy of nicardipine and nitroprusside in preventing poststernotomy hypertension. *J Cardiothorac Anesth* 3:700, 1989.

21. Kataria B, et al. Evaluation of intravenous esmolol for treatment of postoperative hypertension. *J Cardiothorac Anesth* 4:13, 1990.

22. Reves JG, et al. Esmolol for treatment of intraoperative tachycardia and/or hypertension in patients having cardiac operations. *J Thorac Cardiovasc Surg* 100:221, 1990.

23. Sladen RN, et al. Labetalol for the control of elevated blood pressure following coronary artery bypass grafting. *J Cardiothorac Anesth* 4:210, 1990.

24. Cruise CJ, et al. Intravenous labetalol versus sodium nitroprusside

for treatment of hypertension postcoronary bypass surgery. *Anesthesiology* 71:835, 1989.

25. Matthay MA, Wiener-Kronish JP. Respiratory management after cardiac surgery. *Chest* 95:424, 1989.

26. Hammereister KE, et al. Identification of patients at greatest risk for developing major complications at cardiac surgery. *Circulation* 82(Suppl IV):IV-380, 1990.

27. Greenspon AJ, et al. Amiodarone-related postoperative adult respiratory distress syndrome. *Circulation* 84(Suppl III):III-407, 1991.

28. Warner MA, et al. Role of preoperative cessation of smoking and other factors in postoperative pulmonary complications: A blinded study of coronary artery patients. *Mayo Clinc Proc* 64:609, 1989.

29. Young JD, Sykes MK. Artificial ventilation: history, equipment, techniques. *Thorax* 189:753, 1990.

30. Otherson HB Jr. Intubation injuries of the trachea in children. *Ann Surg* 189:601, 1979.

31. Oikkonen M, et al. Comparison of incentive spirometry and intermittent positive pressure breathing after coronary artery bypass graft. *Chest* 99:60, 1991.

32. Utley JR, Stephens DB. Fluid Balance During Cardiopulmonary Bypass. In JR Utley (ed), *Pathophysiology and Techniques of Cardiopulmonary Bypass*, Vol II. Baltimore: Williams & Wilkins, 1983. Pp. 27–35.

33. Elliott MJ. Perfusion for pediatric open heart surgery. *Semin Thorac Cardiothorac Surg* 2:332, 1990.

34. Nordrehaug JE, Johannessen K-A, von der Lippe G. Serum potassium concentration as a risk factor of ventricular arrhythmias early in acute myocardial infarction. *Circulation* 71:645, 1985.

35. Kunau RT, Stein JH. Disorders of hypo- and hyperkalemia. *Clin Nephrol* 7:173, 1977.

36. Gray RJ, et al. Calcium homeostasis during coronary bypass surgery. *Circulation* 62(Suppl I):I-57, 1980.

37. Zaloga GP, Chernow B. Hypocalcemia in critical illness. *JAMA* 256:1924, 1986.

38. Sohmer PR. Transfusion Therapy in Surgery. In LD Petz and SN Swisher (eds), *Clinical Practice of Transfusion Medicine*. New York: Churchill Livingstone, 1989. P. 374.

39. Lum G, Marquardt C, Khuri SF. Hypomagnesemia and low alkaline phosphatase activity in patients' serum after cardiac surgery. *Clin Chem* 35:664, 1989.

40. Surawicz B. Is hypomagnesemia or magnesium deficiency arrhythmogenic? *J Am Coll Cardiol* 14:1093, 1989.

41. Hecker BR, et al. Influence of magnesium ion on human ventricular defibrillation after aortocoronary bypass surgery. *Am J Cardiol* 55:61, 1985.

42. Narins RG, Emmett M. Simple and mixed acid-base disorders: A practical approach. *Medicine* 59:161, 1989.

43. Viitanen A, et al. Pulmonary vascular resistance before and after cardiopulmonary bypass: The effect of $PaCO_2$. *Chest* 95:773, 1989.

44. Ritter JM, Doktor HS, Benjamin N. Paradoxical effect of bicarbonate on cytoplasmic pH. *Lancet* 335:1243, 1990.

45. Kette F, et al. Buffer agents do not reverse intramyocardial acidosis during cardiac resuscitation. *Circulation* 81:1160, 1990.

46. Schiff M, et al. Acquired immunodeficiency syndrome, a complication of cardiothoracic surgery. *J Thorac Cardiovasc Surg* 97:126, 1989.

47. Seidl S, Kuhnl P. Transmission of diseases by blood transfusion. *World J Surg* 11:30, 1987.

48. Peterman TA. Transfusion-associated acquired immunodeficiency syndrome. *World J Surg* 11:36, 1987.

49. Collins JA. Recent developments in the area of massive transfusion. *World J Surg* 11:75, 1987.

50. National Institutes of Health Consensus Conference. Perioperative red cell transfusion. *JAMA* 260:2700, 1988.

51. Kim YD, et al. Effects of hypothermia and hemodilution on metabolism and hemodynamics in patients recovering from coronary artery bypass grafting operations. *J Thorac Cardiovasc Surg* 97:36, 1989.

52. Lociciero J, et al. Aggressive blood conservation in coronary artery surgery: Impact on patient care. *J Cardiovasc Surg* 31:559, 1990.

53. Messmer KFW. Acceptable hematocrit levels in surgical patients. *World J Surg* 11:41, 1987.

54. Utley JR, et al. Correlates of preoperative hematocrit value in patients undergoing coronary artery bypass grafting. *J Thorac Cardiovasc Surg* 98:451, 1989.

55. Cosgrove DM, et al. Determinants of blood utilization during myocardial revascularization. *Ann Thorac Surg* 40:380, 1985.

56. Owings DV, et al. Autologous blood donations prior to elective cardiac surgery. *JAMA* 262:1963, 1989.

57. Britton LW, et al. Predonated autologous blood use in elective cardiac surgery. *Ann Thorac Surg* 47:529, 1989.

58. Love TR, et al. Transfusion of predonated autologous blood in elective cardiac surgery. *Ann Thorac Surg* 43:508, 1987.

59. Scott WJ, Kessler R, Wernly JA. Blood conservation in cardiac surgery. *Ann Thorac Surg* 50:843, 1990.

60. Bashein G, et al. Preoperative aspirin therapy and reoperation for bleeding after coronary artery bypass surgery. *Arch Intern Med* 51:89, 1991.

61. Fullerton DA, Campbell DN, Whitman GJR. Use of human recombinant erythropoietin to correct severe preoperative anemia. *Ann Thorac Surg* 51:825, 1991.

62. Wantanabe Y, et al. Autologous blood transfusion with recombinant

human erythropoietin in heart operations. *Ann Thorac Surg* 51:767, 1991.

63. Bidstrup BP, et al. Reduction in blood loss and blood use after cardiopulmonary bypass with high dose aprotinin (Trasylol). *J Thorac Cardiovasc Surg* 97:364, 1989.

64. Dietrich WD, et al. Reduction of homologous blood requirement in cardiac surgery by intraoperative aprotinin application — clinical experience with 152 cardiac surgical patients. *J Thorac Cardiovasc Surg* 37:92, 1989.

65. Hackmann T, et al. A trial of desmopressin (1-desamino-8-D-arginine vasopressin) to reduce blood loss in uncomplicated cardiac surgery. *N Engl J Med* 321:1437, 1989.

66. Lazenby WD, et al. Treatment with desmopressin acetate in routine coronary artery bypass surgery to improve postoperative hemostasis. *Circulation* 82(Suppl IV):IV-413, 1990.

67. Aris A, et al. Prediction of hematocrit changes in open heart surgery without blood transfusion. *J Cardiovasc Surg* 25:545, 1984.

68. Goodnough LT, et al. Guidelines for transfusion therapy in patients undergoing coronary artery bypass grafting. *Ann Thorac Surg* 50:675, 1990.

69. Delaney VB, Bourke E. Diuretics. In JW Hurst (ed), *The Heart*. New York: McGraw-Hill, 1990. P. 1772.

70. Opie LH (ed). *Drugs for the Heart*. Philadelphia: Saunders, 1991. P. 89.

71. Purdy RE, Boucek RJ. *Handbook of Cardiac Drugs*. Boston: Little, Brown, 1988. P. 171.

72. Hannan EL, et al. Adult open heart surgery in New York State: An analysis of risk factors and hospital mortality rates. *JAMA* 264:2768, 1990.

73. Salomon NW, et al. Diabetes mellitus and coronary artery bypass: Short term risk and long term prognosis. *J Thorac Cardiovasc Surg* 85:264, 1983.

74. Johnson WD, Pedraza PM, Kayser KL. Coronary artery surgery in diabetics: 261 consecutive patients followed four to seven years. *Am Heart J* 104:823, 1982.

75. Seki S. Clinical features of hyperosmolar hyperglycemic nonketotic diabetic coma associated with cardiac operations. *J Thorac Cardiovasc Surg* 91:867, 1986.

76. Woodruff RE, et al. Avoidance of surgical hyperglycemia in diabetic patients. *JAMA* 244:166, 1980.

77. Rich MW, et al. Increased complications and prolonged hospital stay in elderly patients with low serum albumin. *Am J Cardiol* 63:714, 1990.

78. Quinn T, Askanazi J. Nutrition and cardiac disease. *Crit Care Clin* 3:167, 1987.

Postoperative Complications Involving the Heart and Lungs

Despite advances in cardiac surgery and perioperative care, the prevention and treatment of postoperative complications continue to be an integral part of the care of the cardiac surgery patient. As older and sicker adult patients undergo surgery with greater frequency, the incidence of complications has increased [1]. Likewise, infants with congenital heart conditions are undergoing total repair operations at an earlier age than in previous years with a concomitant increase in the potential difficulties encountered in their early postoperative care. Recognition and treatment of perioperative complications are as important as the performance of the surgery itself. A technically perfect operation can be ruined by poor postoperative care, and a less-than-perfect technical operative result can often be "saved" by appropriate management of postoperative problems.

Low Cardiac Output

Low cardiac output occurs during the early postoperative period in approximately 20% of patients who undergo cardiac surgery [2]. The incidence of this complication is dependent on the type and severity of the cardiac lesion undergoing repair, preoperative ventricular function, adequacy of myocardial preservation during the procedure, and the adequacy of the surgical repair. For example, coronary artery bypass procedures on patients with normal left ventricular function have a low incidence of postoperative low cardiac output. In contrast, patients with ischemic mitral valve regurgitation with poor left ventricular function have a notoriously high incidence of low output after mitral valve replacement and coronary bypass surgery.

Although intraoperative technical mishaps or inadequate myocardial protection during surgery can cause damage to a previously normal ventricle, the most important factor determining the incidence of postoperative low output is *preoperative* ventricular function. Thus, preoperative evaluation of ventricular function is important. Careful review of the patient's cardiac catheterization study — both the hemodynamic measurements (cardiac output, left ventricular end-diastolic pressure, and pulmonary artery pressures) and the left ventriculogram — provides a good indication of the presence or absence of preoperative ventricular dysfunction. Other studies, such as radionuclide ventriculography (multigated angiocardiography or MUGA) and echocardiography, also provide valuable information about systolic ventricular function.

Normal systolic function is associated with an ejection fraction of 60 to 75%. Moderate left ventricular dysfunction is present when the ejection fraction is 35 to 50%, and severe impairment of contractility is associated with an ejection fraction below 35%. It must be remembered that the ejection fraction is dependent on preload and afterload; therefore, its meaning must be assessed in the context of the patient's history and other data. The ejection fraction, furthermore, reflects only the systolic (ejection) function of the heart. Diastolic dysfunction, reflected as abnormalities in ventricular relaxation and filling, also can result in heart failure and even pulmonary edema despite the presence of a normal ejection fraction [3]. Patients with ventricular hypertrophy are particularly susceptible to diastolic dysfunction.

Preoperative recognition of poor ventricular function leads to alterations in the management of technical aspects of the operative procedure. In such cases, we routinely use a catheter to vent the left ventricle. Just after cardiopulmonary bypass is begun, the catheter is introduced via the right superior pulmonary vein and advanced through the left atrium into the left ventricle. By applying low suction to the catheter, distention of the ventricle is prevented. During the period of aortic cross-clamping, warm non-coronary blood flow collecting in the left ventricle is evacuated thus helping to keep the heart cool. Likewise, for patients with very poor left ventricular function, a lower cardiopulmonary bypass perfusion temperature (such as 22°C) may be employed. For patients with poor ventricular function (particularly those with very tightly stenotic coronary arteries and those undergoing coronary bypass reoperations or valve procedures) cardioplegia solution may be administered via a small catheter placed in the coronary sinus. This retrograde approach perfuses the myocardium via the coronary venous system thus allowing for an unobstructed route for the cold hyperkalemic cardioplegia solution to cool and cause diastolic arrest of the heart. When used for valve operations, the retrograde cardioplegia delivery route provides convenient, frequent delivery of the cardioplegia solution without the need to cannulate the coronary ostia directly (as in aortic valve replacement) or to interrupt the retraction setup (as in mitral valve procedures). For the patient with poor preoperative ventricular function, we routinely introduce a femoral artery catheter in the operating room just before beginning surgery. This provides access for the guidewire, which allows expeditious introduction of an intraaortic balloon pump should one be required in the operating room or during the early postoperative period.

MANAGEMENT OF LOW CARDIAC OUTPUT

When low cardiac output is present early after cardiac surgery, management should follow a logical order of analysis and treatment (Fig. 4-1). First, consideration should be given to the possibility of reversible mechanical factors causing the poor cardiac performance. This is especially true for the patient who had good preoperative ventricular function and who was weaned from cardiopulmonary bypass without difficulty. Left and right heart filling pressures must be determined to rule out hypovolemia, which is the most common cause of low cardiac output. Filling pressures should be compared with those found optimal in the operating room and before surgery. Cardiac tamponade must be ruled out (see Chap. 5). Consideration should be given to the possibility of technical problems related to the operation; occlusion of bypass grafts, embolic obstruction of a coronary artery, prosthetic valve dehiscence or obstruction, residual shunts, or obstruction of a conduit or baffle among others [4].

4. Postoperative Complications Involving the Heart and Lungs

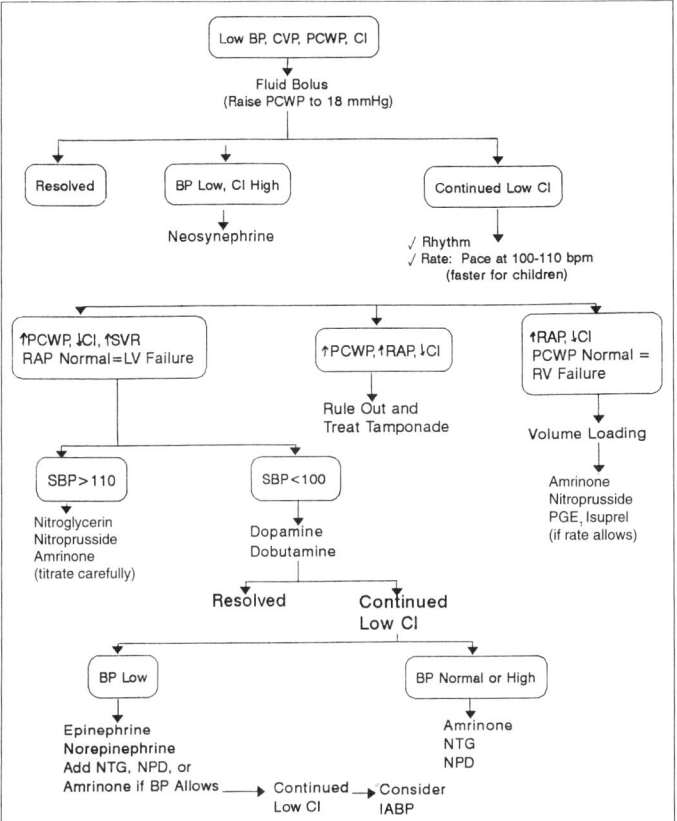

Fig. 4-1. Management algorithm for low cardiac output.
Key: BP = blood pressure; CVP = central venous pressure; PCWP = pulmonary capillary wedge pressure; CI = cardiac index; SVR = systemic vascular resistance; RAP = right atrial pressure; LV = left ventricle; RV = right ventricle; SBP = systolic blood pressure; PGE_1 = prostaglandin E_1; NTG = nitroglycerin; NPD = nitroprusside; IABP = intraaortic balloon pump.
Note: This algorithm is for guidance only. Specific patients may require deviations from this strategy. Also, the specific effects of some medications (such as dopamine and epinephrine) are dose-dependent. See text for details.

The physical examination should be repeated. Patients with low cardiac output have cold, poorly perfused extremities and absent peripheral pulses. In infants, an elevated core temperature is often present. Auscultation should be performed to listen especially for valvular regurgitation murmurs, abnormal prosthetic valve sounds (if one is present), and muffled heart tones. The arterial blood pressure tracing should be inspected for the presence of an abnormally wide pulse pressure indicative of possible aortic valve regurgitation. The pulmonary artery wedge pressure tracing should be examined for the presence of "V" waves suggesting mitral valve regurgitation. The 12-lead ECG should be studied for evidence of ischemia.

Echocardiography provides information about both valvular and ventricular function. In infants, transthoracic echocardiography can be used to visualize the ventricles, assess their contractility, and determine the presence or absence of significant mediastinal blood clots; color flow Doppler can be used to identify residual intracardiac shunts [5]. A bolus of saline injected through a right atrial or central venous catheter will produce a cloud of echo bubbles in the right atrium and ventricle that will appear immediately in the left atrium or ventricle if there is a right-to-left shunt. Conversely, saline injected into the left atrial line will produce echoes in the right side if there is a left-to-right shunt. This valuable technique has reduced the need for cardiac catheterization in an acutely ill baby to decide whether reoperation should be considered [6].

Early after surgery, transthoracic echocardiography is not as useful in adults as it is in infants. Inability to turn the patient, bandages, mediastinal air, chest tubes, and the adult chest configuration combine to make assessment of the heart by this technique difficult. *Transesophageal* echocardiography, however, is easily performed by the experienced operator and provides reliable information regarding ventricular filling and function, valvular function, and the presence or absence of tamponade [7].

Occasionally, particularly in adults, emergency cardiac catheterization, at times including coronary arteriography, may be indicated to rule out reparable abnormalities. If a mechanical cause for the low cardiac output state is identified, immediate surgical repair is usually indicated despite the emotional trauma experienced by both the patient's family and by the surgeon in these situations.

While this evaluation is proceeding, efforts to improve the cardiac output and systemic perfusion are begun. The treatment of low cardiac output involves consideration of the heart rhythm, heart rate, status of the ventricular filling pressure (preload), myocardial contractility, and peripheral (and pulmonary) vascular resistance (afterload).

Early consideration should be given to the patient's cardiac rhythm and rate. Cardiac output decreases with arrhythmias such as heart block, junctional rhythm, atrial fibrillation, and sinus bradycardia. For the severely compromised patient with new-onset atrial fibrillation, synchronized electrical cardioversion is indicated; restoration of normal sinus rhythm or pharmacologic control of a rapid ventricular response to atrial fibrillation will improve cardiac output. For patients with heart block or junctional rhythm, sequential atrioventricular pacing will restore the atrial contribution to the stroke volume, increasing the patient's cardiac output by 15 to 35% [8]. This atrial contraction contribution to ventricular filling is particularly important for the heart in the early period after cardiopulmonary bypass when there may be impaired ventricular diastolic function [9]. Proper capture of the atrium must be ensured, and, for adults, the *atrioventricular interval* (the time between the pacing impulse to the atrium and the impulse to the ventricle) should be set at 150 to 180 msec; shorter intervals are used for pediatric patients. Even for patients in sinus rhythm, if the heart rate is substantially less than 100 beats per minute, pacing at the rate of 100 will result in an improvement in the cardiac output [10]. For patients with intact atrioventricular conduction, this is accomplished best by pacing only the atrium.

Ventricular function is impaired by hypothermia [11,12]. Although rewarming of the patient to 36°C or greater is completed before weaning from cardiopulmonary bypass, this rewarming may be incomplete and further cooling may occur during closure of the incision and transportation of the patient. Thus, the patient frequently becomes cold early after operation and this can contribute significantly to ventricular dysfunction and hemodynamic deterioration [13]. Application of a warming blanket to the patient in the intensive care unit will help return the patient to normal temperature with beneficial effects on cardiac output. For the patient with severe low cardiac output who is cold and shivering, suppression of the shivering with neuromuscular blocking agents will decrease oxygen consumption and improve the hemodynamic status [14,15].

Optimal cardiac output requires adequate return of blood to the heart (preload) for left ventricular filling (Fig. 4-2). Left ventricular preload may be monitored by measurement of the pulmonary artery diastolic pressure, pulmonary capillary wedge pressure, and, if a catheter was placed intraoperatively, left atrial pressure. Although the normal heart functions well with a pulmonary capillary wedge pressure of 6 to 12 mm Hg, failing hearts require higher filling pressures because of poor compliance of the left ventricle. A trial infusion of 250 to 500 ml of crystalloid or colloid fluid to the adult patient, given over a short period, is an important early maneuver in the management of low output [16]. Raising the left ventricular filling pressure to 15 to 18 mm Hg frequently improves the cardiac output. In some patients, very high filling pressures, even up to 25 to 30 mm Hg, are required to optimize left ventricular performance. Knowledge of the preoperative filling pressure can often guide volume administration in the postoperative period. Such volume infusion should be administered with care; overfilling of the heart leads to ventricular distention, worsening of the myocardial performance, and pulmonary edema. Either crystalloid (often as 5% dextrose/one-half normal saline) or colloid may be used for volume expansion. Colloidal solutions may have some advantages when used for volume expansion and are frequently used in cardiac surgery patients whose total body water and sodium are already elevated. This may be in the form of plasma protein fraction, hetastarch, or albumin. Although avoidance of unnecessary blood product transfusion is important, severe anemia in the presence of impaired ventricular function (and loss of ability to compensate for the anemia) results in diminished systemic oxygen delivery. Thus, for these patients, we often transfuse red blood cells to raise the hematocrit to at least 25 to 28% when they are experiencing significant postoperative low cardiac output.

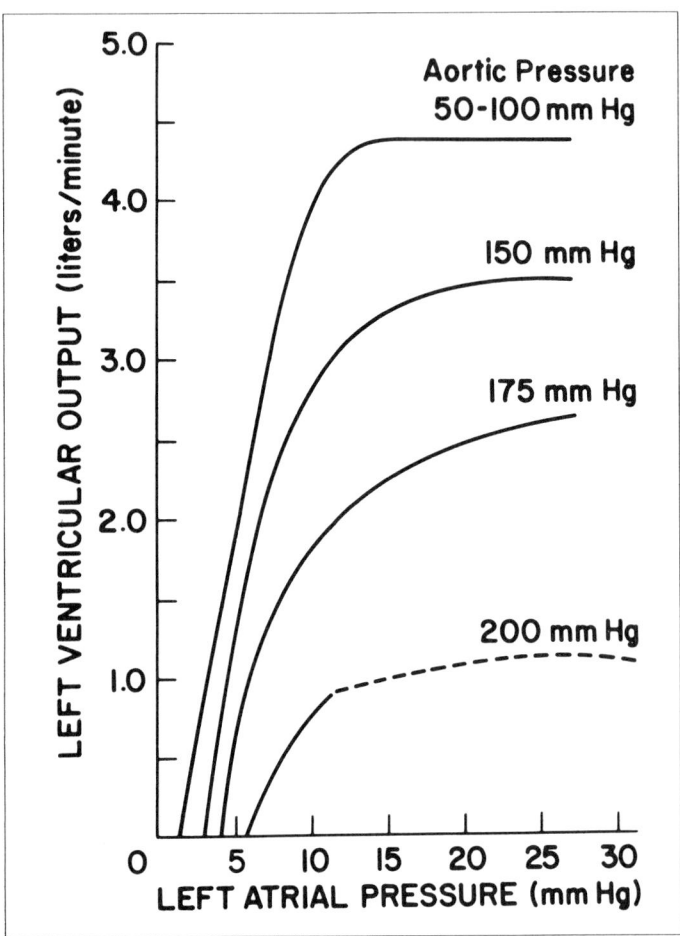

Fig. 4-2. The relationship between left ventricular output, left atrial pressure (preload), and aortic pressure (afterload). Increasing left atrial pressure with aortic pressure constant increases left ventricular output to a limit (Starling relationship). Decreasing aortic pressure with left atrial pressure constant also increases left ventricular output as long as there is sufficient aortic pressure to perfuse the coronary arteries. (Adapted from TC Ruch and HD Patton, *Physiology and Biophysics II*. Philadelphia: Saunders, 1974 p. 179.)

INOTROPIC DRUG TREATMENT OF LOW CARDIAC OUTPUT

Various drugs optimize cardiac output through their effects on myocardial contractility (inotropic effect) or effects on the peripheral resistance (afterload effect) or both. Table 4-1 summarizes the commonly used drugs. Positive inotropic agents act to increase the force and speed of myocardial fiber contraction, and, in general, they also

Table 4-1. Effects of pharmacologic agents used to treat hypotension and low cardiac output

Drug	Inotropic effect	Chronotropic effect	Peripheral resistance	Renal blood flow	Cardiac output	Intravenous dosage range
Amrinone (Inocor)	+	0	−	?	+	5–15 μg/kg/min Load: 0.75 mg/kg
Dobutamine (Dobutrex)	++	+	− or 0	?	++	2–20 μg/kg/min
Dopamine (Intropin)	++	+	− or 0 or + (dose-dependent)	++ (at lower doses)	+	2–15 μg/kg/min
Epinephrine (Adrenalin)	++	++	− or 0 or + (dose-dependent)	−	++	0.01–0.20 μg/kg/min
Isoproterenol (Isuprel)	++	+++	−	+ or 0	++	0.01–0.20 μg/kg/min
Norepinephrine* (Levophed)	++	0 or −	+++	−	++	0.01–0.10 μg/kg/min
Phenylephrine (Neo-Synephrine)	0	0 or −	+++	−	−	0.5–5.0 μg/kg/min

+ = an increase; − = a decrease, 0 = no effect.
*Norepinephrine is often used in conjunction with a vasodilator or in circumstances when peripheral resistance is low.

increase myocardial oxygen consumption. Considerable controversy exists regarding which drug or combination of drugs should be used to treat low cardiac output. Although much experimental and clinical data are available, no one drug is best for all patients with low cardiac output, and several drugs may be equally effective in the same hemodynamic setting. Local institutional custom, personal opinion, and, at times, a bit of superstition often combine to decide which agents are used for which circumstances. Rational selection of drugs to treat low cardiac output requires a basic understanding of the agents available, careful analysis of the hemodynamic abnormalities present, tailoring of the therapy to fit the individual hemodynamic setting, and realization that the patient's state is dynamic and thus alterations in the type of drug support administered may be required with the passage of time [17].

Common to the use of the available positive inotropic drugs is the need for central venous administration to avoid vein irritation and tissue damage in the event of extravasation and to ensure delivery into the circulation. These agents are usually administered via a right atrial catheter, but inactivation of the drug may occur as it traverses the pulmonary circulation. Thus, higher coronary and systemic concentrations and greater drug efficacy may be achieved in particularly difficult situations by administration through a left atrial catheter, if one is present [18]. This may be particularly useful for the infusion of norepinephrine, especially when pulmonary hypertension or right heart failure is present. If the left atrial catheter is used for drug infusion, great care must be taken to avoid the introduction of air emboli. Therefore, we would not attempt this approach unless drug administration to the right side of the circulation appears ineffective or if right heart failure is present.

The sympathetic amines (dopamine, dobutamine, epinephrine, norepinephrine, and isoproterenol) improve cardiac output by a direct beta-adrenergic inotropic effect and have selectively different effects on the peripheral vasculature. Their effects are mediated through the adrenergic receptors. Beta-1 receptors exist predominantly in the myocardium; their activation results in increased speed and force of myocardial contraction, increased rate of automaticity of the sinoatrial node, and faster atrioventricular conduction. The beta-2 receptors are present predominantly in the smooth muscles of blood vessels and bronchi; their activation results in vasodilation and bronchodilation. Alpha-adrenergic receptors exist primarily in the peripheral and pulmonary vasculature. Alpha-receptor stimulation causes vasoconstriction.

Dopamine is frequently used for the treatment of low cardiac output. A unique feature of this agent is that it has distinctly different hemodynamic effects at different doses. When administered at low doses (so-called renal dose dopamine, 1–3 µg/kg/min) dopamine provides stimulation of dopaminergic receptors in the renal, mesenteric, coronary, and cerebral circulations resulting in vasodilation of these vascular beds. Improved renal and mesenteric blood flow results, and urine output usually increases. At moderate doses (3–10 µg/kg/min), dopamine activates beta-1 receptors causing increases in heart rate, myocardial contractility, and cardiac output. At high doses (above 10–15 µg/kg/min), alpha-adrenergic activation predominates resulting in vasoconstriction of most vascular beds. In some patients, significant tachycardia may develop even at moderate doses, thus limiting the effectiveness of dopamine as a positive inotropic agent. Although useful, dopamine is not a strong inotropic agent, probably because it acts indirectly through release of endogenous catecholamines, which may be depleted in the postoperative heart [19]. For the treatment of serious low cardiac output, dopamine is frequently used at low doses for the renal effects with another more potent direct-acting adrenergic agent such as norepinephrine [20].

Dobutamine is a popular, effective short-acting agent for treatment of postoperative low cardiac output syndrome. A synthetic sympathomimetic amine, dobutamine acts through stimulation of beta-1 receptors with no alpha-receptor effects at any dose (unlike dopamine). It has moderate positive inotropic effects and causes a decrease in peripheral vascular and pulmonary vascular resistances. This combination of increased contractility and decreased afterload can be very useful in many patients; thus, dobutamine is often a good first-choice drug for the treatment of mild-to-moderate low output in adults. Dobutamine is preferable to moderate- or high-dose dopamine because it appears to produce a greater increase in cardiac output with less increase in myocardial oxygen consumption, and it may provide greater augmentation of myocardial blood flow [21–25]. Frequently, however, the usefulness of dobutamine is limited by the concomitant tachycardia produced. It is administered in a starting dose of 3 to 5 µg/kg/min, which may be increased to achieve the desired hemodynamic effect (usually up to no more than 12–15 µg/kg/min) or until the heart rate exceeds 100 beats per minute.

Epinephrine (Adrenalin) is the naturally occurring catecholamine released from the adrenal medulla. At low doses (less than 0.02 µg/kg/min), epinephrine activates beta-1 receptors in the heart and beta-2 receptors in skeletal muscle blood vessels causing vasodilation. Cardiac index and heart rate increase while systemic resistance often falls. At low doses, blood may be shunted away from the kidneys and mesentery. At higher doses, the beta-2 effect is lost, and beta-1- and alpha-receptor stimulation predominate. This results in increased myocardial contractility, cardiac index, myocardial oxygen consumption, heart-rate, pulmonary artery pressure, and systemic blood pressure, but at the expense of significant increases in vascular resistance that may seriously compromise kidney and other vital organ perfusion. Vasoconstriction, tachycardia, and arrhythmias limit the usefulness of epinephrine at high doses. Despite these limitations, epinephrine is a popular agent for the treatment of moderate-to-severe low output syndrome, and, for some, it is the inotrope of choice because of its reliable potency, especially in children [19]. Combined with a vasodilator (such as nitroglycerin), the vasoconstriction may be lessened with improvement in the overall hemodynamic state [26]. It also may be useful in very low doses (0.25-0.50 µg/min in adults) for treating bronchospasm.

Norepinephrine, an endogenous neurotransmitter, acts primarily to stimulate beta-1 and alpha receptors with a lesser effect on beta-2 receptors. This results in increased myocardial contractility and constriction of the systemic and pulmonary vascular beds. The effects on the perfusion of different organ systems are variable and depend largely on the relative concentration of alpha receptors. Because the coronary vascular bed has relatively few alpha receptors, norepinephrine results in increased coronary blood flow due to the unopposed effect on coronary beta-2 vasodilator receptors. Additionally, the increase in the myocardial contractile state causes increased myocardial oxygen consumption with a reflex increase in myocardial perfusion. Due to the alpha stimulation of the systemic vascular bed, systemic blood pressure increases dramatically, frequently resulting in a reflex slowing of the heart rate also. Blood flow is redistributed so as to increase heart and brain perfusion, while blood flow to skeletal muscle, skin, and splanchnic beds decreases. Norepinephrine is less arrhythmogenic than epinephrine.

These qualities make norepinephrine a particularly useful drug for treating severe low cardiac output states, especially when associated with hypotension. A starting dose of 0.05 µg/kg/min is increased as needed to raise the blood pressure and cardiac index. High doses (above 0.5 µg/kg/min) or prolonged use may result in ischemia of vital organs (liver and kidneys) or digits because of the alpha-stimulation effect. To overcome this and to maintain organ flow, norepinephrine is sometimes used in conjunction with the vasodilator phentolamine, an alpha-blocking agent. Experimental studies and clinical experience have found this combination to be of value [27,28]. Similarly, the addition of nitroglycerin or nitroprusside to norepinephrine infusion seems logical, although the physiologic effects are not well documented. The combination of norepinephrine and low-dose dopamine appears to have beneficial effects on renal blood flow [20].

Isoproterenol acts predominantly to stimulate beta-1 receptors in the heart and beta-2 receptors in the peripheral vasculature, resulting in increases in heart rate, contractility, cardiac output, and myocardial oxygen consumption with a decrease in peripheral vascular resistance. The result is an increase in the cardiac index, largely due to the increased heart rate, with little change in blood pressure [29]. In general, isoproterenol is not recommended for the treatment of postoperative myocardial dysfunction, especially in patients with ischemic heart disease, because it causes a significant increase in myocardial oxygen consumption and is very arrhythmogenic [17]. One benefit of isoproterenol is that it lowers pulmonary vascular resistance, an especially helpful action when reactive pulmonary hypertension and right heart dysfunction are present. This is particularly useful in children with pulmonary hypertension in whom isoproterenol can be infused constantly into a central vein at 0.01 to 0.05 µg/kg/min if the heart rate is not excessive. It is also used in cardiac transplant recipient patients who tend to have a slow heart rate and diminished contractility for 2 to 3 days, and in other situations where elevated pulmonary vascular resistance and right heart failure can be an issue.

Amrinone is an effective inotropic agent and vasodilator that does not act by stimulation of adrenergic receptors. This bipyridine agent inhibits intracellular phosphodiesterase activity, resulting in increased cyclic adenosine monophosphate and calcium entry into the cells. This causes a positive inotropic response in the myocardium and relaxation in vascular smooth muscle. There is little chronotropic effect. The net result is increased myocardial contractility and cardiac output, with decreased peripheral vascular resistance. Myocardial oxygen consumption does not increase [30]. It has been observed that this drug acts much like the combination of dobutamine (direct inotrope with little vascular effect) and nitroprusside (peripheral vascular dilator) [31]. This favorable set of hemodynamic alterations increases cardiac output at lower filling pressures [32]. Amrinone also appears to lower pulmonary vascular resistance in patients with pulmonary hypertension; therefore, it may have a unique value in the treatment of right ventricular failure [33,34]. Amrinone is administered intravenously first as a loading dose (0.75 mg/kg) over 2 to 3 minutes followed by constant infusion (5–10 µg/kg/min). Some authorities recommend the administration of a second loading dose (0.75 mg/kg) 30 minutes after the first, while others recommend doubling the initial loading dose. Side effects of amrinone include thrombocytopenia, elevation of hepatic enzyme levels, and arrhythmias. Thrombocytopenia may become a particular problem for patients who are receiving amrinone while also being supported by an intraaortic balloon pump. Although not usually employed as a first-line drug for the treatment of postoperative low cardiac output because of its relatively weak inotropic effects, amrinone is a valuable addition to the more frequently used and more potent catecholamine agents for the treatment of severely compromised patients [35–37]. It is especially useful in those infants and children with increased pulmonary vascular resistance. Other phosphodiesterase inhibitors that may be given orally (enoximone and milrinone) have also shown utility in the management of impaired cardiac function in the postoperative patient, but they are not available for routine use in the United States [38,39].

Calcium chloride administered by slow intravenous bolus (10 mg/kg) will raise the patient's blood pressure associated with increases in peripheral vascular resistance and myocardial contractility. This effect, however, is transient, and sustained improvement in the hemodynamic state is not achieved [19]. Continuous infusion does not result in sustained improvement in the cardiac index and risks dangerous hypercalcemia. There are several potential adverse effects of bolus calcium administration: ventricular irritability, coronary vasospasm, bradycardia, sinus arrest, exacerbation of myocardial reperfusion injury, and possibly pancreatitis [40]. Furthermore, in experimental animal studies, pretreatment with calcium blocks the ability of administered epinephrine to raise cardiac output and blood pressure [41]. We recommend calcium administration only for documented hypocalcemia or hyperkalemia or in the treatment of calcium channel blocker overdose [42]. Frequently, the ionized calcium concentration will be depressed as a result of cardiopulmonary bypass. Calcium is often administered after reperfusion of the heart and before termination of bypass; in this situation calcium administration is often guided by measurement of the ionized calcium concentration. Other than in this situation, we do not routinely use calcium in the treatment of postoperative low cardiac output in adults. We have found calcium to be more effective in children and, accordingly, we use it more often in the younger patient.

Digitalis preparations are frequently first-line drugs for the treatment of *chronic* congestive heart failure, but they have little or no role in the management of acute postoperative low cardiac output (with the exception of the treatment of atrial arrhythmias). *Digoxin* has a relatively slow onset of action. It has a narrow margin between therapeutic and toxic levels. Toxicity occurs at lower serum levels in the presence of hypokalemia, hypomagnesemia, or hypoxia — all conditions that may arise during the early postoperative period [43]. Digoxin has vasoconstrictor effects on the splanchnic circulation and causes constriction of normal and atherosclerotic human coronary arteries [44]. Also, digoxin has multiple, potentially hazardous interactions with a number of drugs commonly used in the perioperative period (including amiodarone, verapamil, quinidine, calcium chloride, diuretics, ibuprofen, and succinylcholine chloride) [45]. For these reasons, the use of digoxin as a first-line agent to treat acute low cardiac output is not recommended in adults. We are more likely to administer digoxin early in treating low output states in infants.

Other inotropic agents have been described for use in cardiac surgical patients with postoperative low cardiac output, although their use is not widespread. Triiodothyronine, administered postoperatively to patients with impaired left ventricular function, is reported to increase cardiac output while decreasing peripheral and pulmonary vascular resistances and reducing the need for other inotropic agents [46]. The combination of glucose (50% dextrose), insulin (80 units/liter), and potassium (100 mEq/liter) infused intravenously at 1.0 ml/kg/hr has been reported to improve cardiac output, decrease the need for other inotropic drugs, decrease the need for intraaortic balloon pump support, and perhaps improve survival in postoperative adult patients with cardiogenic shock [47]. Additionally, the glucose-insulin-potassium ("GIK") infusion has been shown to have myocardium-sparing effects on patients suffering acute myocardial infarction. Despite these potential benefits, these agents are used infrequently, and, by far, most clinical experience involves the use of the adrenergic agents for the treatment of postoperative low cardiac output.

VASOACTIVE DRUGS IN THE MANAGEMENT OF LOW CARDIAC OUTPUT

Drugs that act to alter the degree of systemic vascular resistance and, thus, the patient's blood pressure, are used frequently in the treatment of low cardiac output. Vasodilating agents are most often employed. By decreasing peripheral vascular constriction, these drugs decrease the resistance against which the left ventricle ejects (the afterload), thus increasing the cardiac output. If the ventricular preload is adequate, little or no reduction in systemic arterial pressure should result. However, if the blood volume is low, hypotension may occur. This potential complication of vasodilator therapy is, of course, reversible by blood volume expansion. It is important to remember that blood volume may be low even when central venous or left atrial pressure is normal in the vasoconstricted patient. Afterload reduction results in a decrease in the pulmonary capillary wedge pressure, reflecting a decrease in ventricular filling pressure and myocardial wall tension. Afterload-reducing drugs should be used only when ventricular preload is adequate, generally with the pulmonary capillary wedge (or left atrial) pressure being 10 to 15 mm Hg. Because of the risk of hypotension, continuous blood pressure monitoring is employed when using vasodilators.

The agents most commonly used for afterload reduction in the setting of acute low cardiac output are *nitroglycerin* and *nitroprusside*. Both are administered by continuous intravenous infusion and have very short half-lives. Nitroprusside acts to cause relaxation of both capacitance and resistance vessels. Nitroglycerin has a dose-related response, with relaxation of venous capacitance vessels occurring at low doses and relaxation of the resistance arteries and arterioles occurring at high doses. Nitroprusside is relatively more effective than nitroglycerin in increasing cardiac output because it is a more potent arterial vasodilator. On the other hand, nitroglycerin is generally preferable to nitroprusside in the setting of acute myocardial ischemia because it increases coronary artery flow and has possible favorable effects on internal mammary artery bypass graft flow rates [48]. Nitroprusside is administered as a continuous infusion of 0.5 to 8.0 µg/kg/min. Long-term (>48–74 hour) use of nitroprusside may result in cyanide toxicity and should be avoided, particularly in patients with impaired renal function [49]; thiocyanate levels can be monitored if prolonged use is required. Nitroglycerin is begun at 0.1 µg/kg/min and increased by 0.1 to 0.2 µg/kg/min until the desired effect is reached (which may be up to 200–300 µg/min in an average-sized adult) or until hypotension occurs.

Phentolamine is a vasodilating agent that acts by alpha-adrenergic blockade. Used alone infrequently, it is sometimes employed concurrently with a strong inotropic and vasoconstricting drug such as norepinephrine. The usual dose is 0.5 to 1.0 µg/kg/min by continuous intravenous infusion.

Prostaglandin E_1 (PEG_1) is a very potent vasodilator used infrequently in adults. It is used mainly as a direct infusion into the pulmonary artery in transplant or mitral valve patients with elevated pulmonary vascular resistance, as part of the treatment for right heart failure [50], and in infants with pulmonary hypertension. The usual starting dose is 0.01 µg/kg/min and this may be increased up to 0.10 µg/kg/min to achieve the desired effect. It is used infrequently in adults to lower systemic vascular resistance.

Frequently, the use of vasodilators alone in the treatment of low cardiac output is limited by hypotension; most often these drugs are used with an inotropic agent to augment cardiac output and thus maintain the systemic arterial pressure. Various combinations of inotrope plus vasodilator are used with clinical success, including epinephrine plus nitroglycerin, dopamine plus nitroprusside, norepinephrine plus nitroglycerin, and norepinephrine plus phentolamine [51–53].

Drugs that cause peripheral vasoconstriction are occasionally useful in the management of patients early after cardiac surgery. These drugs are usually used when the arterial pressure is low, the systemic vascular resistance is low, and the cardiac output is relatively normal or high. Agents with alpha-adrenergic agonist properties increase peripheral vascular resistance and arterial pressure. Although the arterial pressure may rise, the cardiac output may fall, which results in decreased organ perfusion. Thus, the use of such agents as *phenylephrine* (which has only alpha-stimulation properties) is limited to those instances where the peripheral vascular resistance is abnormally low. These instances are very infrequent in the setting of low cardiac output. More often, phenylephrine is useful in "high output" hypotensive states where the arterial pressure is low but cardiac output is above normal. This state is encountered occasionally immediately after weaning the patient from cardiopulmonary bypass in the operating room, in the setting of septic shock, or as a result of a drug reaction. Phenylephrine is administered as a bolus (for adults, 0.1–0.5 mg IV push) or, more commonly, as a constant infusion (1–5 µg/kg/min). *Norepinephrine*, besides its beta-adrenergic stimulating effects, also has potent alpha-stimulating properties and causes increased arterial pressure. This combination of alpha-vasoconstriction and beta-inotropic stimulation is useful in patients with low cardiac output but a normal or low state of peripheral vascular resistance. Vasoconstrictors should be avoided in the patient who is "clamped down" in a state of high vascular resistance associated with low cardiac output. Further elevation of the afterload may result in increased blood pressure but also increased work for the heart and decreased vital organ perfusion.

Overall, drug therapy for low cardiac output requires assessment of the hemodynamic situation based on physical examination and invasive measurements. Some patients with postoperative mild-to-moderate low cardiac output have a depressed cardiac index and normal peripheral vascular resistance. Many of these are successfully treated with moderate-dose dopamine or dobutamine or a low-dose epinephrine infusion. More severe states of low output may require higher-dose epinephrine or norepinephrine with the addition of a vasodilator. For patients with coronary artery disease, nitroglycerin is preferred to nitroprusside as the initial agent for afterload reduction. The treatment of the very severe low output state may require the simultaneous use of several inotropic drugs including both a catecholamine agent (e.g., epinephrine) and a phosphodiesterase inhibitor (e.g., amrinone) in addition to low-dose dopamine to augment renal blood flow, and possibly a vasodilator such as nitroprusside.

Remember that all patients do not react uniformly to the same inotropic agents and that the patient's hemodynamic status may change over the course of hours. Thus, flexibility, often with some experimentation, is necessary to determine the most suitable agent or combination of agents for a given patient. The recovering patient is weaned from the drugs one by one with careful monitoring of hemodynamic parameters.

INSTITUTION OF MECHANICAL SUPPORT FOR LOW CARDIAC OUTPUT

The most commonly used form of mechanical support for the failing heart after cardiac surgery is intraaortic balloon counterpulsation (somewhat erroneously called a "balloon pump"). The intraaortic balloon pump provides afterload reduction (decreased impedance to ventricular emptying in early systole) with a resultant increase in cardiac output. Elevation of the aortic diastolic pressure with inflation of the balloon results in increased coronary artery perfusion pressure. In contrast to the effects of most inotropic drugs, myocardial oxygen consumption is not increased and, in fact, may be decreased. Intraaortic balloon pump support is also very useful for patients with mitral valve regurgitation because it may decrease mitral annular size and lessen the severity of regurgitation by favoring the forward ejection of left ventricular blood into a lowered resistance circuit. Patients with left-to-right shunting through postinfarction ventricular septal defects benefit from a reduction in the magnitude of the shunt in addition to augmentation of coronary blood flow. Thus, the intraaortic balloon pump is frequently used in adult cardiac surgery patients suffering from low cardiac output. Although such support is usually for one to a few days to allow for recovery of the myocardium, support for long periods (even weeks) is possible, although rarely indicated.

In general, an intraaortic balloon pump is inserted when the patient's cardiac index is less than 1.8 to 2.0 liter/min/m^2 despite moderate doses of inotropic drugs (such as dobutamine at 10 mg/kg/min) in the absence of hypovolemia or reversible conditions such as tamponade. It may also be indicated in ischemic states in poorly revascularized patients. The most frequent complications involve injury to the femoral artery, iliac artery, or aorta; these occur in up to 10% of patients who require such support [54].

For selected patients, other forms of mechanical assist are used to support the circulation while awaiting recovery of the native heart or procurement of a suitable donor heart for transplantation. Ventricular assist devices have been most successful when employed as a "bridge" to emergency transplantation. These forms of mechanical assist include the nonpulsatile centrifugal pump (Biomedicus) and external pulsatile devices such as the Abiomed BVS 5000 and Thoratec (not currently approved for noninvestigational use) ventricular assist device systems [55]. Appropriate patient selection is very important for the successful use of these devices, and the decision to employ such support must be made early, before irreversible end-organ damage develops. Commonly accepted hemodynamic parameters indicating the need for ventricular assist device implantation are: (1) cardiac index less than 1.8 liter/min/m^2 despite use of inotropic drug support and the intraaortic balloon pump, (2) systolic aortic pressure less than 90 mm Hg, and (3) left atrial pressure greater than 20 to 25 mm Hg [56]. Contraindications include the presence of ongoing infection, severe bleeding diathesis, pulmonary hemorrhage, and significant renal insufficiency. For those who might be candidates for transplantation, standard transplant criteria and contraindications apply. We would not recommend the use of such devices unless ventricular dysfunction is acute and potentially reversible or the patient is a cardiac transplant candidate.

LOW CARDIAC OUTPUT DUE TO RIGHT VENTRICULAR FAILURE

Not all instances of postoperative low cardiac output are secondary to failure of the left ventricle. Inadequate output from the right ventricle results in inadequate filling of the left ventricle, decreased left ventricular cardiac output, and poor systemic perfusion. Patients with preexisting pulmonary hypertension (such as those with long-standing mitral valve disease, some transplant patients, or those with chronic left-to-right shunts) or right ventricular hypertrophy are at particular risk for right ventricular failure. Inadequate protection of the right ventricle during aortic cross-clamping may also result in postoperative right ventricular dysfunction [57]. Other causes of right ventricular injury include the performance of a right ventriculotomy necessary for cardiac repair (as in the correction of tetralogy of Fallot), right ventricular infarction, inadequate maintenance of right ventricular hypothermia due to the warming effects of overhead lights, poor delivery of cardioplegia if right coronary artery obstruction is present, and air embolism into the right coronary artery during the early period of left ventricular ejection. Since the right coronary ostium is anterior on the aorta, any air present in the ascending aorta will tend to rise to that location in the supine patient. Elevation of pulmonary artery pressure produces increased afterload to ejection of the right ventricle with a detrimental effect on the right ventricular output.

The diagnosis of right ventricular failure is based on the demonstration of a low cardiac output with elevated right-sided filling pressures (central venous or right atrial) and relatively normal or decreased left-sided filling pressures (pulmonary capillary wedge or left atrial). If the potential for right ventricular failure is suspected at the time of surgery, direct continuous measurement of left atrial pressure is very useful. An *increase* in right atrial pressure with a *decrease* in left atrial pressure is a particularly ominous sign. Echocardiography can be confirmatory by demonstrating poor right ventricular contractility in the presence of relatively normal left ventricular wall motion. The basis of treatment of right ventricular failure is volume loading and inotropic support without increasing pulmonary vascular resistance and the maintenance of coronary perfusion pressure [37]. In the absence of severe pulmonary hypertension, right ventricular output is very dependent on its preload [58]. It may, therefore, be necessary to increase the right heart output. The goal of inotropic drug support is to improve right ventricular contractility and right ventricular myocardial perfusion without increasing pulmonary vascular resistance. Isoproterenol infusion results in improved contractility and a decrease in pulmonary vascular resistance. The usefulness of this agent is frequently limited, however, by the tachycardia and systemic vasodilation it causes. Dobutamine is often useful as it frequently does not cause elevation of the pulmonary artery pressure, and, if the systemic blood pressure is adequate, nitroprusside may be added to decrease the pulmonary vascular resistance. Amrinone, by providing inotropic support to the myocardium while simultaneously decreasing pulmonary vascular resistance, is particularly useful for postoperative right ventricular failure.

PGE_1 also lowers pulmonary vascular resistance and is efficacious for the treatment of severe right heart failure after mitral valve replacement and cardiac transplantation [50]. Infusion is begun at 0.01 µg/kg/min and increased to 0.10 µg/kg/min. Although PGE_1 is a potent pulmonary vasodilator, frequently enough will reach the systemic circulation to cause hypotension that can adversely affect right ventricular function by impairing its coronary perfusion [59] It is often necessary to maintain systemic pressure and vascular resistance by concomitant infusion of norepinephrine via a left atrial catheter. Since air embolism is a potential risk of left-sided infusion, care must be taken with this method of drug administration [60]. In patients with severely compromised right ventricular function, this process is facilitated by the use of a second left atrial catheter dedicated to norepinephrine infusion. Finally, even though left ventricular function may be normal, the use of intraaortic balloon counterpulsation may prove helpful, probably due to its beneficial effects on septal wall motion and left ventricular filling pressure.

When adequately treated, the low cardiac output due to right ventricular failure will frequently be temporary and abate over a period of a few days. Pharmacologic support of the right ventricle should not be removed too rapidly; it will often be required during the patient's emergence from anesthesia and weaning from the ventilator.

Cardiac Arrest

Cardiac arrest may occur in the postoperative patient unexpectedly (as in sudden development of ventricular fibrillation) or as the terminal event after a progressive downhill course (such as refractory low cardiac output syndrome). Patients who suffer unexpected cardiac arrest have the best chance of successful resuscitation, but the complication must be managed quickly and appropriately. Thus, the ECG and blood pressure are monitored constantly in all patients early after surgery (when the risk of cardiac arrest is the greatest) with alarm systems in place to alert the nursing staff if dangerous abnormalities occur. These alarms are lifesaving and must not be silenced. If false alarms are occurring due to a poor-quality ECG signal, then the skin electrodes should be changed and the connections should be checked. Solving the problem by silencing the alarm system can lead to failure to recognize the development of a potentially reversible, but otherwise fatal, arrhythmia.

Despite the many possible underlying causes of cardiac arrest in the postoperative patient (including arrhythmia, ischemia, pulmonary embolism, abrupt mechanical obstruction of a prosthetic valve, and tamponade), the initial management is the same and follows the basic protocol outlined by the Advanced Cardiac Life-Support (ACLS) guidelines [61].

In postoperative patients, ventricular fibrillation is the most common arrhythmia at the time of cardiac arrest. Prompt defibrillation is imperative; delays in defibrillation decrease the chance of successful resuscitation. Even if the patient is not being monitored, a witnessed cardiac arrest can be treated initially with an attempt at "blind" defibrillation, as it is likely that ventricular fibrillation is the underlying rhythm. The need for "blind" defibrillation has, however, been reduced by the increasing use of defibrillation devices that allow for "through-the-paddle" monitoring. The recommended initial defibrillation energy dose is 200 joules. It is important to place the paddles across the patient's chest in a position that will optimize the amount of energy delivered to the heart (i.e., so that the paddles face each other as well as possible with the center of the mass of the heart between them). An unsuccessful defibrillation attempt should be followed immediately by a second shock of 200–300 joules and, if this is unsuccessful, then immediately by a 360-joule shock. Delays in shock delivery, even for administering drugs, decrease patient survival [62].

If defibrillation is not immediately successful, or if more than 1 or 2 minutes have elapsed, closed CPR should begin. A bedboard should be placed beneath the patient to improve the effectiveness of closed chest cardiac massage. An adequate endotracheal airway is established, ventilation with 100% oxygen is begun, and closed chest massage performed. Moderate hyperventilation is best; frequent determinations of the arterial blood gases should be performed if an arterial catheter is present. ECG monitoring is established if not already in progress. Secure intravenous access is essential, preferably through a central or femoral venous route.

Experimental evidence shows that standard closed chest cardiac massage restores perfusion to less than 25% of normal [63]. Although a normal systolic blood pressure (70–90 mm Hg) may be generated, the mean perfusion pressure is frequently far below normal during CPR. Adequacy of massage may be determined by observing the arterial blood pressure monitor (if an arterial catheter is in place), palpating the peripheral pulses, and examining the patient's pupils, which, if previously dilated, will frequently decrease to normal size.

For some postoperative patients, adequate perfusion pressure cannot be generated by closed chest massage because of instability of the sternum. In others, the presence of a compressing blood clot within the mediastinum may prevent effective CPR. Also, the presence of a prosthetic valve may make closed massage more hazardous because the myocardium can be perforated when compressed against the rigid prosthesis. In these instances, the chest incision should be reopened for open cardiac massage using the sterile thoracotomy instruments readily available in all properly equipped cardiac surgical intensive care units. Open chest (or "internal") cardiac massage is often more effective than closed chest massage, especially if tamponade is relieved on opening the chest. Great care must be taken in reopening the sternotomy incision, particularly if the patient has coronary bypass grafts.

Open massage is performed by placing one hand behind the heart and one hand on the anterior surface of the right atrium and ventricle. The hands should be kept flat while pressing them together at a rate of about 80 to 90 times per minute for adults. Compression begins at the apex and is advanced toward the ventricular outflow tracts. The heart should not be kneaded or squeezed by the fingers as this may cause perforation of the myocardium. Open cardiac massage allows for direct visualization of the heart, safer compressions in the presence of a prosthetic valve, less trauma to mediastinal structures, inspection for causative factors (such as an occluded bypass graft), direct application of pacing wires or internal defibrillation paddles, and direct injection of drugs into the heart. Fear of infection should not prevent the surgeon from reopening the patient's chest for open resuscitation, as the infection rate among those who survive is low (about 5%) [64].

Changes have been made in the American Heart Association recommendations for drug administration during cardiac arrest, but *epinephrine remains the agent of choice for cardiac arrest of almost any cause* [65]. The combined alpha- and beta-adrenergic agonist properties of epinephrine result in increased systemic vascular resistance which directs more of the cardiac output to the brain and heart; also, the drug increases myocardial contractility and heart rate. Epinephrine may facilitate defibrillation of the heart by converting "fine" fibrillation to "coarse" fibrillation. The adult dose is a 1.0-mg intravenous bolus, and this may be repeated every 3 to 5 minutes as needed. Some authorities suggest that even larger doses of epinephrine should be used when treating cardiac arrest [66]. In the event that an intravenous catheter is not present, 1.0 to 2.0 mg of epinephrine can be mixed with 10 ml of normal saline (for adults) and injected down the patient's endotracheal tube [67]. The pediatric dose of intravenous epinephrine for cardiac arrest is 0.1 µg/kg. Sodium bicarbonate is no longer recommended for routine administration in the early treatment of the patient who suffers cardiac arrest and who did not have prearrest metabolic acidosis [62]. Adverse effects of bicarbonate administration in this setting include paradoxical intracellular acidosis, impairment of oxygen delivery by increasing hemoglobin's affinity for oxygen, hyperosmolality with possible detrimental neurologic effects, and alkalemia-induced reduction of cerebral blood flow. The acidosis of mixed venous blood that accompanies cardiac arrest is essentially entirely respiratory in etiology, although this may not be accurately reflected by the arterial blood gases. Administration of sodium bicarbonate in this setting probably increases the carbon dioxide tension of the mixed venous blood and the PCO_2 of the tissues, thus worsening the state of tissue acidosis [68]. Actually, it takes 20 to 30 minutes before metabolic acidosis develops during cardiac arrest unless the patient had acidosis before the arrest [66]. When a preexisting metabolic acidosis (such as from prolonged low cardiac output prior to the cardiac arrest) is present, then conservative bicarbonate administration is recommended as discussed in Chapter 3. Prompt and frequent arterial blood gas determinations will provide guidance for the administration of bicarbonate.

The indications for calcium administration during cardiac arrest have also undergone modification. We do not routinely use calcium in this setting except for the treatment of severe hypocalcemia, hyperkalemia, or calcium channel-blocking drug toxicity [62]. Adverse effects of routine calcium used during cardiac arrest include ventricular irritability, coronary vasospasm, bradycardia or sinus arrest, and possible exacerbation of myocardial ischemic injury [42].

After successful resuscitation from cardiac arrest, an arterial cannula should be introduced and the patient should be monitored in the intensive care unit. If the cause of the arrest is thought to be ischemia, and the ischemia is continuing, then further stabilization can be achieved by the addition of intraaortic balloon pump support. A nasogastric tube is often placed, and a pulmonary artery catheter for measurement of cardiac output may be indicated. Serial ECGs and measurements of cardiac enzymes to rule out a myocardial infarction should be ordered. Coronary arteriography should be considered if an occluded coronary bypass graft is suspected. Patients are then managed as indicated by their hemodynamic condition.

ELECTROMECHANICAL DISSOCIATION

Electromechanical dissociation (EMD), also known as "pulseless electrical activity" (PEA) is a usually fatal cause of cardiac arrest characterized by lack of ejection of blood from the heart despite relatively normal ECG complexes [69]. The underlying pathophysiology of EMD is not well understood. Treatment is administration of epinephrine; calcium is not recommended unless hypocalcemia, hyperkalemia, or calcium channel-blocking drug toxicity is present

[70]. Although primary EMD is difficult to treat successfully, secondary EMD (where loading conditions of the heart are such that there is little or no cardiac output in the presence of adequate ventricular complexes) may be reversible. Reversible causes of EMD include severe hypovolemia, severe hypoxia, hypothermia, massive pulmonary embolism, tamponade, tension pneumothorax, and prosthetic valve dysfunction resulting in obstruction to inflow or outflow of the heart. When one is confronted with a patient with EMD, these possibly reversible causes must be kept in mind. For example, we have encountered patients with acute EMD whose mitral valve prostheses become jammed open by a left atrial catheter that had migrated through the valve orifice.

Postoperative Cardiac Arrhythmias

Abnormalities of the heart rhythm occur in more than one-third of patients after open heart surgery and, thus, the management of these arrhythmias is an almost daily part of the care of the cardiac surgery patients. Although sometimes only a benign event, postoperative arrhythmias may be life-threatening and may contribute significantly to both short- and long-term morbidity. The high frequency of postoperative arrhythmias and the potential for serious adverse sequelae make it important to identify quickly and treat appropriately. Most of the common arrhythmias are successfully managed by routine measures (Table 4-2). Table 4-3 summarizes the parenterally administered drugs useful in treating postoperative arrhythmias.

POSTOPERATIVE BRADYARRHYTHMIA

A slow heart rate may lead to a significant decrease in the cardiac output. The most effective combination of rate and ventricular filling time for adults is approximately 100 to 110 beats per minute. The cardiac output of infants is particularly rate-dependent, and bradycardia (less than 80 beats per minute) should be treated even if the arterial pressure is normal. Sinus bradycardia (heart rate less than 70 beats per minute) is not unusual in adult patients who are receiving beta-adrenergic antagonists in the perioperative period. Other drugs that can cause bradycardia include verapamil, diltiazem, and amiodarone. It is standard practice to attach temporary atrial and ventricular pacing wires to the heart at the time of operation; thus, the treatment of sinus bradycardia is simply the institution of pacing. Pacing the atrium alone usually suffices (since conduction through the atrioventricular nodes is usually preserved), and atrial pacing is more physiologic than sequential atrioventricular pacing.

If the pacing wires fail to capture and do not provide satisfactory atrial or ventricular pacing, symptomatic bradycardia can be treated emergently with atropine (adult dose, 0.5–1.0 mg IV, may repeat every 3–5 minutes to a total dose of 3.0 mg; pediatric dose, 0.02 mg/kg, may repeat every 5 minutes to a total dose of 1.0 mg in a child, 2.0 mg in an adolescent). Longer-term treatment includes continuous intravenous infusion of isoproterenol (adult dose, 1–2 µg/min; pediatric dose, 0.01-0.10 µg/kg/min), dopamine infusion (5–

Table 4-2. Management strategies for postoperative arrhythmias

Arrhythmia	Treatment

Premature ventricular contractions	1. Observe if infrequent or chronic
	2. Check blood gases and potassium
	3. If new, or frequent, consider:
	   a. Overdrive pacing
	   b. Lidocaine
	   c. Magnesium
	   d. Beta-adrenergic blocking agent
	   e. Procainamide (caution: may have proarrhythmic effect)

Sinus bradycardia, some nodal bradycardias	1. Atrial pacing 2. Atropine 3. Isoproterenol
Ventricular tachycardia	1. Lidocaine 2. Countershock if sustained and unstable 3. Bretylium 4. Magnesium 5. Procainamide
Complete heart block, slow nodal rhythm	1. Sequential atrioventricular pacing 2. Ventricular pacing 3. Isoproterenol
Nodal rhythm	1. Pacing (atrial if possible) 2. Not treated if rate is reasonable and blood pressure satisfactory
Atrial fibrillation	Not always treated if ventricular rate is reasonable and cardiac index remains satisfactory. If rate is fast: 1. Verapamil (may cause hypotension), or, 2. Diltiazem 3. Digoxin (slow onset of therapeutic effect) 4. Cardioversion if unstable 5. Beta blocker 6. Procainamide (to convert to sinus rhythm)
Atrial flutter	1. Rapid atrial pacing. If ineffective 2. Adenosine 3. Diltiazem or verapamil 4. Digoxin 5. Procainamide 6. Beta blocker 7. Cardioversion
Atrial premature beats	1. Not usually treated 2. Beta blocker
Paroxysmal supraventricular tachycardia	1. Verapamil or diltiazem 2. Adenosine 3. Beta blocker 4. Digoxin (rule out digoxin toxicity first) 5. Atrial pacing
Sinus tachycardia	1. Treat underlying cause 2. Beta blocker

Table 4-3. Parenteral drugs used to treat postoperative arrhythmias

Drug	Adult dose		Indications	Side effects
Adenosine	*IV bolus:*	6 mg; may repeat with 12 mg if indicated	Paroxysmal supraventricular tachycardia	Bronchoconstriction, flushing, atrioventricular block
Bretylium	*IV load:*	5–10 mg/kg over 15 min for ventricular tachycardia 5–10 mg/kg IV push for ventricular fibrillation	Ventricular tachycardia/fibrillation	Hypotension, nausea
	IV infusion:	1–2 mg/min		
Digoxin	*IV load:*	1.0 mg in divided doses over 4–8 hr	Atrial fibrillation/flutter (slows ventricular response)	Arrhythmias, anorexia, nausea, vomiting, diarrhea, confusion, colored vision, depression
	Oral load:	2.0 mg in divided doses over 48 hr		
	Maintenance:	0.125–0.250 mg q day		
Diltiazem	*IV bolus:*	0.25 mg/kg over 2 min may repeat in 15 min	Atrial fibrillation/flutter	Hypotension, atrioventricular block, decreased cardiac output
	IV infusion:	5–15 mg/hr		
Esmolol	*IV bolus:*	500 µg/kg over 1 min (may omit bolus dose)	Tachycardia, atrial fibrillation/flutter	Hypotension, bronchospasm, decreased cardiac output (transient due to short half-life)
	IV infusion:	50–200 µg/kg/min		
Lidocaine	*IV bolus:*	1.0–1.5 mg/kg; repeat with 0.5–1.5 mg/kg in 5–10 min	Ventricular tachycardia, ventricular fibrillation, symptomatic premature ventricular contractions	Confusion, coma, seizures
	IV infusion:	1–4 mg/min		

Table 4-3 (continued)

Drug	Adult dose		Indications	Side effects
Phenytoin (Dilantin)	IV load:	10 mg/kg over 1 hr	Digoxin toxicity, ventricular arrhythmias in children	Dysarthria, pulmonary infiltrates, lupus, gingivitis, macrocytic anemia
	Oral:	300–600 mg/day, 2–4 mg/kg/day in children		
Procainamide	IV load:	500–1000 mg (up to 17 mg/kg) at 20–30 mg/min	Ventricular tachycardia, ventricular fibrillation, symptomatic premature ventricular contractions, atrial fibrillation/flutter	Hypotension, drug fever, lupus-like syndrome
	IV infusion:	1–4 mg/min		
Propranolol	IV:	0.5–1.0 mg q5min up to 2–5 mg	Atrial fibrillation/flutter, ventricular irritability, sinus tachycardia	Hypotension, decreased cardiac output, bronchospasm
Quinidine gluconate	Oral:	324–648 mg tid	Atrial fibrillation/flutter, ventricular tachycardia, ventricular fibrillation	Nausea, diarrhea, headache, dizziness, fever, thrombocytopenia
Quinidine sulfate	Oral:	200–400 mg qid	Same as quinidine gluconate	Same as above
Verapamil	IV bolus:	2.5–10.0 mg; repeat in 10–20 min	Paroxysmal supraventricular tachycardia, rate control of atrial fibrillation/flutter	Hypotension, bradycardia, nausea, decreased cardiac output, constipation, increases serum digoxin levels
	Oral:	80–120 mg tid		

10 µg/min), epinephrine infusion (2–10 µg/min), external cardiac pacing (which is often painful for the patient), and passage of a temporary transvenous pacing wire.

Various degrees of heart block may develop after surgery, most frequently after valve replacement and congenital procedures that involve manipulations near the atrioventricular conduction system. First-degree block (PR interval greater than 200 msec) is not uncommon, causes no symptoms, usually disappears spontaneously, and requires no treatment. We frequently leave a ventricular-demand pacemaker in place as a backup, should the first-degree block worsen. Second-degree block occurs when only some atrial impulses are conducted to the ventricle. If this results in a significant bradycardia, treatment is sequential atrioventricular pacing via the temporary epicardial leads.

Third-degree (complete) heart block is a serious problem since, in the postoperative patient, the ventricular escape rate may be only 30 to 40 beats per minute. It is often encountered immediately after cardiopulmonary bypass, possibly as a side effect of the cardioplegic solution. Complete heart block infrequently persists in coronary bypass surgery patients (occurring in about 4%), is usually self-limiting, and rarely occurs after the first postoperative day [71]. It is, however, much more common in patients after aortic or mitral valve replacement than in coronary bypass patients, occurring in up to 15% of the former [72]. Thus, at the time of surgery, secure placement and testing of the pacing wires are of prime importance for patients undergoing valve procedures. Institution of pacing (preferably sequential atrioventricular) is the treatment of choice. Most of these patients will regain normal atrioventricular conduction within hours to days after valve replacement, although a few (presumably due to irreversible injury to the conduction system during surgery) will require placement of a permanent pacemaker prior to discharge from the hospital. No patient with surgically induced complete heart block should be discharged from the hospital without pacemaker implantation.

Management of Temporary Cardiac Pacing Systems

Use of temporary pacing for bradyarrhythmia (sinus or heart block) can be lifesaving for the postoperative patient, and, for that reason, it is the current standard of care to attach temporary ventricular (and usually atrial) pacing electrodes to the heart at the time of operation. Optimal placement involves separation of the electrodes by 2 cm; good contact with the myocardium; and avoidance of contact with coronary arteries, bypass grafts, and mediastinal drainage tubes [73]. The pacing leads exit through the chest wall and are attached to an external pulse generator.

The generator may be one of several types that have the ability to sense native myocardial depolarization and to deliver current to the leads for pacing. Sequential generators provide for both atrial and ventricular pacing and for adjusting the length of time between the atrial and ventricular impulses. The external pulse generator allows for adjusting the amount of current delivered to the heart (in milliamperes) and the sensitivity of sensing. The demand mode of pacing causes the pacemaker to deliver current to the heart only when the sensed rate is below the rate set by the operator. The asynchronous mode provides a pacing current to the heart irrespective of the native heart rate. Most frequently, the demand mode is used with the backup rate setting at 60 beats per minute. The sensitivity of sensing is also adjustable. Failure of pacing (failure to capture) may be due to poor contact between the pacing electrode and the heart, failure to turn on the pulse generator, battery failure, setting the milliamperage too low, or poor contact between the pacing leads and the generator. Failure of the device to sense appropriately indicates a loose connection, too low a sensitivity setting, or early battery failure [74]. Also, an inadequate potential difference between the two epicardial electrodes may result in poor sensing. This problem may be diagnosed by attaching the two leads to the right and left arm leads of an ECG machine. If less than 1mV deflection is recorded in lead I, a ground lead can be inserted in the skin to provide a greater voltage difference and allow proper sensing.

Recently, we have, at times, employed a temporary, external, dual chamber demand mode (DDD) pacemaker (Pace Medical, Inc., Model 4578) for postoperative pacing. This may offer some advantages when a rapid atrial rate is present with atrioventricular block or when conduction system function and atrial rate are continuously changing.

POSTOPERATIVE TACHYARRHYTHMIAS

Approximately one-third of patients who undergo open heart procedures suffer postoperative tachyarrhythmias. Most of these are supraventricular (atrial fibrillation and flutter) and are easily recognized as such. Occasionally, however, a wide QRS tachycardia occurs, and it may be difficult to determine the exact nature of the arrhythmia.

Wide QRS Tachycardia

A wide complex tachycardia may be either supraventricular or ventricular in origin; misdiagnosis may lead to improper treatment. For example, if a tachycardia interpreted as supraventricular is actually ventricular in origin, treatment with verapamil may cause disastrous hypotension resulting in ventricular fibrillation [75]. Determining the origin of a wide QRS tachycardia is usually difficult and, in some cases, impossible without sophisticated electrophysiologic study procedures. Clues to the diagnosis of ventricular tachycardia in this setting are a history of prior myocardial infarction and the presence of atrioventricular dissociation on the ECG (although this is frequently impossible to demonstrate even in documented ventricular tachycardia). Recording the electrogram from the atrial wires, if present, may help in this diagnosis.

The safest course to follow when confronted with a patient with a wide QRS tachycardia is to *assume the wide complex tachycardia is ventricular tachycardia* and treat it as such. The first drug of choice for wide complex tachycardia of uncertain type is lidocaine (1.0-1.5 mg/kg). If lidocaine does not terminate the arrhythmia, adenosine (6 mg rapid IV infusion, followed by 12 mg in 1–2 minutes if required) is recommended. While adenosine's action is very short-lived, it will frequently terminate broad complex supraventricular tachycardia without much effect in ventricular tachycardia. Thus, if the tachycardia is supraventricular, adenosine is useful both as a diagnostic and therapeutic agent. If these measures are not successful, procainamide should be administered. This type IA antiarrhythmic agent is often effective treatment for ventricular tachycardia. Also, although not specifically approved by the Food and Drug Administration for this purpose, it is frequently used for the treatment of supraventricular arrhythmias. Procainamide may convert atrial fibrillation to sinus rhythm and slows conduction in accessory bypass tracts if such are involved in the tachycardia. Procainamide is administered to adults at a rate of 100 mg IV every 5 to 10 minutes, up to a total loading dose of 1 g. Careful monitoring of the blood pressure and ECG is performed during the loading procedure. It may then be given by continuous infusion at 2 to 4 mg/min (adult dose) with monitoring of blood levels and the ECG QT interval. Finally, refractory wide complex tachycardia may respond to bretylium (initial dose 5 mg/kg).

Supraventricular Tachycardia

Supraventricular tachycardia is very common during the first few days after open heart surgery. The most frequently encountered tachycardias are sinus tachycardia, atrial fibrillation, and atrial flutter.

Sinus Tachycardia

Sinus tachycardia may be the result of hypovolemia, anemia, fever, agitation, or inadequate pain relief. It may, however, be a compensatory response to compromised cardiac function and may indicate a serious problem such as ongoing myocardial ischemia or tamponade. Thus, when sinus tachycardia is present, evaluation should be undertaken to rule out the presence of a low cardiac output state. This would include a physical examination, measurement of arterial pH, and, if necessary, placement of a pulmonary artery catheter for thermodilution measurement of cardiac output.

During the first few hours after surgery, occasional adult patients exhibit sinus tachycardia (heart rate greater than 110 beats per minute) often associated with hypertension. This hyperdynamic state is more common in younger male adults and may be related to a greater-than-normal catecholamine response to the stress of operation. Sinus tachycardia in the intubated patient early after operation may suggest a patient who is awake and feeling pain but who cannot move because of continued muscle paralysis.

For patients with uncomplicated sinus tachycardia, the initial treatment is assurance of adequate cardiac filling pressures and adequate pain control. If correction of hypovolemia and pain does not alleviate the tachycardia (and low output is not present), treatment with a beta-blocking agent may be indicated. Esmolol is particularly well suited for this purpose because of its very short half-life and rapid reversibility on discontinuation. The initial loading dose is 500 µg/kg administered intravenously followed by continuous infusion of 50 to 200 µg/kg/min, adjusting the infusion to lower the heart rate to around 100 beats per minute. Caution must be used because hypotension or bradycardia may result, necessitating abrupt discontinuation of the drug [76]. Some patients, especially those undergoing coronary bypass surgery, may experience mild sinus tachycardia (rate 110–120 beats per minute) postoperatively for no apparent reason. Treatment with a beta-adrenergic blocking agent may be indicated to reduce myocardial oxygen demands.

Atrial Fibrillation and Flutter

The most common postoperative tachyarrhythmia is atrial fibrillation, although atrial flutter is not rare, and combinations of the two also occur. Atrial fibrillation and flutter are much less frequent in children. Risk factors for atrial fibrillation complication include: age (more than 65 years), history of atrial arrhythmia, preoperative left ventricular end-diastolic pressure greater than 20 mm Hg, and premature atrial contractions noted on the preoperative ECG [77–79]. Most commonly, atrial fibrillation or flutter or both develop on the second day after surgery. Although the cause of these arrhythmias is unknown, contributing factors probably include manipulation and cannulation of the atrium, intraoperative ischemia, and the effects of endogenous and administered catecholamines. For most patients, the ventricular response to atrial fibrillation or flutter is usually 130 to 160 beats per minute, and this rate is hemodynamically well tolerated. With the onset of tachycardia, however, the patient frequently feels warm, becomes diaphoretic, and may be anxious. Thus, it is useful to warn patients preoperatively about the possibility (and the generally benign nature) of postoperative atrial fibrillation. Patients with marginal cardiac function may suffer hemodynamic deterioration due to loss of the normal synchronized "atrial kick" that contributes about 10 to 15% to the cardiac output. Rare patients suffer extreme tachycardia (more than 200 beats per minute) with severe hypotension. Postoperative atrial fibrillation and flutter often contribute to prolongation of hospital stay and may be associated with postoperative stroke [80]. Atrial fibrillation is usually recognized by the irregular nature of the ventricular response. Analysis of the patient's arterial blood pressure monitor tracing usually aids in the diagnosis. If the ventricular response is uniform, making the diagnosis more difficult, an atrial electrogram may be obtained by recordings from the atrial pacing wires that were implanted at surgery (Fig. 4-3). This will reveal the atrial complexes that are irregular in rhythm, amplitude, and polarity. Intravenously administered adenosine can be used to cause transient slowing of the ventricular rate so that atrial activity can be analyzed. Its action is rapid but evanescent; hence it is useful mainly for diagnostic, not therapeutic, purposes.

Atrial flutter is usually characterized by a regular ventricular response with a rate of about 150 beats per minute. This represents an atrial contraction rate of about 300 per minute with 2 : 1 atrioventricular block allowing for only every other atrial complex to be conducted and to result in ventricular contraction. The degree of block may, however, be variable resulting in an irregular ventricular response. In atrial flutter, the atrial electrogram will demonstrate regular atrial complexes, usually at 230 to 350 beats per minute, with uniform amplitude and polarity. These atrial "flutter waves" are usually recognizable on the standard ECG tracing and facilitate the diagnosis of atrial flutter. Occasional patients will have faster atrial flutter rates in the range of 340 to 430 beats per minute.

Because atrial arrhythmias are so common after cardiac surgery, many investigations have been conducted to determine if prophy-

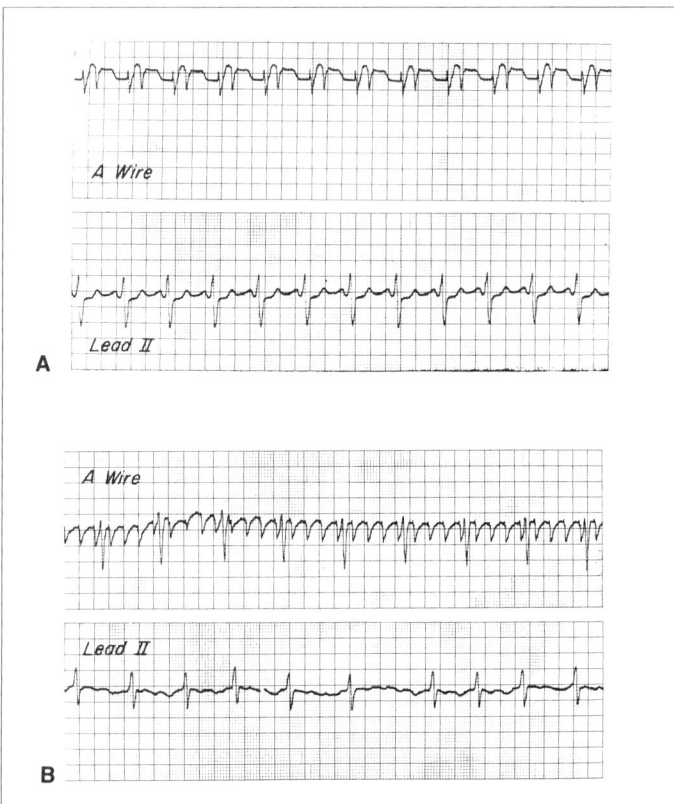

Fig. 4-3. Atrial electrode tracings. Recordings made from atrial electrodes (A wire) and corresponding lead II for a patient with normal sinus rhythm (A) and a patient with atrial flutter-fibrillation (B). Atrial activity is much more easily analyzed in the atrial wire tracing than in conventional leads.

lactic drug treatments will prevent their occurrence. In various studies, prophylactic digoxin, beta blockers, and calcium channel blockers have been shown to reduce the incidence of postoperative atrial fibrillation and flutter [81–88]. The most experience is probably with beta blockers, and, at low doses, this class of drugs is clearly useful for the prevention of atrial dysrhythmias after cardiac surgery [89–91]. Thus, the early postoperative administration of *propranolol* (10–20 mg PO every 6 hours), or *atenolol* (25 mg PO each day) should be considered for those patients who have no contraindications (such as poor left ventricular function or bronchospastic disease). This prophylaxis may be especially beneficial for patients at increased risk, such as those older than 65 years.

The method of management of atrial fibrillation or flutter depends on the status of the patient. If the patient is hemodynamically compromised, electrical cardioversion is the treatment of choice. This is especially useful for the patient who develops atrial fibrillation or flutter during the first few hours after surgery and is still intubated and under the effect of general anesthesia. Synchronous cardioversion is performed with external paddles, placed a bit more cephalad across the chest wall than for ventricular defibrillation (to place the atria directly in the path of the delivered energy), and begun using 20 to 50 joules (0.2–1.0 joule/kg for infants). It is important to ensure that the synchronization circuit of the cardioversion energy source is used to prevent discharge during the T wave of the patient's ECG, as this might result in the initiation of ventricular fibrillation. If the patient is awake, pretreatment with a short-acting barbiturate or sedative is desirable to prevent pain and memory of the event. If one is not successful at the initial energy setting, a higher energy level may be tried, but there is probably no advantage to exceeding 100 joules for cardioversion of supraventricular tachycardia. Although frequently successful, electrical cardioversion of postoperative atrial arrhythmias often provides only temporary restoration of sinus rhythm, probably because the underlying precipitating factors leading to the development of the arrhythmia remain unchanged. Thus, some form of drug therapy (such as procainamide or a beta blocker) is useful to help maintain sinus rhythm.

Atrial flutter (but not fibrillation) may be treated by rapid atrial pacing. This is performed by using a special pacemaker that can deliver up to 800 electrical impulses per minute. The pacemaker is connected to the atrial pacing electrodes (*not the ventricular,* as this may result in ventricular fibrillation) and the atrium is captured by pacing at a rate about 20% faster than the underlying atrial rate (which is usually either 2 or 3 times the ventricular rate). When monitoring lead II, evidence of atrial capture is seen when the atrial depolarization wave reverses polarity. Rapid atrial pacing is maintained for 10 to 15 seconds and then abruptly stopped. Frequently, this results in conversion of atrial flutter to atrial fibrillation, a rhythm generally more easily controlled by medications.

Most patients who develop supraventricular tachycardia after cardiac surgery experience atrial fibrillation, and this most frequently occurs on the second or third day after operation. By this time, the patient is usually extubated and alert. Drug treatment is preferable to electrical cardioversion in this situation. If the patient's average ventricular rate is less than 110 beats per minute and he or she is comfortable without evidence of hemodynamic compromise, no treatment is necessary. Most of these patients will spontaneously convert to normal sinus rhythm in 1 to 2 days.

For many years, the mainstay of drug treatment for postoperative atrial fibrillation and flutter has been *digoxin,* although recently we rely more often on agents such as verapamil or diltiazem in the early postoperative period. The adult loading ("digitalization") dose is 0.25 to 0.50 mg IV digoxin with subsequent doses of 0.25 mg every 4 to 6 hours until a total dose of 1.25 mg has been administered. The maintenance dose is 0.125 to 0.250 mg per day. Digitalization of pediatric patients begins with 10 µg/kg of an intravenous loading dose followed by 5 µg/kg 8 hours and again 16 hours later. The pediatric maintenance dose is 4 µg/kg administered intravenously every 12 hours. Serum digoxin levels should be followed, as digoxin has a narrow therapeutic-toxic ratio. It is excreted nearly entirely by the kidneys, so toxic levels may accumulate rapidly in patients with renal insufficiency. Side effects include dangerous arrhythmias (ventricular tachycardia and fibrillation, atrioventricular block, and accelerated junctional rhythm), gastrointestinal complaints (anorexia, nausea, and vomiting), and visual disturbances. Digoxin toxicity is potentiated by hypokalemia; serum digoxin levels are increased in the presence of quinidine, verapamil, and amiodarone. The main action of digoxin is to slow atrioventricular conduction thereby decreasing the ventricular response rate; it probably does not, by itself, cause cardioversion from atrial arrhythmia to sinus rhythm [92]. Even so, many patients with postoperative atrial arrhythmias treated by digoxin (or treated by nothing for that matter) will spontaneously convert to sinus rhythm within 24 to 48 hours. Once begun, digoxin is continued for 4 to 6 weeks after operation. One drawback of using digoxin to treat atrial fibrillation or flutter is that its rate-controlling effect is not usually apparent for 1 to 2 hours. Frequently, it is desirable to provide more rapid control of the patient's heart rate, and newer drugs are available for that purpose.

Verapamil is effective in slowing the ventricular response to atrial fibrillation and flutter [93]. Occasional patients will revert to sinus rhythm with verapamil administration. For adults, 2.5-mg boluses are given intravenously every 5 to 10 minutes until the desired effect (or total dosage of 15–20 mg) is achieved. Verapamil, however, may cause hypotension due to the drug's negative inotropic effects and must be used with caution in patients with poor ventricular function. When administering verapamil intravenously, it is necessary to monitor the patient's blood pressure continuously by an intraarterial cannula or very frequently with a blood pressure cuff. The hypotensive response to verapamil may be effectively prevented by pretreatment with calcium [94,95]. For this purpose, 500 mg of calcium chloride is slowly administered intravenously followed by the verapamil boluses. The rate-slowing effect of intravenously administered verapamil is, however, short-lived, with the heart rate often returning to tachycardia levels within 30 minutes. For longer-term control, orally administered verapamil may be added (40–80 mg every 6–8 hours). Sometimes, early after surgery, it is useful to digitalize the patient for longer-term rate control and to use small intravenous doses of verapamil while waiting for the digoxin to take effect. Because of the risk of heart block secondary to combined administration of both drugs, it is recommended that a temporary pacemaker, in the demand mode (VVI), be connected to the patient's ventricular electrodes to provide backup pacing should severe bradycardia occur.

Diltiazem, another calcium antagonist, is an effective agent for the treatment of postoperative atrial fibrillation. When administered intravenously, it reliably lowers the ventricular response to atrial fibrillation and flutter [96,97]. Treatment is begun with a bolus infusion of 0.25 mg/kg (adult dose) over 2 minutes. This can be repeated if necessary and then followed by a constant infusion of 5 to 15 mg/hr. This agent may prove to be preferable to verapamil as it has less of a negative inotropic effect and less frequently causes hypotension. Hypotension, when it does occur, can be reversed with calcium.

An alternative class of drugs for treatment of atrial fibrillation or flutter is the beta-adrenergic antagonists. These agents will provide effective slowing of the ventricular rate. With careful monitoring (preferably for the patient still in the intensive care unit), *esmolol* is very useful for quick control of the rapid response to atrial tachycardia [98]. Again, caution must be used in patients with impaired ventricular function or other contraindications to beta blockade (such as bronchospastic lung disease). For patients taking by mouth, propranolol (10–20 mg every 6 hours) or atenolol (25–50 mg per day), given orally will provide rate control. However, they require time to exert an effect.

Although postoperative atrial fibrillation or flutter is usually self-limiting and conversion to sinus rhythm often occurs within a few days, some patients remain in the arrhythmia. It is generally preferable to restore sinus rhythm before discharge from the hospital. For these patients, antiarrhythmic agents of the IA class are employed to effect "chemical" cardioversion. *Quinidine* or *procainamide* may be administered orally to the patient who already has satisfactory rate control with digoxin to effect cardioversion to sinus rhythm. Procainamide is usually better tolerated because it has a lower incidence of side effects and because of its major active metabolite, *N*-acetylprocainamide (NAPA), can be measured conveniently. Since the duration of procainamide treatment is usually limited to a few weeks, the risk of its most serious side effect, a drug-induced lupuslike syndrome, is minimized.

Other newer (and more expensive) drugs are being used occasionally to treat postoperative atrial arrhythmias. Two drugs of the IC class with demonstrated effectiveness are *propafenone* and *flecainide* [99–101]. Both drugs appear to be more effective than conventional therapy (i.e., digoxin) in converting atrial fibrillation to sinus rhythm. *Sotalol*, a new class III beta-blocking agent, has demonstrated prophylactic effectiveness in preventing supraventricular arrhythmias after myocardial revascularization [102].

Junctional Ectopic Tachycardia

Postoperative junctional ectopic (nodal) tachycardia is a potentially dangerous arrhythmia that occurs most commonly after congenital heart surgery in neonates and infants [103]. This may be due to enhanced automaticity in the bundle of His during low cardiac output. Hypotension and vagolytic drugs are contributing factors for the development and maintenance of this arrhythmia. The atrial rate is typically slower than the ventricular rate resulting in atrioventricular dissociation. Severe hemodynamic instability may result and treatment can be difficult. The diagnosis is based on demonstration of a narrow complex tachycardia with atrioventricular dissociation. The loss of atrioventricular synchrony serves to lower cardiac output even further, and adrenergic stimulation (by exogenous drugs or by patient anxiety and stimulation) frequently increases the heart rate and worsens the situation.

Treatment is directed at optimizing the patient's metabolic state (correcting acidosis, hypokalemia, and hypocalcemia) and minimizing adrenergic stimulation. Drugs that will increase adrenergic tone by direct stimulation (such as dopamine or isoproterenol) or by reflex actions (such as nitroprusside) should be avoided because they will increase the junctional rate. Likewise, vagolytic and negative inotropic agents should not be administered. Sedation with morphine and atrial pacing at a rate slightly above the junction rate are indicated. Adenosine may have a role in the management of this arrhythmia [104,105].

Ventricular Tachyarrhythmias

Premature ventricular contractions (PVCs) are common in adult patients with heart disease both before and after surgery; they are uncommon in children. When present postoperatively, PVCs are usually not a problem in themselves but they may serve as an indicator of less obvious disturbances such as metabolic and electrolyte abnormalities (especially hypokalemia, hypoxia, myocardial ischemia, poor ventricular function, acidosis, alkalosis, or digoxin toxicity). Thus when new-onset PVCs occur early after surgery, especially at a frequency of greater than 4 to 6 per minute, the patient's blood gases and digoxin (if receiving the drug) and serum potassium levels should be checked. PVCs occurring with more than one morphology (multifocal PVCs), couplets, or short runs of VT are of greater concern and should be promptly evaluated. A 12-lead ECG is indicated to rule out ischemia. If this is normal and the patient is otherwise stable, specific treatment is not usually required for unifocal, single PVCs. Due to the potential proarrhythmic side effect of most antiarrhythmic drugs, treatment of asymptomatic PVCs can lead to the development of more dangerous arrhythmias in up to 10% of patients. One safe way to eliminate PVCs is by overdrive pacing, in which the atrium is paced at a rate of 5 to 10 beats per minute faster than the native heart rate. When the heart rate increases in this way, there is less time for ectopic pacemakers to become depolarized to threshold levels and to initiate premature beats.

More serious ventricular tachyarrhythmias are not common after cardiac surgery (an incidence of 1.4% of 1251 patients in one series [106]). They can, however, lead to immediate hemodynamic decompensation and rapid death of the patient if not quickly recognized and appropriately treated. Patients undergoing ventricular aneurysm resection or endocardial resection and those with left ventricular hypertrophy are at greatest risk for this complication. Prophylactic administration of antiarrhythmic agents (such as lidocaine or procainamide) does not always prevent the development of postoperative ventricular arrhythmias in this group of patients and because of their proarrhythmic effects (particularly procainamide), may be counterproductive in this regard.

As discussed previously, a wide QRS tachycardia should be treated as ventricular in origin until proven otherwise. Even if well tolerated, ventricular tachycardia should generally be treated expeditiously because deterioration to ventricular fibrillation may suddenly occur. If the patient is hemodynamically stable, treatment of ventricular tachycardia may be begun with lidocaine (1 mg/kg) followed by subsequent doses of 0.5 mg/kg every 8 to 10 minutes until a total dose of 3 mg/kg is reached. If this does not result in resolution of ventricular tachycardia, procainamide is administered (100 mg every 5 to 10 minutes up to a total dose of 1.0 g). If ventricular tachycardia persists, electrical cardioversion is performed.

If the patient with ventricular tachycardia is hypotensive, immediate cardioversion is indicated. This is accomplished using external paddles applied to the chest wall facing each other to maximize the current flow through the heart. For patients with a permanent pacemaker in place, the paddles should be kept at least 5 inches away from the pacemaker generator to prevent pacemaker malfunction. The initial energy dose should be 100 joules and, if this is unsuccessful, subsequent attempts are made using 200, 300, and, if required, up to 360 joules. The pediatric electrical dose is 0.5 to 4.0 joules/kg. Lidocaine infusion should be begun as soon as possible.

Ventricular fibrillation results in sudden total cessation of the cardiac output and must be treated immediately by electrical defibrillation. For this purpose, the initial adult dose is 200 joules (2 joules/kg for infants and children). The standard external paddle position is with one anterior to the right of the sternum at the second intercostal space and the other below and lateral to the left of the left nipple [107]. If a 200-joule shock is unsuccessful, a 300-joule dose is used (followed by 360 joules, if required); repositioning of the external paddles may improve the current flow to the heart. The first drug to be administered is lidocaine. Cardiac massage is required to effect myocardial delivery of medications administered during ventricular fibrillation. If defibrillation has still not been accomplished, bretylium (adult dose, 5–10 mg/kg IV bolus), magnesium sulfate (adult dose, 1.0–2.0 g IV bolus over 1 to 2 min, repeat in 5 to 10 min), or procainamide may be of benefit. Epinephrine (1.0 mg IV push) may be required if ventricular fibrillation is not "coarse."

Management of the Patient with an Automatic Implantable Cardioverter Defibrillator (ICD)

ICD implantation has become an important part of the medical and surgical therapies for patients who suffer life-threatening cardiac arrhythmias. During the early postimplantation period, special considerations apply to these patients. Although the ICD has the capability of recognizing ventricular tachycardia and fibrillation, some centers do not activate the device until 2 to 3 days after surgery at which time final device programming is done: This is to prevent the delivery of shocks to the heart triggered by electrocautery in the operating room or by early postoperative supraventricular tachyarrhythmias. Thus, all persons involved in the early postoperative care of these patients must be aware when the ICD is *nonfunctional* and that serious ventricular tachyarrhythmias should be treated immediately just as they are in any other patient. If this approach is used, a sign is prominently displayed above the patient's bed stating this information. If the device is activated at the time of implantation, the rate cutoff (the heart rate at which the device will deliver a shock) should be set at a high rate so that rapid atrial arrhythmias will not cause the device to deliver an inappropriate shock to the heart.

If transthoracic cardioversion of ventricular tachycardia or defibrillation is required for the patient with an ICD in place, it may be difficult to deliver sufficient energy to the heart [108]. This is due to interference caused by the metal mesh patch leads that are components of the ICD system. If the initial attempt at external defibrillation is unsuccessful, it is important to change the orientation of the external paddles. Moving one paddle to an anterior (apex of the heart) position and the other to a posterior position will likely allow for successful conversion of ventricular fibrillation. Awareness of this potential problem and knowing how to deal with it will help prevent a fatal outcome. Since the ICD does not change the propensity to develop ventricular arrhythmias, it is important to restart the antiarrhythmic agents that the patient was receiving before surgery. In our experience, the postoperative use of epidural catheters for the administration of anesthetic and analgesic drugs has decreased the morbidity of implantation surgery in these patients, particularly if a thoractomy approach is used.

Postoperative Ischemia and Perioperative Infarction

Myocardial ischemia, either transient or irreversible leading to infarction, may occur during and after cardiac surgery. This complication is most frequently associated with coronary artery bypass procedures. In fact, up to 40% of coronary artery bypass surgery patients exhibit some evidence of postoperative ischemia with the highest incidence occurring within 6 hours of weaning the patient from cardiopulmonary bypass [109]. Early recognition of the presence of myocardial ischemia can lead to treatment to limit the damage that occurs or, in the case of coronary spasm, to effect a complete reversal of the condition.

PERIOPERATIVE INFARCTION

Depending on the diagnostic criteria used, the incidence of new myocardial infarctions associated with myocardial revascularization procedures ranges from 5 to 25% [110]. The incidence in congenital and valvular procedures is lower, but the potential for this complication is present with all open heart operations. Unless extensive ECG, enzymatic, and radionuclide testing is performed, many perioperative myocardial infarctions go unnoticed. Not surprisingly, the operative mortality in those with perioperative infarcts is increased significantly and the long-term survival also may be affected adversely [111–113]. Efforts to identify preoperative factors predictive of perioperative myocardial infarction have had conflicting results.

Release of myocardial creatine kinase MB (CK-MB) isoenzyme is the most sensitive method to detect perioperative myocardial ischemia [114]. Of the various diagnostic enzyme tests available (including lactate dehydrogenase and aspartate aminotransferase), CK-MB analysis is the most useful for detecting perioperative myocardial infarctions [115]. Analysis of this information is complex due to creatine kinase kinetics and because the enzyme is released to some extent during surgical manipulation (without infarction) of the heart and infarctions occur at various times (a significant proportion do not occur during surgery but rather in the first 24 hours postoperatively). The usual pattern of CK-MB release results in a peak of serum enzyme concentrations at 12 to 16 hours after surgery; some release occurs in nearly all patients who undergo cardiac surgery of any type. A significantly greater peak serum level and a more prolonged period of enzyme elevation, however, are observed in those patients who, by other tests, are found to suffer perioperative infarction. As a rule, perioperative myocardial infarction must be considered as likely in patients whose peak CK-MB (at 12–16 hours after surgery) is above 50 IU/liter and as unlikely in those with peak levels below 15 IU/liter.

Significant myocardial infarction is usually (but not always) associated with ECG changes. The patterns of ECG changes according to the location of the infarct are summarized in Table 4-4. The postoperative ECG is not nearly as sensitive as cardiac enzyme analysis for the diagnosis of perioperative infarction, but the presence of new Q waves is essentially 100% diagnostic. A significant number of patients will have "diagnostic" elevations of CK-MB but will not demonstrate new Q waves. Nearly all patients with new Q waves, however, will have high CK-MB peaks. Patients who suffer perioperative infarctions as diagnosed by new Q waves have a significantly greater mortality rate than those with probable infarcts (by enzymes) but no new Q waves. This indicates that the amount of muscle lost sufficient to cause the ECG changes has a more detrimental effect on cardiac function than the amount of infarcted muscle required to cause enzyme changes alone.

The technetium-99m scan is both highly sensitive and specific. The scan is performed 2 to 4 days postoperatively. Uptake of technetium by the area of infarcted muscle at an intensity equal to or greater

Table 4-4. Electrocardiographic (ECG) identification of acute myocardial infarction (MI) location

ECG changes associated with transmural MI:
1. Hyperacute or inverted T waves
2. ST-segment elevation
3. New Q wave (longer than 0.04 second duration or greater than ⅓ the height of the QRS complex)

ECG changes associated with non–Q-wave (subendocardial) MI:
1. ST-segment depression
2. Inverted T waves

Location of infarction	ECG leads demonstrating ECG changes listed above
Anteroseptal	V_1, V_2
Anteroapical	V_2, V_3
Anterolateral	$V_4–V_6$, I, aVL
Large anterior	$V_1–V_6$
Lateral	I, aVL, V_5, V_6
Inferior	II, III, aVF
Posterior*	V_1, V_2, V_3

*The changes in a posterior MI are mirror images of anterior infarctions, i.e., inverted hyperacute T waves and ST-segment depression.

than the intensity of uptake by the sternum or nearby ribs is considered abnormal and positive [116,117]. The scan is not reliable early (less than 36 hrs) after infarction, which limits its clinical utility in the acute setting. It does, however, provide a method by which a perioperative infarct can be ruled in or out for the patient with conflicting or nondiagnostic enzymatic and ECG results.

Patients who suffer an uncomplicated perioperative infarction are treated essentially the same as those who experience a normal, uncomplicated postoperative course, although nitroglycerin is administered intravenously for 24 to 48 hours if the patient's blood pressure will allow. Systemic nitroglycerin will improve perfusion to ischemic myocardium in patients with bypass grafts in place [118]. Complications such as low cardiac output and arrhythmias are managed as described elsewhere in this chapter. Prophylactic lidocaine administration is of no proven benefit following myocardial infarction and is not used at our institutions in this setting. After recovery, it is often useful to obtain some measure of the patient's ejection fraction (by nuclear angiography or echocardiography) to allow for determination of the extent of damage incurred. It often is determined that no significant decrease in the ejection fraction has occurred, a finding that can be reassuring for the patient and the surgeon alike.

CORONARY ARTERY SPASM

Coronary artery spasm during the early postoperative period after coronary artery bypass surgery can be an unrecognized cause of sudden, severe cardiovascular collapse that may be fatal [119]. This complication often presents as acute hypotension with the ECG demonstrating ST-segment elevation, although ventricular tachycardia, fibrillation, or atrioventricular block also may occur as initial manifestations. When this happens in the operating room, nitroglycerin may be injected directly into vein grafts for relief of the spasm. When it occurs in the postoperative patient, calcium channel-blocking agents are administered (nifedipine sublingually in 10-mg increments or verapamil intravenously in 2.5-mg increments). Intravenously administered nitroglycerin is usually not effective for the acute situation. Table 4-5 outlines the strategy for the prevention and treatment of early postoperative coronary artery spasm. Although the prevalence of this problem among coronary bypass patients was previously as high as 2.5%, it is our impression that this has declined, possibly because of the common perioperative administration of calcium channel-blocking agents to these patients [120].

Pulmonary Complications

Abnormalities of gas exchange or ventilation are not unusual after cardiac surgery. In fact, nearly all patients develop atelectasis to various degrees. Preoperative identification of patients at risk for pulmonary complications (as discussed in Chap. 3) and proper attention to postoperative pulmonary care will help minimize the incidence and severity of these pulmonary complications. Some patients, however, because of preexisting disease such as asthma or because of acquired disorders such as phrenic nerve injury, may

Table 4-5. Management of early postoperative coronary artery spasm

Situation	Management
Preoperative	1. Identify patients at risk 2. Maintain oral calcium channel-blocking drugs until time of operation
Intraoperative	1. Inject intragraft nitroglycerin (0.2-mg increments) 2. Administer sublingual nifedipine (10-mg increments) or intravenous diltiazem (10-mg increments) or verapamil (2.5–5.0 mg increments) 3. Avoid vasoconstricting agents
Postoperative Patient stable	1. Perform cardiac catheterization 2. If spasm present, inject nitroglycerin directly into coronary artery or vein bypass graft
Patient unstable	1. Quickly exclude other causes of deterioration 2. Administer sublingual nifedipine or intravenous diltiazem or verapamil 3. If patient is severely hypotensive or arrested, perform emergency sternotomy for open cardiac massage and direct injection into vein grafts

Source: Adapted from JH Lemmer, MM Kirsh. Coronary artery spasm following coronary artery surgery. *Ann Thorac Surg* 46:108–115, 1988.

develop serious pulmonary complications requiring management after cardiac surgery.

Patients with acquired heart disease requiring surgery often have been heavy cigarette smokers and suffer significant chronic obstructive lung disease. Despite the increased risk of pulmonary complications in these patients, even those with severe pulmonary impairment can successfully undergo cardiac operations [121,122]. Thus, even severe preoperative pulmonary dysfunction is not usually a contraindication to cardiac surgery when the benefits of the planned operation are judged to outweigh the increased risk.

ATELECTASIS

Radiographic evidence of atelectasis is present during the early postoperative period in 80 to 90% of patients who have undergone heart surgery [123]. Most commonly, the left lower lobe is affected, the degree of atelectasis is subsegmental, and the radiographic appearance is exacerbated after the patient is extubated.

Although the sternotomy incision is less painful and less debilitating than the lateral thoracotomy incision, a significant decrease in pulmonary function still occurs after open heart surgery via this approach. Cardiopulmonary bypass increases lung water content thus resulting in further abnormalities of ventilation and gas exchange early after surgery. In adults undergoing coronary bypass procedures, there is a reduction of at least 25 to 50% in forced vital capacity (FVC) and forced expiratory volume in 1 second (FEV_1) postoperatively. This decrease is larger in patients who have undergone mobilization of the internal mammary artery than those who have not [124–126]. Vigorous pulmonary toilet, with frequent use of the incentive spirometer and early ambulation, is generally effective treatment for postoperative atelectasis. Bronchoscopy is rarely necessary.

BRONCHOSPASM

Bronchospasm is occasionally encountered either intra- or postoperatively. Patients at increased risk are those with preexisting asthma and those who suffer chronic obstructive lung disease with a reactive component. When present during closure of the sternum, hyperinflation of the lungs may cause hypotension due to compression of the heart as the sternal halves are being brought together. If present during the early postoperative period in the ventilated patient, severe bronchospasm may result in hypoxemia and high ventilatory pressures.

Treatment of bronchospasm is by intravenously and inhalation administered agents. For the acute situation when the patient is suffering hemodynamic compromise due to lung hyperinflation, intravenous low-dose epinephrine (0.25-0.50 μg/min for adults) provides both bronchodilation and inotropic support. Corticosteroids, although slower to act, are also effective and do not result in wound-healing problems when used as a short course during the perioperative period [127]. For patients with known severe reactive airway disease, we frequently administer steroids several hours preoperatively and for a few days postoperatively. Theophylline is a mainstay of treatment for chronic bronchospasm, but we use it infrequently in the early postoperative period. Tachycardia very frequently results from intravenously administered theophylline, and serious arrhythmias may result even at nontoxic serum concentrations [128]. When theophylline is needed, we frequently digitalize patients in anticipation of the increased likelihood of atrial fibrillation. Severe, life-threatening bronchospasm may be observed in certain settings, such as in patients with asthma or as a manifestation of drug allergy or reaction to blood products. In these instances, when conventional measures are not effective, we have used intravenous PGE_1 as a very effective and potent bronchodilator.

Various inhaled agents are useful for the treatment of bronchospasm. If the patient is on a ventilator, these agents may be administered directly via a nebulizer into the delivered oxygen-air mixture. For this purpose, we prefer albuterol. This drug has relatively selective beta-2 agonist properties associated with a short onset of action and effectiveness of 4 to 6 hours. Arrhythmias are rare. After extubation, albuterol can be given as nasal mist treatments by the respiratory therapist or self-administered with an inhaler.

It should be remembered that bronchospasm may be a manifestation of early pulmonary edema, in which case diuresis will be beneficial.

PHRENIC NERVE INJURY

Temporary or permanent injury to one or both phrenic nerves may occur during cardiac surgery. In some patients, this occurs as the result of direct trauma (such as during mobilization of the internal mammary artery or during a difficult dissection in a patient undergoing reoperation). In others, it may be the result of cold thermal injury from the ice-saline slush placed within the pericardial sac during aortic cross-clamping for the purpose of myocardial protection.

In adults undergoing surgery using topical ice slush, radiographic evidence of phrenic nerve injury may occur in up to 25% of patients. This is associated with an increased incidence of postoperative atelectasis and the appearance of an elevated (usually left) hemidiaphragm on postoperative chest radiographs [129,130]. Most patients are asymptomatic, but this diaphragmatic paralysis can be of critical importance to patients with preexisting pulmonary dysfunction. If both phrenic nerves are injured, severe morbidity may result [131]. Use of a foam pad placed between the ice and the pericardium to insulate the left phrenic nerve from the slush can effectively lower the incidence of this complication [132]. Thus, some use an insulating pad routinely and others use cold saline irrigation instead of slush. In most adults, cold injury to the phrenic nerve does not result in serious consequences and phrenic nerve function appears to return with time, although up to 20% of those affected may have persistent diaphragm elevation 1 year after surgery [131].

In children, phrenic nerve paralysis can be a serious problem. In a series of 7670 pediatric cardiac procedures, the incidence was 1.6% [133]. Infants do not tolerate loss of effective hemidiaphragmatic function as well as adults and may not be weaned from mechanical ventilation as the result of the injury. Definitive diagnosis is based on the demonstration of paradoxical movement of the diaphragm during fluoroscopic or ultrasound examination. In the patient who is receiving positive-pressure ventilation, the paralyzed diaphragm may appear normal on the chest x-ray; thus, one of these tests is necessary to confirm the diagnosis of phrenic nerve paralysis. This problem should be suspected in the pediatric patient who cannot be weaned from the ventilator as expected. In most patients, diaphragmatic function will return, but if ventilatory dependency lasts more than 2 weeks, consideration should be given to performing a diaphragmatic plication procedure, especially for children less than 2 years old. This procedure will often allow extubation of the previously ventilator-dependent patient [134].

PROLONGED RESPIRATORY INSUFFICIENCY

Abnormal respiratory function is frequently associated with heart disease, either acquired or congenital, and it may prevent prompt discontinuance of mechanical respiratory support and extubation.

Perioperative complications (such as severe neurologic injury or pneumonia) may also interfere with weaning the patient from mechanical ventilation. In some patients, pulmonary function is adequate but cardiac function is tenuous, and prolonged ventilatory support is desirable while the heart is allowed to recover. Thus, techniques of respiratory support are crucial to postoperative care.

Patients who need prolonged positive-pressure ventilation require careful management. **No patient dependent on a respirator for his or her life should be left unattended.** Ventilator alarm systems must remain activated at all times. Periods off the respirator (required for tracheal care, x-ray films, etc.) must be limited to 1 or 2 minutes at a time, and the monitor should be watched for the appearance of ventricular irritability or bradycardia indicative of hypoxia. A self-inflating bag (Ambu bag) connected to an oxygen supply must be at each bedside. Whenever a patient appears to be ventilated improperly or if there is any question of machine malfunction, the nurse, respiratory therapist, or physician in attendance should immediately begin hand ventilation while the problem is being resolved.

Determining the adequacy of mechanical ventilation is based on both physical examination and arterial blood gas analysis. The patient who "looks comfortable" may be hypoxic or hypercarbic or both; thus periodic measurements of the blood gases are required. We frequently use a pulse oximeter that provides a continuous estimate of the patient's degree of arterial oxygenation. This oxygen saturation monitor, however, gives no information regarding carbon dioxide and acid-base status. Thus, although useful, the pulse oximeter cannot be relied on as the sole method of monitoring the ventilator-dependent patient.

A precise method of quantitating the lung's ability to oxygenate the blood is to determine the arterial-alveolar (A-a) gradient:

$$\text{A-a gradient} = 760 - P_{H_2O} - P_{CO_2} - (\text{arterial } P_{O_2} \text{ on an } F_{IO_2} \text{ of } 1.0)$$

The A-a gradient can be measured daily to provide a valuable objective index of progress in patients who cannot undergo extubation early after surgery. When the gradient is less than 350 mm Hg, and if the patient's hemodynamic condition is stable, steps toward extubation (such as a trial of breathing on pressure support or a T-tube setup) are made.

An early goal of prolonged ventilatory management is to reduce the patient's inspired oxygen concentration (F_{IO_2}) to below 50%. Concentrations above this level are associated with detrimental changes in the lungs. Thus, we use the lowest F_{IO_2} that will yield an arterial oxygen saturation of 92 to 94%. The addition of PEEP will frequently allow for improved oxygenation at lower F_{IO_2}. Patients who are fluid-overloaded (as are many cardiac surgery patients early after operation) should undergo vigorous diuresis as long as adequate cardiac function is maintained. For some patients, especially those with concomitant renal insufficiency, continuous arteriovenous hemofiltration can be useful. This technique provides for the removal of excess fluid in addition to the elimination of cardiopulmonary toxic substances that may be contributing to the respiratory failure [135].

The patient undergoing prolonged ventilatory support must not be allowed to starve. Failure to maintain nutrition may impair respiratory muscle function and further hamper efforts at weaning the patient from the ventilator [136]. If it is anticipated that extubation and normal feeding are more than a few days away (or if a few days have already passed), then nutrition must begin. If bowel activity is present, a soft small-bore nasogastric tube may be used for enteral feedings; if not, central venous hyperalimentation is begun.

Preferences for the route of endotracheal intubation differ among institutions. In general, the oral route is preferred when the period of intubation is expected to be short. This route of intubation is often easier to perform but can cause trauma to the mouth and is uncomfortable for the awake patient. The nasal route is more comfortable but is associated with sinusitis and pressure necrosis of the skin of the nares (contributed to, in some patients, by low cardiac output).

Prolonged endotracheal intubation is uncomfortable and has the potential for local complications. The presence of the endotracheal tube between the vocal cords is associated with cord ulceration and posterior commissure stenosis, both of which occur with increasing frequency as the length of time the tube is present increases. This has led some authorities to recommend performance of a tracheostomy in ventilator-dependent patients after a set period (such as 10 or 14 days) [137]. A policy of performing a tracheostomy after a specified period of intubation may not, however, be applicable to all cardiac surgery patients. For one thing, the complication rate associated with a tracheostomy may be comparable to that associated with prolonged translaryngeal intubation [138,139]. Complications of a tracheostomy include tracheal ulceration, bleeding, tracheoinnominate fistula, and late tracheal stenosis. Important for the patient with a recent sternotomy incision is the risk of mediastinal contamination, which may occur during the tracheostomy. To decrease this risk, we wait at least 10 days (and often longer) after the original cardiac procedure before proceeding with a tracheostomy. For those patients who clearly are not going to be weaned from the ventilatory in the near future, however, a tracheostomy is recommended. The tracheostomy tube is more comfortable for the patient, allows for more convenient management of pulmonary secretions, and is useful during a slow weaning protocol. This latter feature is particularly valuable as the patient may be disconnected from the ventilator (or placed on a positive-pressure support system) for increasingly longer periods of time as the ability to breathe on his or her own improves. This avoids the trials of extubation and, sometimes, reintubation, which are traumatic and dangerous for the patient and may be required to wean the patient from prolonged endotracheal intubation.

In patients who require airway access only for pulmonary toilet, we have found the percutaneous "mini-tracheostomy" to be of use. This allows for the introduction of small-bore catheters for suctioning of secretions and cough stimulation.

ADULT RESPIRATORY DISTRESS SYNDROME (ARDS)

This poorly defined syndrome, also known as "noncardiogenic pulmonary edema" or "increased permeability pulmonary edema," is characterized by severe respiratory insufficiency with relatively normal cardiac function. It is likely a primary alveolar endothelial disorder with increased capillary permeability resulting in extravasation of protein-containing fluid in the alveolar space. The major physiologic result is hypoxia. The patient's chest x-ray demonstrates bilateral fluffy infiltrates. Frothy, protein-rich secretions are copious and require frequent suctioning. Important disorders to rule out in this situation include blood product transfusion reaction and sepsis.

Treatment of postoperative ARDS is largely supportive [140]. PEEP is used to lower the FIO_2 to below 60% while maintaining the arterial saturation above 90%, if possible. Frequently, the amount of PEEP used is limited by the reduction in cardiac output and blood pressure that often occurs when 10 cm or more of PEEP is utilized. There are no medications currently used for the specific treatment of ARDS; steroids are of no benefit.

PNEUMOTHORAX

Pneumothorax may occur in patients after open heart surgery, especially when they are receiving positive-pressure ventilation. It is more common in those with preexisting obstructive or bullous disease and those requiring significant levels of PEEP. Tension pneumothorax may develop quickly in the mechanically ventilated patient; this possibility should be kept in mind during the evaluation of a patient who has suddenly decompensated. Although breath sounds may be diminished on the affected side, the noise produced by the ventilator and other noise in the intensive care unit may cause the breath sounds to appear equal despite the presence of a large pneumothorax. Other clues to the presence of tension pneumothorax include distended neck veins and tracheal deviation away from the involved hemithorax. If the patient is severely hypotensive and a pneumothorax is strongly suspected, treatment is begun by inserting a 16-gauge intravenous catheter (cannula-over-needle type, e.g., Intracath) into the pleural space. A rush of air exiting from the chest through the cannula, associated with hemodynamic improvement of the patient, confirms the diagnosis. If the patient is sufficiently stable, then a chest x-ray may be obtained before definitive therapy. This will reveal collapse of the lung and, if tension is present, shifting of the mediastinal structures away from the affected side. Definitive therapy is the placement of a chest tube (Fig. 4-4).

We do not recommend chest tubes with integral sharp stylets for general use because damage may result from uncontrolled insertion. For pneumothorax the insertion site may be at the second intercostal space anteriorly (lateral to the mammary vessels) or through the fourth intercostal space and directed superiorly, which will result in a more cosmetic appearance when the insertion site is healed. For adequate drainage of blood or fluid, the tube should be placed in the dependent portion of the chest through the fourth or fifth intercostal space, either in the posterior gutter or along the diaphragm. Pleural fluid or blood generally collects dependently so the chest tube should be placed inferiorly in the pleural space. The midaxillary line is preferred because more posteriorly located tubes are more uncomfortable. The diaphragm rises as high as the sixth intercostal space laterally; therefore, the insertion site should not

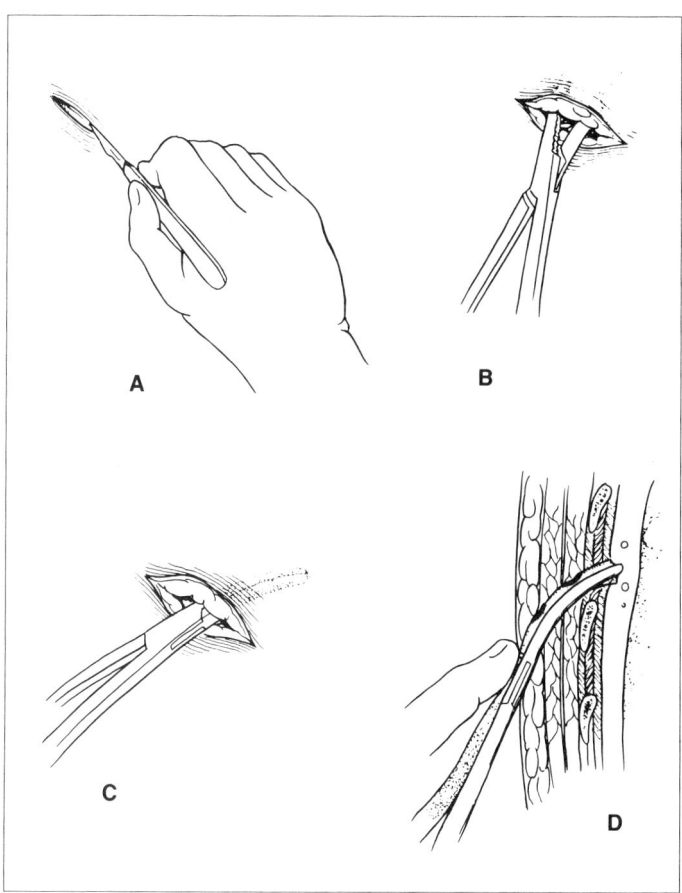

Fig. 4-4. Insertion of a chest tube. A chest tube may be inserted safely even in patients with coagulopathy who are on ventilators if proper technique is used. Under local anesthesia, a small incision is made and a tunnel dissected bluntly through the subcutaneous tissues to the rib (A). A tract through the intercostal muscles is created bluntly *over* the superior surface of the rib selected to avoid trauma to the intercostal vessels that follow the inferior edge (B, C). A gloved finger may be inserted into the pleural space to verify that the lung is not adherent if in doubt. A pleural tube of adequate caliber (*not* a Foley catheter) is guided into the pleural space with a clamp (D), attached to a water seal drainage system, and sutured securely.

be lower than this interspace, and, if possible, the tube should be inserted during full inspiration.

PLEURAL EFFUSIONS

All patients undergoing cardiac surgical procedures are at risk for developing significant postoperative effusions. Patients with chronic congestive heart failure frequently have pleural effusions before surgery. Although these may be drained during surgery, it is not unusual for the effusions to recur. As cardiac function improves postoperatively, the effusions often resolve. If not, or if symptoms recur, drainage may be necessary by thoracentesis or chest tube placement.

Children who undergo the Fontan-Kreutzer operation (right atrial-to-pulmonary artery anastomosis for single-ventricle lesions) are especially likely to develop troublesome postoperative effusions, particularly if the patient's central venous pressure exceeds 15 mm Hg. These fluid collections are sometimes chylous in nature, and continued drainage of the protein-rich fluid may result in malnutrition. Efforts to lower right atrial pressure with nitroglycerin, diuresis, and optimization of blood gases will help diminish the effusions. In some patients, the problem is a major one and may require treatment by thoracic duct ligation, tetracycline pleurodesis, or pleuroperitoneal shunt [141]. Adults who undergo cardiac surgery also develop postoperative pleural effusions, especially patients who have undergone coronary artery bypass procedures using the (usually left) internal mammary artery. These patients have increased volumes of mediastinal and pleural tube drainage (of both bloody and serous fluid) during the early postoperative period and develop pleural effusions more frequently than patients who do not undergo mobilization of the internal mammary artery. The use of ice slush resulting in phrenic nerve dysfunction and left lower lobe atelectasis contributes to pleural effusion development. Bilateral effusions may result from the use of both mammary arteries. Occasionally patients who have undergone mammary artery mobilization develop symptomatic pleural effusions weeks or even months after surgery [142]. The presentation is that of dyspnea with exertion; physical examination reveals dullness to percussion and absent breath sounds on the affected side. A chest x-ray confirms the diagnosis. Treatment is thoracentesis to remove the usually clear, amber-colored fluid and allow for full expansion of the lung. In some patients, the fluid collection recurs, and repeat thoracentesis is required.

References

1. Naunheim KS, et al. The changing profile of the patient undergoing coronary artery bypass surgery. *J Am Coll Cardiol* 11:494, 1988.

2. Kumon K, et al. Organ failures due to low cardiac output syndrome following open heart surgery. *Jpn Circ J* 50:329, 1986.

3. Apstein CS, Lorell BH. The physiological basis of left ventricular diastolic dysfunction. *J Cardiac Surg* 3:475, 1988.

4. Doty DB. The surgeon's response to a low-output state after cardiopulmonary bypass: Etiologies and remedies. *J Cardiac Surg* 3:256, 1990.

5. Matsuzaki M, Toma Y, Kusukawa R. Clinical applications of transesophageal echocardiography. *Circulation* 82:709, 1990.

6. Valdes-Cruz LM, et al. Recognition of residual postoperative shunts by contrast echocardiography. *Circulation* 55:148, 1977.

7. Reichert SL, et al. Transesophageal echocardiography in hypotensive patients after cardiac surgery. Comparison with hemodynamic parameters. *J Thorac Cardiovasc Surg* 104:321, 1992.

8. Hartzler GO, et al. Hemodynamic benefits of atrioventricular sequential pacing after cardiac surgery. *Am J Cardiol* 40:232, 1977.

9. Wehlage DR, Bohrer H, Ruffman K. Impairment of left ventricular diastolic function during coronary artery bypass grafting. *Anesthesia* 45:549, 1990.

10. Eichorn EJ, et al. Left ventricular inotropic effect of atrial pacing after coronary artery bypass grafting. *Am J Cardiol* 63:687, 1989.

11. Greene PS, et al. Systolic and diastolic left ventricular dysfunction due to mild hypothermia. *Circulation* 80(Suppl III):III-44, 1989.

12. Boldt J, et al. Myocardial temperature during cardiac operations: Influence on right ventricular function. *J Thorac Cardiovasc Surg* 100:562, 1990.

13. Czer L, et al. Transient hemodynamic dysfunction after myocardial revascularization. *J Thorac Cardiovasc Surg* 86:226, 1983.

14. Zwischenberger JB, et al. Suppression of shivering decreases oxygen consumption and improves hemodynamic stability during postoperative rewarming following cardiopulmonary bypass. *Surg Forum* 3:11, 1985.

15. Holtzclaw BJ. Postoperative shivering after cardiac surgery: A review. *Heart Lung* 15:292, 1986.

16. American College of Cardiology/American Heart Association Task Force. Management of acute myocardial infarction. *Circulation* 82:664, 1990.

17. DiSesa VJ. The rational selection of inotropic drugs in cardiac surgery. *J Cardiac Surg* 2:385, 1987.

18. Hochberg MS, et al. Pulmonary inactivation of vasopressors following cardiac operations. *Ann Thorac Surg* 41:200, 1986.

19. Tinker J. Potent inotropes are the drugs of choice after cardiopulmonary bypass. *J Cardiothorac Anesth* 1:256, 1987.

20. Schaer GL, Fink MP, Parrillo J. Norepinephrine alone versus norepinephrine plus low-dose dopamine: Enhanced renal blood flow with combination pressor therapy. *Crit Care Med* 13:492, 1985.

21. Ward HB, et al. Enhanced cardiac efficiency with dobutamine after global ischemia. *J Surg Res* 33:21, 1982.

22. Leier CV, Unverferth DV. Dobutamine. *Ann Intern Med* 99:490, 1983.

23. Mueller HS. Inotropic agents in the treatment of cardiogenic shock. *World J Surg* 9:3, 1985.

24. Fowler MB, et al. Dobutamine and dopamine after cardiac surgery: Greater augmentation of myocardial blood flow with dobutamine. *Circulation* 70(Suppl I):I-103, 1984.

25. DiSesa VJ, et al. Hemodynamic comparison of dopamine and dobutamine in the postoperative volume-loaded, pressure-loaded and normal ventricle. *J Thorac Cardiovasc Surg* 82:256, 1982.

26. Balderman SC, Aldridge J. Pharmacologic support of the myocardium following aortocoronary bypass surgery: A comparative study. *J Clin Pharmacol* 26:175, 1986.

27. Lemmer JH Jr, et al. Norepinephrine plus phentolamine improves regional blood flow during experimental low cardiac output syndrome. *Ann Thorac Surg* 38:108, 1984.

28. Gray R, et al. Low cardiac output states after open heart surgery: Comparative hemodynamic effects of dobutamine, dopamine, and norepinephrine plus phentolamine. *Chest* 80:16, 1981.

29. Holloway EL, et al. Action of drugs in patients early after cardiac surgery: I. Comparison of isoproterenol and dopamine. *Am J Cardiol* 35:656, 1975.

30. Baim DS. Effect of phosphodiesterase inhibition on myocardial oxygen consumption and coronary blood flow. *Am J Cardiol* 63:23A, 1989.

31. Jessup M. Weaning from cardiopulmonary bypass: Theory and practice. *Chest* 98:7, 1990.

32. Benotti JR, et al. Hemodynamic assessment of amrinone. *N Engl J Med* 299:1373, 1978.

33. Deeb GM, et al. Amrinone versus conventional therapy in pulmonary hypertensive patients awaiting cardiac transplantation. *Ann Thorac Surg* 48:665, 1989.

34. Hines RA. Management of acute right ventricular failure. *J Cardiac Surg* 5:285, 1990.

35. Goenen M, et al. Amrinone in the management of low cardiac output after cardiac surgery. *Am J Cardiol* 56:33B, 1985.

36. Guimond JG, et al. Augmentation of cardiac function in end-stage heart failure by combined use of dobutamine and amrinone. *Chest* 90:302, 1986.

37. Olsen KH, Kluger J, Fieldman A. Combination high dose amrinone and dopamine in the management of moribund cardiogenic shock after open heart surgery. *Chest* 94:503, 1988.

38. Boldt J, et al. Efficacy of the phosphodiesterase inhibitor enoximone in complicated cardiac surgery. *Chest* 98:53, 1990.

39. Zeplin HE, Dieterich HA, Stegmann T. The effect of enoximone and dobutamine on hemodynamic performance after open heart surgery. *J Cardiovasc Surg* 31:574, 1990.

40. Fernandez-del Castillo C, et al. Risk factors for the development of pancreatic injury following cardiopulmonary bypass. *N Engl J Med* 325:382, 1991.

41. Zaloga GP, et al. Calcium attenuates epinephrine's beta adrenergic effects in postoperative heart surgery patients. *Circulation* 81:196, 1990.

42. Paraskos JA. Cardiovascular pharmacology III: atropine, calcium, calcium blockers, and beta-blockers. *Circulation* 74(Suppl IV):IV-86, 1986.

43. Bhatia SJS, Smith TW. Digitalis toxicity: mechanisms, diagnosis, and management. *J Cardiac Surg* 2:453, 1987.

44. Indolfi C, et al. Effect of digoxin on epicardial coronary artery diameter in man. *Circulation* 82(Suppl III):III-149, 1990.

45. Purdy RE, Boucek RJ. Congestive Heart Failure. In RE Purdy and RJ Boucek (eds), *Handbook of Cardiac Drugs*. Boston: Little, Brown, 1988, Pp. 42–47.

46. Novitzky D, et al. Triiodothyronine as an inotropic agent after open heart surgery. *J Thorac Cardiovasc Surg* 98:972, 1989.

47. Coleman GM, et al. Efficacy of metabolic support with glucose-insulin-potassium for left ventricular pump failure after aortocoronary bypass surgery. *Circulation* 80(Suppl I):I-91, 1989.

48. Jett GK, et al. Vasoactive drug effects on blood flow in internal mammary artery and saphenous vein grafts. *J Thorac Cardiovasc Surg* 94:2, 1987.

49. Patel CB, et al. Use of sodium nitroprusside in post-coronary bypass surgery. *Chest* 89:663, 1986.

50. D'Ambra MN, et al. Prostaglandin E_1: A new therapy for refractory right heart failure and pulmonary hypertension after mitral valve replacement. *J Thorac Cardiovasc Surg* 89:567, 1985.

51. Balderman SC, Aldridge J. Pharmacologic support of the myocardium following aortocoronary bypass surgery: A comparative study. *J Clin Pharmacol* 26:175, 1986.

52. Sturm JT, et al. Combined use of dopamine and nitroprusside therapy in conjunction with intra-aortic balloon pumping for the treatment of postcardiotomy low-output syndrome. *J Thorac Cardiovasc Surg* 82:13, 1981.

53. Miller DC, et al. Postoperative enhancement of left ventricular performance by combined inotropic-vasodilator therapy with preload control. *Surgery* 88:108, 1980.

54. Scheidt S, et al. Mechanical circulatory assistance with the intraaortic balloon pump and other counterpulsation devices. *Prog Cardiovasc Dis* 25:55, 1982.

55. Miller LW. Mechanical assist devices in intensive cardiac care. *Am Heart J* 121:1887, 1991.

56. Pae WE, et al. Long-term results of ventricular assist pumping in postcardiotomy cardiogenic shock. *J Thorac Cardiovasc Surg* 93:434, 1987.

57. Christakis GT, et al. Right ventricular function and metabolism. *Circulation* 82(Suppl IV):IV-332, 1990.

58. Reuse C, Vincent J-L, Pinsky MR. Measurements of right ventricular volumes during fluid challenge. *Chest* 98:1450, 1990.

59. Vlahakes GJ, Turley K, Hoffman JIE. The pathophysiology of failure in acute right ventricular hypertension: Hemodynamic and biochemical correlations. *Circulation* 63:87, 1981.

60. D'Ambra MN, Beller JP. Pulmonary Circulation: Pharmacologic

Management. In HC Grillo, et al. (eds), *Current Therapy in Cardiothoracic Surgery*. Toronto: B C Decker, 1989. Pp. 278–282.

61. Standards and guidelines for cardiopulmonary resuscitation (CPR) and emergency cardiac care (ECC). *JAMA* 255:2843, 1986.

62. Weaver WD, et al. Effect of epinephrine and lidocaine on outcome after cardiac arrest due to ventricular fibrillation. *Circulation* 82:2027, 1990.

63. Bircher N, Safar P, Stewart R. A comparison of standard, "MAST"-augmented and open-chest CPR in dogs: A preliminary investigation. *Crit Care Med* 8:147, 1980.

64. McKowen RL, et al. Infectious complications and cost-effectiveness of open resuscitation in the surgical intensive care unit after cardiac surgery. *Ann Thorac Surg* 40:388, 1985.

65. Otto CW. Cardiovascular Pharmacology II: The use of catecholamines, pressor agents, digitalis, and corticosteroids in CPR and emergency cardiac care. *Circulation* 7(Suppl IV):IV-80, 1986.

66. Callaham M. Advances in the management of cardiac arrest. *West J Med* 145:670, 1986.

67. Raehl CL. Endotracheal drug therapy in cardiopulmonary resuscitation. *Clin Pharm* 5:572, 1986.

68. Weil MH, et al. Difference in acid-base state between venous and arterial blood during cardiopulmonary resuscitation. *N Engl J Med* 315:153, 1986.

69. Charlap S, et al. Electromechanical dissociation: diagnosis, pathophysiology, and management. *Am Heart J* 118:355, 1989.

70. Thompson BM, et al. Calcium: limited indications, some danger. *Circulation* 74(Suppl IV):IV-90, 1986.

71. Baerman JM, et al. Natural history and determinants of conduction defects following coronary bypass surgery. *Ann Thorac Surg* 44:150, 1987.

72. Keefe DL, et al. Atrioventricular conduction abnormalities in patients undergoing isolated aortic or mitral valve replacement. *PACE* 8:393, 1985.

73. Del Nido P, Goldman BS. Temporary epicardial pacing after open heart surgery: complications and preventions. *J Cardiac Surg* 4:99, 1989.

74. Finkelmeier BA, O'Mara SR. Temporary pacing in the cardiac surgical patient. *Crit Care Nurse* 4:108, 1984.

75. Steinman RT, et al. Wide QRS tachycardia in the conscious adult — ventricular tachycardia is the most frequent cause. *JAMA* 261:1013, 1989.

76. Gray RJ, et al. Esmolol: A new ultrashort-acting beta-adrenergic blocking agent for rapid control of heart rate in postoperative supraventricular tachyarrhythmias. *J Am Coll Cardiol* 5:1451, 1985.

77. Hashimoto K, Ilstrup DM, Schaff HV. Influence of clinical and hemodynamic variables on risk of supraventricular tachycardia

after coronary artery bypass. *J Thorac Cardiovasc Surg* 101:56, 1991.

78. Leitch JW, et al. The importance of age as a predictor of atrial fibrillation and flutter after coronary artery bypass grafting. *J Thorac Cardiovasc Surg* 100:338, 1990.

79. Douglass PS, Hirshfeld JW, Edmunds LH. Clinical correlates of atrial tachyarrhythmias after valve replacement for aortic stenosis. *Circulation* 72(Suppl II):II-159, 1985.

80. Taylor GJ, et al. Usefulness of atrial fibrillation as a predictor of stroke after isolated coronary artery bypass grafting. *Am J Cardiol* 60:905, 1987.

81. Mohr R, Smolinsky A, Goor DA. Prevention of supraventricular tachyarrhythmia with low-dose propranolol after coronary bypass. *J Thorac Cardiovasc Surg* 81:840, 1981.

82. Johnson LW, et al. Prophylactic digitalization for coronary artery bypass surgery. *Circulation* 53:819, 1976.

83. Tyras DH, et al. Supraventricular tachyarrhythmias after myocardial revascularization: A randomized trial of prophylactic digitalization. *J Thorac Cardiovasc Surg* 77:310, 1979.

84. Csicsko JF, Schatzlein MH, King RD. Immediate postoperative digitalization in the prophylaxis of supraventricular arrhythmias following coronary artery bypass. *J Thorac Cardiovasc Surg* 81:419, 1981.

85. Matangi MF, Neutze JM, Graham IC. Arrhythmia prophylaxis after aorta-coronary bypass: The effect of minidose propranolol. *J Thorac Cardiovasc Surg* 89:439, 1985.

86. Stephenson LW, et al. Propranolol for prevention of postoperative cardiac arrhythmias: A randomized study. *Ann Thorac Surg* 29:113, 1980.

87. Silverman NA, Wright R, Levitksy S. Efficacy of low-dose propranolol in preventing postoperative supraventricular tachyarrhythmias. *Ann Surg* 196:194, 1982.

88. Ferraris VA, et al. Verapamil prophylaxis for postoperative atrial dysrhythmias: A prospective, randomized double-blind study using drug level monitoring. *Ann Thorac Surg* 43:530, 1987.

89. Lauer MS, et al. Atrial fibrillation following coronary artery bypass surgery. *Prog Cardiovasc Dis* 31:367, 1989.

90. Andrews TC, et al. Prevention of supraventricular arrhythmias after coronary artery bypass surgery: A meta-analysis of randomized control trials. *Circulation* 84(Suppl III):III-236, 1991.

91. Kowey PR, et al. Meta-analysis of the effectiveness of prophylactic drug therapy in preventing supraventricular arrhythmia early after coronary artery bypass grafting. *Am J Cardiol* 69:963, 1992.

92. Falk RH, et al. Digoxin for converting recent-onset atrial fibrillation to sinus rhythm — a randomized, double-blinded trial. *Ann Intern Med* 106:503, 1987.

93. Plumb VJ, et al. Verapamil therapy of atrial fibrillation and atrial

flutter following cardiac operation. *J Thorac Cardiovasc Surg* 83:590, 1982.

94. Haft JI, Habbab MA. Treatment of atrial arrhythmias; effectiveness of verapamil when preceded by calcium infusion. *Arch Intern Med* 146:1085, 1986.

95. Barnett JC, Touchon RC. Short-term control of supraventricular tachycardia with verapamil infusion and calcium pretreatment. *Chest* 97:1106, 1990.

96. Salerno DM, et al., and the Diltiazem-Atrial Fibrillation/Flutter Study Group. Efficacy and safety of intravenous diltiazem for treatment of atrial fibrillation and atrial flutter. *Am J Cardiol* 63:1046, 1989.

97. Ellenbogen KA, et al. A placebo-controlled trial of intravenous diltiazem infusion of 24-hour heart rate control during atrial defibrillation and atrial flutter: A multicenter study. *J Am Coll Cardiol* 18:891, 1991.

98. Schwartz M, et al. Esmolol: Safety and efficacy in postoperative cardiothoracic patients with supraventricular tachyarrhythmias. *Chest* 93:705, 1988.

99. Suttorp MJ, et al. The value of class IC antiarrhythmic drugs for acute conversion of paroxysmal atrial fibrillation or flutter to sinus rhythm. *J Am Coll Cardiol* 16:1722, 1990.

100. Connolly SJ, et al. Randomized placebo controlled trial of propafenone for treatment of atrial tachyarrhythmias after cardiac surgery. *J Am Coll Cardiol* 10:1145, 1987.

101. Wafa SS, et al. Efficacy of flecainide acetate for atrial arrhythmias following coronary bypass grafting. *Am J Cardiol* 63:1058, 1989.

102. Suttorp MJ, et al. Effectiveness of sotalol in preventing supraventricular tachyarrhythmias shortly after coronary artery bypass grafting. *Am J Cardiol* 68:1163, 1991.

103. Gillette PC. Diagnosis and management of postoperative junctional ectopic tachycardia. *Am Heart J* 118:192, 1989.

104. Camm AJ, Garratt CJ. Adenosine and supraventricular tachycardia. *N Engl J Med* 325:1621, 1991.

105. Lerman BB, Belardinelli L. Cardiac electrophysiology of adenosine. *Circulation* 83:1500, 1991.

106. Kron IL, et al. Unanticipated postoperative ventricular tachyarrhythmias. *Ann Thorac Surg* 38:317, 1984.

107. Aylward PE, Kerber RE. The technique of electrical countershock. *J Crit Illness* 1:47, 1986.

108. Walls JT, et al. Adverse effects of permanent cardiac internal defibrillator patches on external defibrillation. *Am J Cardiol* 64:1144, 1989.

109. Mangano DT and the Study of Perioperative Ischemia (SPI) Research Group. Myocardial ischemia following surgery: Preliminary findings. *J Cardiac Surg* 5:288, 1990.

110. Chaitman BR, et al. Participating CASS Medical Centers. Use of

survival analysis to determine the clinical significance of new Q waves after coronary bypass surgery. *Circulation* 67:302, 1983.

111. Val PG, et al. Diagnostic criteria and prognosis of perioperative myocardial infarction following coronary bypass. *J Thorac Cardiovasc Surg* 86:878, 1983.

112. Namay DL, et al. Effect of perioperative myocardial infarction on late survival in patients undergoing coronary artery bypass surgery. *Circulation* 65:1066, 1982.

113. Force T, et al. Perioperative myocardial infarction after coronary bypass surgery. *Circulation* 82:903, 1990.

114. Baur HR, et al. Serum myocardial creatine kinase (CK-MB) after coronary arterial bypass surgery. *Am J Cardiol* 44:679, 1979.

115. Van Lente F, et al. The predictive value of serum enzymes for perioperative myocardial infarction after cardiac operations. *J Thorac Cardiovasc Surg* 98:704, 1989.

116. Berger HJ, Zaret BL. Nuclear cardiology. *N Engl J Med* 305:799, 1981.

117. Burns RJ, et al. Myocardial infarction determined by technetium-99m pyrophosphate single-photon tomography complicating elective coronary artery bypass grafting for angina pectoris. *Am J Cardiol* 63:1429, 1989.

118. Klein RC, et al. Evaluation of the effects of systemic nitroglycerin on perfusion of ischemic myocardium in coronary heart disease assessed intraoperatively by antegrade blood flow through intact saphenous vein bypass grafts. *Am Heart J* 101:292, 1981.

119. Lemmer JH Jr, Kirsh MM. Coronary artery spasm following coronary artery surgery. *Ann Thorac Surg* 46:108, 1988.

120. Skarvan K, et al. Coronary artery spasms after coronary artery bypass surgery. *Anesthesiology* 61:323, 1984.

121. Carter AR, et al. Thoracic alterations after cardiac surgery. *AJR* 140:475, 1983.

122. Bevelaqua F, et al. Complications after cardiac operations in patients with severe pulmonary impairment. *Ann Thorac Surg* 50:602, 1990.

123. Banaszak EF, et al. Radiological manifestations of pulmonary complications following coronary artery bypass grafting. *Chest* 96:240S, 1989.

124. Shapira N, et al. Determinants of pulmonary function in patients undergoing coronary bypass. *Ann Thorac Surg* 50:268, 1990.

125. Ferdinande PG, et al. Pulmonary function tests after different techniques for coronary artery bypass surgery. *Intensive Care Med* 14:623, 1988.

126. Berrizbeitia LD, et al. Effect of sternotomy and coronary bypass surgery on postoperative pulmonary mechanics. *Chest* 96:873, 1989.

127. Matthay MA, Wiener-Kronish JP. Respiratory management after cardiac surgery. *Chest* 95:424, 1989.

128. Bittar G, Friedman HS. The arrhythmogenicity of theophylline. *Chest* 99:1415, 1991.

129. Curtis JJ, et al. Elevated hemidiaphragm after cardiac operations: Incidence, prognosis, and relationship to the use of topical ice slush. *Ann Thorac Surg* 48:764, 1989.

130. Wheeler WE, et al. Etiology and prevention of topical cardiac hypothermia-induced phrenic nerve injury and left lower lobe atelectasis during cardiac surgery. *Chest* 88:680, 1985.

131. Chandler KW, et al. Bilateral diaphragmatic paralysis complicating local cardiac hypothermia during open heart surgery. *Am J Med* 77:243, 1984.

132. Esposito RA, Spencer FC. The effect of pericardial insulation on hypothermic phrenic nerve injury during open heart surgery. *Ann Thorac Surg* 43:303, 1987.

133. Watanabe T, et al. Phrenic nerve paralysis after pediatric cardiac surgery. *J Thorac Cardiovasc Surg* 94:383, 1987.

134. Shoemaker R, et al. Aggressive treatment of acquired phrenic nerve paralysis in infants and small children. *Ann Thorac Surg* 32:251, 1981.

135. Coraim FG, et al. Acute respiratory failure after cardiac surgery: Clinical experience with the application of continuous arteriovenous hemofiltration. *Crit Care Med* 14:714, 1986.

136. Hamilton-Farrell MR, Hanson GC. General care of the ventilated patient in the intensive care unit. *Thorax* 45:962, 1990.

137. Whited RE. A prospective study on laryngotracheal sequelae in long-term intubation. *Laryngoscope* 94:367, 1984.

138. Marsh HM, Gillespie DJ, Baumgartner AE. Timing of tracheostomy in the critically ill patient. *Chest* 96:190, 1989.

139. Stauffer JL, Olsen DE, Petty TL. Complications and consequences of endotracheal intubation and tracheostomy: A prospective study of 150 critically ill adult patients. *Am J Med* 70:65, 1981.

140. Mathay WA, Wiener-Kronish JP. Respiratory management after cardiac surgery. *Chest* 95:424, 1989.

141. Murphy MC, Newman BM, Rodgers BM. Pleuroperitoneal shunts in the management of persistent chylothorax. *Ann Thorac Surg* 48:195, 1989.

142. Kollef MH, et al. Delayed pleuropulmonary complications following coronary artery revascularization with the internal mammary artery. *Chest* 94:68, 1988.

Postoperative Complications Involving Other Organ Systems

Bleeding After Cardiac Surgery

Management of early postoperative bleeding is a familiar task for those who care for cardiac surgical patients. Some bleeding occurs after all cardiac operations that utilize cardiopulmonary bypass, and it is significant enough to require early reoperation to control hemorrhage in 2 to 5% of patients. Postoperative blood losses are often unusually excessive in reoperations, in cyanotic patients, and in patients who have experienced prolonged cardiopulmonary bypass times [1]. Excessive bleeding after open heart surgery may be the result of one or several of many factors including: inadequate surgical hemostasis (so-called surgical bleeding), platelet dysfunction, platelet depletion, plasma clotting factor deficiency, residual heparin effect (incomplete reversal by protamine), primary fibrinolysis, and consumption coagulopathy. In a patient suffering excessive bleeding early after open heart surgery, the major problem is determining whether the bleeding is secondary to a reversible coagulation abnormality or whether it is due to mechanical (surgical) causes such as a leaking suture line.

Mediastinal drainage tubes are routinely placed at the completion of the operation and are attached to suction collection receptacles. These allow for periodic determination of the rate of bleeding by simply observing how fast blood is collecting in the calibrated receptacle. Although there is no strict definition of "excessive" postoperative bleeding, serious concern should be raised when the mediastinal-tube output exceeds 4 to 5 ml/kg/hr during the first few hours after operation. Early postoperative bleeding typically decreases significantly during the first 3 to 4 hours after surgery and becomes relatively minimal (less than 0.5 ml/kg/hr) by 6 hours. When postoperative bleeding exceeds these general guidelines, efforts must be made to determine the presence or absence of treatable conditions (e.g., coagulopathy) and whether to return the patient to the operating room for surgical exploration. When the rate of bleeding is massive (i.e., more than 8 to 10 ml/kg/hr), the prompt return of the patient to the operating room for exploration is usually indicated.

Platelet abnormalities are the most common cause of nonsurgical postoperative bleeding [2]. Postoperative thrombocytopenia may be present in patients who have required intraaortic balloon or ventricular assist device placement before surgery. Patients treated with heparin before surgery may also have heparin-associated thrombocytopenia [3,4]. Hemodilution due to the priming volume of the cardiopulmonary bypass circuit results in a decrease in the patient's platelet count, but usually not below 100,000 platelets/mm^3; long bypass times may result in a greater decrease in the platelet count. More important, a reversible loss of platelet function accompanies surgery using cardiopulmonary bypass. The cause for the dysfunction is not clear, but it is likely related to platelet activation and degranulation during bypass from contact with the nonendothelialized surfaces of the bypass circuit (tubing and oxygenator) or to direct trauma to platelet membrane receptors. Hypothermia may contribute to the temporary impairment of platelet function. Whatever the cause, a definite transient decrease in platelet function occurs, prolonging the patient's bleeding time early after cardiac surgery; this abnormality usually disappears within 2 to 4 hours after the procedure [5]. Aspirin is an effective adjunct in the treatment for unstable angina and is frequently administered after thrombolytic therapy for acute myocardial infarction. Patients who take aspirin before open heart surgery experience a further insult to effective platelet function and have an increased risk of abnormal postoperative bleeding, an increased need for postoperative blood transfusion, and an increased incidence of reoperation for hemorrhage [6,7]. When administered for the purpose of improving coronary artery bypass patency, aspirin should be given only postoperatively (within 6 hours of surgery); this will avoid the increased bleeding effects while maintaining the beneficial effects on early graft patency [8].

Hemodilution cardiopulmonary bypass results in significant decreases in plasma clotting factor concentrations, but the postoperative levels usually remain well above the level (25–30% of normal) required for normal hemostatic function [5]. Thus, clotting factor deficiency is not a frequent cause of postoperative bleeding. It would, however, be expected to play a role in patients who have received massive transfusions of packed red blood cells, due to further dilution of the clotting factors, and in very polycythemic patients whose plasma volume is reduced. Assessment of the plasma clotting factor function is by measurement of the prothrombin time (PT). This test of the extrinsic portion of the clotting system has a normal upper-limit value of 13 seconds, although values of up to 16 seconds usually indicate sufficient clotting factor concentration to effect relatively normal clotting under most circumstances. Treatment of clotting factor deficiency (when the patient is bleeding) consists of the administration of a sufficient quantity of fresh frozen plasma over a short period of time. Thus 15 ml/kg of fresh frozen plasma (3–4 units for the average-size adult) are administered quickly while attending to the patient's filling pressures (central venous and pulmonary artery diastolic or wedge pressure) to avoid fluid overload.

In order to prevent thrombosis within the cardiopulmonary bypass circuit during operation, large doses of heparin are administered to the patient. Heparin, a negatively charged polysaccharide, enhances the efficacy of the naturally occurring coagulation inhibitor, antithrombin III [9]. Heparin sensitivity is quite variable among individuals and is lower in pediatric patients as compared with adults. At the end of the cardiopulmonary bypass period, the heparin effect is reversed by the administration of protamine. Protamine, a positively charged polypeptide, binds with heparin, removing it from antithrombin III, and the ability of the blood to coagulate is restored. During the cardiopulmonary bypass, the adequacy of heparinization is measured by the activated clotting time (ACT) or heparin quantification based on protamine neutralization (Hepcon system). Various protocols for maintenance of adequate intraoperative anticoagulation are utilized [10]. After completion of bypass and the neutralization of heparin, the reappearance of circulating heparin in the blood with resultant bleeding (the so-called heparin rebound) has been described [11]. This is attributed to the return of administered heparin from the extravascular to the intravascular space and to the shorter half-life of protamine as compared with heparin. The incidence of heparin rebound and its relation to the problem of postoperative bleeding is not known. During the postoperative period, the presence of unneutralized heparin is suggested by a prolongation of the ACT or the activated partial thromboplastin time (APTT), although these tests are not specific for heparin. Performance of the thrombin time (TT) using blood drawn directly from the patient's vein (to avoid contamination by heparin flush solution) will confirm the presence or absence of heparin. In practice, it is customary to administer additional protamine (25–50 mg) to the bleeding patient who has a prolonged ACT or APTT, even without confirmation of heparin presence by the TT. The risk of additional protamine is minimal, although it should be given slowly to avoid hypotension.

Primary fibrinolysis, once thought to be a common contributor to bleeding early after cardiac surgery, is now believed to be a rare cause, although it may occur occasionally, especially in patients with cyanotic heart disease. Laboratory studies suggestive of fibrinolyis — such as a shortened euglobulin clot lysis time, decreased fibrinogen level, and elevated level of fibrinogen degradation products (FDP) — usually reflect hemodilution, normal factor consumption due to surgical trauma to tissues, and secondary fibrinolysis, rather than a primary consumptive process [5]. The presence of low-to-moderate levels of FDP is common after open heart surgery and does not indicate pathologic lysis. When significant, fibrinolysis may be treated with aminocaproic acid (Amicar), but caution is urged in the use of this agent, which, if infused intravenously at a rapid rate, may rarely result in hypotension and arrhythmias. For adults, a loading dose of 5.0 g Amicar is given over 1 hour followed by continuous infusion of 1.0 g/hr for 5 to 8 hours. When administered to the patient who is not anticoagulated, uncontrolled thrombosis can potentially occur. For most patients with postoperative bleeding, aminocaproic acid is not indicated and presents certain hazards.

Serious consumption coagulopathy (or disseminated intravascular coagulation) is also an unlikely cause of early postoperative bleeding [5]. Significant decreases in fibrinogen and plasminogen levels occur with open heart surgery due to hemodilution, but these return to normal after 12 to 24 hours. Sufficient plasma levels of fibrinogen are, however, required for normal hemostasis. Hemodilution (especially if large amounts of blood have been transfused) and prolonged bypass time (with subclinical consumption of fibrinogen occurring in the oxygenator) may lead to insufficient levels of plasma fibrinogen in the absence of pathologic consumption. For the bleeding patient with a low fibrinogen level (below 100 mg/dl), administration of cryoprecipitate is indicated. Each unit of cryoprecipitate contains about 250 mg of fibrinogen, and this will raise the adult plasma fibrinogen level by about 10 mg/dl. The usual adult dose is 10 units. The pediatric dose is 1 unit of cryoprecipitate per 5 kg of body weight.

MANAGEMENT OF THE BLEEDING PATIENT

When excessive bleeding is present, replacement of the blood loss at a rate sufficient to maintain the patient's red cell volume and intravascular volume at desired levels is required. Although blood conservation and avoidance of blood product transfusion are important, overzealous application of these principles may result in dangerous anemia or hypovolemia, particularly if the rate of blood loss suddenly increases. Thus, in the bleeding patient, it is wise to maintain a margin of safety with regard to the hematocrit (28–30%) and intravascular volume level (keep at a level appropriate to the patient's ventricular function and cardiac lesion).

Massive bleeding mandates prompt reoperation. There are no identified criteria to assist in the recognition of patients with surgically correctable causes of excessive mediastinal bleeding other than a high rate of early bleeding [12]. If the patient is sufficiently stable for transport, reentry may be performed in the operating room. This is preferable, as recannulation and cardiopulmonary bypass occasionally are required to correct a bleeding site on the back of the heart. If the patient is unstable, reexploration may be performed in the intensive care unit with only a relatively few instruments being required. It is important for every cardiac surgical intensive care unit to have a sterile set of instruments (including wire cutters and sternal retractor) and a good light source ready at all times for this purpose. Often the bleeding site can be repaired in the intensive care unit. If not, it is usually possible at least to control the bleeding with digital pressure and transfuse the patient until he or she is sufficiently stable for transfer to the operating room for definitive repair. Open resuscitation in the intensive care unit results in surprisingly few infections if sterile technique is used and antibiotics are administered [13].

When the rate of bleeding is excessive, but not massive, the decision whether to reoperate is sometimes a difficult one. The approach to this situation is to correct the hemostatic abnormalities as best as possible and, if bleeding continues, then to perform exploration. A useful algorithm for the management of the bleeding patient is shown in Figure 5-1.

An examination of the patient provides some clues to the nature of the patient's bleeding. Diffuse oozing from the skin incision and intravenous catheter sites suggests a platelet abnormality; failure of blood within the mediastinal tubes to clot suggests a platelet or coagulation factor abnormality or both; and the presence of clotted blood in the patient's tubes suggests relatively normal hemostatic function and the presence of surgical bleeding.

Laboratory studies are essential. When the patient is bleeding excessively, the following studies should be drawn, preferably by a new venipuncture: PT, APTT, platelet count, and fibrinogen level.

Treatment of the bleeding patient may be initiated by providing 5 to 10 cm of positive end-expiratory pressure (PEEP) to the ventilator settings. Although conflicting data are available, this maneuver may reduce bleeding through a tamponade effect [14]. Care must be taken, however, as excessive PEEP may decrease cardiac output (especially in the presence of hypovolemia), and overexpansion of the lungs may be detrimental to internal mammary artery bypass

5. Postoperative Complications Involving Other Organ Systems 161

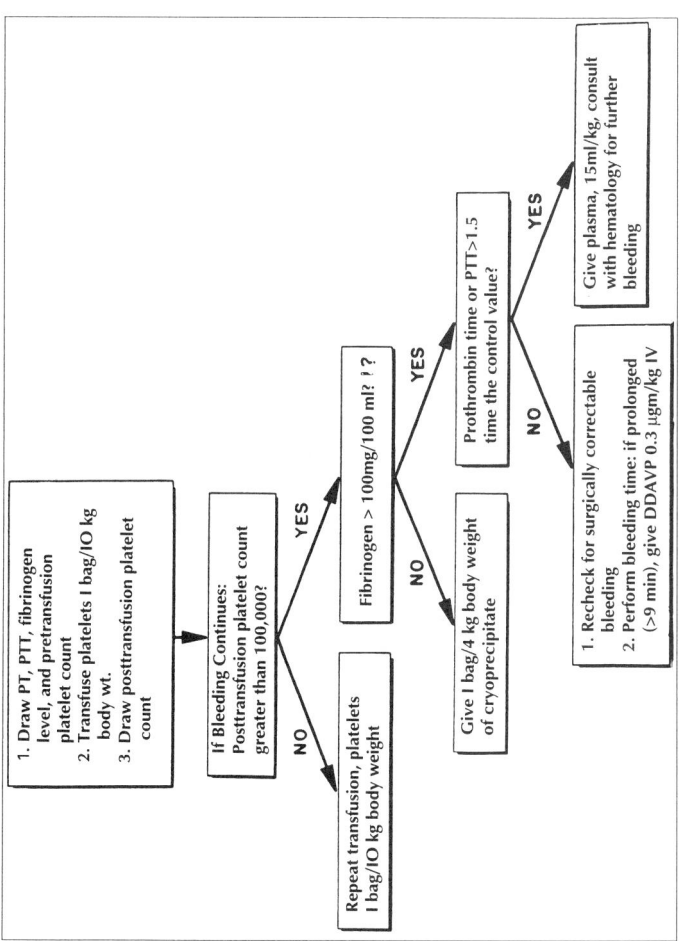

Fig. 5-1. An algorithm for management of the patient who is bleeding excessively early after cardiac surgery. *Key:* PT = prothrombin time; PTT = partial thromboplastin time; DDAVP = deamino-D-arginine vasopressin (also known as desmopressin acetate). (Reprinted with permission from the Society of Thoracic Surgeons. LT Goodnough, et al. Guidelines for transfusion support in patients undergoing coronary artery bypass grafting. *Ann. Thorac Surg* 50:675, 1990.)

grafts, if present. An empiric dose of 25 to 50 mg of protamine may be given (slowly) while awaiting the results of the laboratory studies. Control of hypertension, if present, will help reduce the rate of bleeding. For this purpose, an intravenous infusion of a short-acting agent such as nitroglycerin or nitroprusside is chosen.

Since platelet abnormalities are the most common identifiable cause of nonsurgical postoperative bleeding, transfusion of platelets is performed, even if the platelet count has not yet been reported from the laboratory or if it is in the relatively normal range (above 100,000/mm^3). Although the quantity of platelets may be relatively normal, those present may be dysfunctional and may not provide adequate clot formation. Children receive 5–10 ml/kg of platelet concentrate, whereas adults receive 1 plasmapheresis unit (equal to about 6 individual platelet units). After transfusion, the platelet count should be repeated. If bleeding continues and the count is less than 100,000/mm^3, a repeat platelet transfusion should be performed.

If the patient's PT is greater than 17 to 18 seconds (or 1.5 times the laboratory control), then a plasma clotting factor deficiency is likely present and treatment with fresh frozen plasma (15 ml/kg) is indicated. Studies suggest clotting factor replacement is not required at a PT of less than 16 seconds [15]. Many surgeons, however, will administer fresh frozen plasma to the bleeding patient whenever the PT is abnormal. If the APTT is significantly prolonged (twice normal or greater), consideration should be given to the possibility of a continued heparin effect and to the administration of more protamine. If the fibrinogen level is less than 100 mg/dl, transfusion of cryoprecipitate is indicated.

As discussed in chapter 2, desmopressin acetate has not been demonstrated to be effective for routine use in open heart surgery. It may, however, have a role in the treatment of the bleeding patient to improve platelet function (especially for patients who receive preoperative aspirin) or following complex operations [16]. Although the role of desmopressin remains undefined at this time, it is a relatively safe agent having rare major adverse effects — hyponatremia and seizures [17]. Treatment consists of an intravenous dose of 0.3 µg/kg (in 50 ml of normal saline for adults or 10 ml of normal saline for infants) given over 30 minutes.

Excessive postoperative bleeding results in the need for red cell transfusion. This can be minimized by the use of autotransfusion blood collection systems, but this blood is devoid of platelets and plasma coagulation factors. For every 4 to 5 units of red blood cells transfused (or retransfused) to the patient, 2 units of fresh frozen plasma usually should be given to prevent coagulation factor dilution to levels below those needed for adequate hemostasis function. Massive blood transfusions may result in elevated bilirubin and liver enzyme levels, which become apparent several days later.

CARDIAC TAMPONADE

The most serious acute result of excessive postoperative mediastinal bleeding is the development of cardiac tamponade. Frequently, this develops in the patient who is bleeding rapidly initially, but then suddenly slows as coagulation defects have been corrected. Tamponade is a potentially fatal complication that may develop slowly or rapidly and may be difficult to diagnose.

Of the possible causes of shock early after cardiac surgery, tamponade may occur as frequently as ventricular dysfunction and may be treated more easily [18]. In the early postoperative setting, tamponade occurs due to blood in the pericardial space causing impairment of heart filling (usually by compression of the right atrium or ventricle or both). Tamponade results in decreased cardiac output. In a postoperative patient with low cardiac output, tamponade must always be considered and ruled out. The classic physical examination signs of tamponade (muffled heart sounds, jugular venous distention, Kussmaul's sign, and pulsus paradoxus) may be difficult to discern or may be absent in the intubated patient in the noisy intensive care unit environment. Hypotension, narrowed pulse pressure, tachycardia, low mixed venous oxygen saturation, and elevated venous pressures are nonspecific and may be present as the result of either tamponade or ventricular dysfunction. Hemodynamic measurements will demonstrate elevation of the central venous pressure to the level of the left heart filling pressure (left atrial, pulmonary artery capillary wedge, or pulmonary artery diastolic pressure), referred to as *equalization of filling pressures*. In many patients, the chest x-ray will reveal a widened mediastinal shadow, although this is also common in postoperative patients without tamponade [19].

Echocardiography may be useful in determining the presence of cardiac tamponade. In general, the finding of right ventricular diastolic collapse in patients with pericardial effusion is sensitive and specific in the diagnosis of tamponade, although this echocardiographic finding may be less useful in early postoperative patients [20,21]. In this setting, transesophageal echocardiography is often superior to transthoracic echocardiography [22]. Occasional patients will suffer regional cardiac tamponade with a loculated blood collection located posterior or lateral to the heart. In these patients, right ventricular collapse will be absent but impairment of left ventricular filling will be suggested by echocardiography [23].

Even if echocardiography does not demonstrate tamponade, a high index of suspicion still must be maintained; immediate decompression may be lifesaving for the patient who decompensates acutely. Frequently, if urgent decompression is needed, it may be accomplished by opening the inferior portion of the patient's wound and introducing a gloved finger into the mediastinal space. If the diagnosis of tamponade is correct, the surgeon (and patient) will be rewarded by an outpouring of bloody fluid and rapid improvement in the patient's hemodynamic status. If this does not produce relief, a sternotomy may be required in the intensive care unit. If the diagnosis is incorrect, the morbidity from this is generally minimal. Patients with tamponade who are relatively stable may be transferred to the operating room for a reentry sternotomy and clot removal, generally with minimal complications and no increase in the length of hospital stay. *The greatest danger is that cardiac tamponade may go unrecognized and untreated.*

Renal Failure

Despite the hemodynamic perturbations caused by cardiac surgery utilizing cardiopulmonary bypass, significant changes in renal function are unusual [24]. In one report, oliguric acute renal failure occurred in 1.5% of 752 patients who underwent cardiac operations, and the mortality of the complication was 27% [25]. Less severe renal insufficiency may develop in 5 to 10% of cardiac surgery patients [26,27]. Preoperative variables associated with postoperative renal failure include elevated serum creatinine levels, concurrent coronary bypass and valve surgery, and advanced age [28]. Additionally, prolonged periods of cardiopulmonary bypass, aortic cross-clamping, and total duration of operation correlate with an increased incidence of postoperative renal insufficiency [29].

Renal failure after cardiac surgery is usually secondary to acute tubular necrosis as the result of impaired kidney perfusion. Drug toxicity and cholesterol emboli are other potential causes. Acute tubular necrosis is frequently a reversible process, although proper management is required to prevent secondary complications (hyperkalemia, fluid overload, and uremia) until renal function returns.

The diagnosis should be suspected in the patient with little urinary output (less than 30 ml/hr for 2–3 consecutive hours) and rising creatinine levels in the early postoperative period. It is first necessary to be sure that the patient's bladder catheter is not obstructed by irrigating it with 30 to 60 ml of sterile saline. Palpation of the lower abdomen to exclude bladder distention is important. Next, it must be ensured that the patient has adequate intravascular volume and cardiac output. Hypovolemia and low cardiac output will further contribute to kidney injury. If filling pressures are low or normal (central venous or pulmonary capillary wedge pressure less than 15–18 mm Hg), a fluid challenge should be given. If the hematocrit is low, the red blood cell volume should be increased with packed red blood cell transfusion. Otherwise, a bolus infusion of 500 to 1000 ml of crystalloid solution may be administered over 30 to 60 minutes (10 ml/kg for pediatric patients).

If there is little or no response to the fluid challenge, a large dose of furosemide (100–200 mg IV for adults; 2–4 mg/kg IV for infants) is sometimes successful in initiating urine flow. At Massachusetts General Hospital, an infusion of furosemide with mannitol is utilized (1.0 g of furosemide in 500 ml of 20% mannitol). The infusion is begun at 5 to 10 ml/hr in adults (0.1 ml/kg/hr for pediatric patients). The infusion rate is adjusted according to response. Low-dose dopamine (2–3 µg/kg/min IV) infusion also should be started. Presumably by improving total renal blood flow and intrarenal blood flow distribution, low-dose dopamine has been demonstrated to improve urine output and associated renal function variables with acute postoperative renal insufficiency [30].

Despite these measures, oliguric renal failure may develop, and even very high doses of loop diuretics will not be effective in maintaining urine output. Should oliguric renal failure occur, efforts are directed to preventing complications of the oliguric state. Fluid intake should be limited to daily output plus about 500 ml in adults. Frequent physical examination will help to follow the state of hydration of the patient. Potassium should not be administered unless the serum level falls below 3.5 mEq/liter. Even then, replacement should be done cautiously, in small amounts, and frequent determinations of the serum potassium level are required to recognize hyperkalemia early. Magnesium-containing antacids should be discontinued and replaced with aluminum hydroxide antacids (Basaljel or Amphojel, 15–30 ml 3 times daily) to prevent hypermagnesemia and to decrease intestinal absorption of phosphate. Patients on drugs eliminated by renal excretion must be monitored carefully, and dosages should be changed as indicated. Aspirin should be discontinued. Serum levels of aminoglycoside antibiotics, digoxin, antiarrhythmic agents, and other drugs should be followed closely (Appendix 4), and doses should be decreased as indicated. Appendix 5 lists some of the commonly used drugs that should be considered for adjusted doses in the presence of renal failure.

For most oliguric patients, intervention will be required at some point to treat hyperkalemia, acidosis, fluid overload, or complications of uremia, such as lethargy and pericarditis. Peritoneal dialysis can be performed conveniently at the bedside, and it is particularly useful for infants with renal failure. Hemodialysis is usually the preferred method, although it may not be well tolerated by patients with recent cardiac surgery because of the possibility of hypotension and cardiovascular collapse. For adult patients, continuous arteriovenous hemofiltration has proven to be very successful for the management of postoperative renal failure [31–33]. In this technique, gradual filtration of the blood is accomplished at a rate slower than hemodialysis (blood flow rate through the hemofilter being 50–100 ml/min). The mechanism of fluid removal is by hydrostatic pressure. Solutes (such as potassium) accompany the fluid, and the removed fluid is replaced with physiologic (potassium-free) solution as needed. Up to 500 ml/hr of fluid may be removed. Hemofiltration is simpler than hemodialysis but requires longer periods of use in order to accomplish the same degree of fluid or solute removal. The important advantage of continuous hemofiltration is that it does not result in the hemodynamic instability that commonly occurs with conventional hemodialysis. Such instability, predominantly hypotension, may result in arrhythmias and myocardial ischemia, thus limiting the use of conventional dialysis in some cardiac surgery patients.

Occasional patients will suffer nonoliguric renal failure after cardiac surgery; this form of kidney failure is generally much easier to manage. When the patient urinates in satisfactory or even excessive amounts, it is important to monitor accurately urine output, daily weight, and serum electrolyte concentrations. Replacement should be provided as indicated to prevent hypovolemia and electrolyte abnormalities, usually by matching the urine output with administration of one-half normal saline.

Acute renal failure requiring dialysis after cardiac surgery is a complication associated with high mortality, but most of the patients who die also suffer complications of other organ systems. Patients with isolated renal failure, however, can have a very hopeful prognosis with a survival rate of 80% [34].

Infectious Complications

As with any type of surgery, infectious complications of cardiac surgery can lead to considerable morbidity and mortality. The economic implications in terms of a prolonged hospital stay, increased hospital bill to the patient, and increased cost to the hospital are considerable [35]. Although rather rare in pediatric patients, serious infectious problems complicate cardiac operations in a significant proportion of adult patients [36,37]. Pneumonia and wound infections remain the most common among the potential postoperative infections.

PNEUMONIA

Although only occurring in 1 to 4% of patients, postoperative pneumonia carries with it a mortality rate of 25% [38]. Patients found to be at increased risk for the development of postoperative pneumonia include those with chronic obstructive lung disease, those requiring more than 2 days of mechanical ventilation after operation, and those who were prophylactically administered gastric acid inhibitors (antacids or H_2 blockers). The diagnosis of pneumonia is based on the presence of fever, the development of an infiltrate on chest x-ray, and a sputum culture that grows a predominant organism. Treatment is by administration of specific antibiotics, aggressive pulmonary toilet, and ventilator support as required.

WOUND INFECTIONS AND MEDIASTINITIS

Wound infections after a sternotomy incision may be superficial, involving only the skin and subcutaneous fat, or they may be deep, involving the sternum and underlying mediastinal structures.

Superficial infections are characterized by serosanguineous drainage and local inflammation with the underlying sternum remaining stable. In this instance, removal of the overlying skin sutures, culture of the drainage, administration of antibiotics, and local dressings are often successful treatment.

Deep infections, however, are usually associated with great morbidity in terms of patient pain, the need for reoperations, prolonged hospitalization, and death. Bacterial mediastinitis occurs in 0.8 to 2.0% of adult patients undergoing open heart surgery. In our experience, the incidence in children is much lower. In various published reports, the risk factors identified for the development of serious postoperative sternal wound complications include: bilateral internal mammary artery bypass grafting in diabetics, prolonged operative time, obesity, the need for blood transfusion greater than 5 units, history of emphysema, prolonged postoperative mechanical ventilation, reoperations, early chest reexploration for postoperative bleeding, and prolonged postoperative low cardiac output [39–42]. Patients with tracheostomies are also at increased risk for sternal incision infections due to the close proximity of the incision to the tracheal stoma, which is colonized by bacteria. If the tracheostomy is present before the sternotomy, all efforts should be made to isolate the stoma from the incision during the procedure and to avoid connecting the mediastinal dissection with the plane of the pretracheal fascia. If the tracheostomy is required postoperatively, the skin incision should be placed as high as possible, taking care to limit the dissection so that it does not communicate with the previous substernal dissection. The sternal wound should be protected from the tracheostomy by dressings.

Prophylactic antibiotic administration for cardiac surgery is the standard of care, although solid scientific evidence demonstrating the effectiveness of such treatment does not exist [43]. At our institutions, the prophylactic antibiotic of choice is a cephalosporin, such as cefazolin (Kefzol or Ancef) [44,45]. The intravenous infusion is begun in the operating room during preparations for surgery but before making the incision. The adult dose is 1.0 g and the pediatric dose is 15.0 mg/kg of body weight. A similar dose should be added to the prime solution of the cardiopulmonary bypass pump circuit. For patients undergoing implantation of foreign material (such as prosthetic valve or defibrillator implantation), some surgeons use vancomycin in addition to cefazolin for prophylactic antibiotic coverage. Postoperatively, the patient receives the same dose of cefazolin every 8 hours for 24 to 48 hours. Patients who are allergic to cefazolin and those with serious penicillin allergies (due to the real but low incidence of cross-reactivity) receive vancomycin instead of cephalosporin (adult dose, 1.0 g IV every 12 hours; pediatric dose, 15.0 mg/kg IV every 12 hours). It is important to administer vancomycin slowly because rapid infusion results in vasodilation and hypotension.

The early diagnosis of sternal infection and mediastinitis after cardiac surgery can be difficult. The standard chest radiograph is of little value in predicting infection or sternal dehiscence. A vertical sternal lucency (the so-called sternal stripe) is frequently seen on early postoperative chest x-ray but is not a sensitive indicator of infection or dehiscence in the absence of other findings [19]. In some patients, fever, leukocytosis, and a positive blood culture will be the first manifestations of the hidden infection that only later becomes obvious [46]. Most cases of postoperative sternal infection and mediastinitis occur within 2 weeks of surgery. The most common early sign is drainage from the wound; sternal instability usually develops subsequently. Sterile sternal dehiscence sometimes occurs, requiring rewiring, but this is not an infectious complication. In some patients, the diagnosis of sternal infection and mediastinitis may not be clear-cut. In such instances, we have found the chest CT to be of value. If infection is present, there may be an excessive amount of mediastinal fluid with air-fluid levels, bone destruction, and separation of the sternum. Needle aspiration of the mediastinum under CT scan guidance for Gram stain and culture of the fluid obtained may also be performed to aid in the diagnosis of mediastinitis.

Treatment of serious sternotomy wound infections depends on the stage of the process at the time of diagnosis. If early, when the sternum is infected but not destroyed, success is often achieved by prompt reoperation, debridement of the sternal edges, copious irrigation of the mediastinum, placement of retrosternal irrigation and drainage catheters, rewiring of the sternum, and closure of the fascia and skin. Appropriate intravenous antibiotics are administered for at least 7 days. A dilute antibiotic solution (such as vancomycin 15 mg in 1 liter of saline or gentamycin 5 mg in 1 liter of saline), chosen according to Gram-stain results, is infused through the irrigating catheters (we use flat Jackson-Pratt drains) at 100 to 200 ml/hr with the fluid exiting via the drainage catheters (32-Fr. chest tubes). The irrigations are continued until the drainage fluid is sterile by culture (usually 3–5 days). Although frequently successful, this method has potential associated complications such as erosion of the catheters into mediastinal structures, superinfection by *Candida*, and systemic toxicity from absorption of the irrigating antibiotic [33].

More long-standing, advanced infections are associated with large amounts of suppurative fluid in the mediastinum, loss of integrity of the sternum, and diffuse cellulitis of the skin and subcutaneous tissues. In the past, these patients frequently were treated by opening the sternum, exposing and draining the mediastinum, packing the wound with gauze, and allowing granulation tissue to form before secondary closure or skin grafting. This method, however, requires a very extended hospitalization and risks hemorrhage from mediastinal structures secondary to the dressing changes. More recently, a variety of methods have been developed to deal with serious mediastinal infection. These include the use of the omentum as a vascular pedicle for obliteration of the dead space after debridement and the use of various muscle flaps (especially the pectoralis and rectus muscles) for primary closure [47–50]. Some authorities have recently advocated the use of pectoralis musculocutaneous flaps for the initial management of all sternal wound infections, avoiding the use of mediastinal irrigation [50]. Our experience with the early aggressive use of muscle flap closure of the seriously infected mediastinum has been excellent. Attention to the patient's nutritional state is important.

CATHETER SEPSIS

Infection of an intravenous catheter can lead to fever, bacteremia, toxicity, shock, endocarditis, and bacterial seeding of the patient's fresh sternotomy incision. Patients who have been hospitalized for a period of time before surgery should be closely inspected to rule out the preoperative presence of phlebitis. Catheters or sheaths placed via the groin into the femoral artery or vein at the time of cardiac catheterization should be removed preoperatively if other access sites are possible, the patient is not heparinized, and surgery will not be performed for 12 to 24 hours. If surgery is imminent, we remove these groin cannulas postoperatively as soon as hemostatic function has returned. Prolonged postoperative use of groin catheters that were placed preoperatively appears to be associated with an increased incidence of venous thrombosis as well as an increased incidence of infectious complications, including sternal wound infections. If an infected peripheral intravenous catheter site is found preoperatively, it is best to postpone the surgery and treat the patient with antibiotics (and vein excision if required) for several days, unless the planned procedure is urgent in nature. The use of sterile technique is mandatory when monitoring lines are introduced by the anesthesiologist or surgeon in the operating room. Physicians placing central lines should scrub briefly and wear a sterile gown, gloves, and mask for the procedure.

When a postoperative patient develops a fever, atelectasis is the most likely cause. Catheter sepsis, however, can also occur very early after surgery, and this must be kept in mind. Infected central lines are usually *not* associated with redness or drainage at the insertion site. Thus, if the fever persists, blood cultures should be drawn, the catheter should be removed, and its tip should be cultured. In general, if central venous access is still needed for the care of the patient, this should be achieved through a new site rather than by exchanging the suspect catheter with a new one over a guidewire [51].

Gastrointestinal Complications

Gastrointestinal complications occur infrequently after cardiac surgery (incidence of 0.5 to 2.0%); they are often insidious in onset, difficult to diagnose, and severe in their consequences [52,53]. The cause of most gastrointestinal complications is likely relative hypoperfusion during the period of cardiopulmonary bypass [54]. Other contributing factors include postoperative low cardiac output, postoperative bleeding, use of vasopressors, narcotic administration, and preexisting vascular disease. Gastrointestinal complications requiring surgery have a mortality rate of 40% in cardiac surgical patients [55]. Clinical manifestations of gastrointestinal problems may be subtle in the patient who has recently undergone open heart surgery. Thus, a high index of suspicion is required.

ACUTE PANCREATITIS

Acute pancreatitis is probably the most common gastrointestinal complication to occur in the early postoperative period, although it is often very mild or subclinial. In fact, asymptomatic elevation of both the serum pancreatic and nonpancreatic isoamylase levels occurs in about one-third of patients after cardiopulmonary bypass [56–59]. It is speculated that the relative hypoperfusion of the pancreas during the period of cardiopulmonary bypass, calcium administration, high-dose narcotic anesthesia, and vasoconstriction secondary to vasopressors may contribute to the development of acute pancreatitis. Although the pancreatitis is usually mild, severe hemorrhagic pancreatitis does develop rarely [60]. Clinically evident pancreatitis in the postoperative patient often becomes apparent on the second or third postoperative day when the patient complains of abdominal pain and nausea, vomiting, or anorexia. The diagnosis may be confirmed by an elevated serum amylase level. Treatment consists of withholding oral feedings and, if an ileus is present, placement of a nasogastric tube for suction drainage of the stomach. Postoperative pancreatitis is usually self-limiting, and most patients are able to restart a clear liquid diet within a few days.

GASTROINTESTINAL TRACT BLEEDING

Significant gastrointestinal tract bleeding occurs surprisingly rarely after cardiac surgery (incidence less than 0.4%). Thus, for patients who do not have a history of ulcer disease, we do not routinely administer prophylactic histamine-receptor antagonists unless it appears that the patient will be severely ill for a long time. For patients with a history of ulcer disease, prophylactic H_2 blockers are given in addition to antacids via the nasogastric tube in sufficient quantities to keep the gastric pH above 5.0. When an H_2

blocker is indicated, ranitidine is preferable to cimetidine because it has fewer interactions with cardiovascular drugs [61]. Alternatively, Carafate (1 g qid) may be used for prophylaxis. Gastrointestinal bleeding will be manifest by the appearance of blood in the nasogastric tube drainage or by the development of melanotic stools (or both). When a significant amount of bleeding has occurred, the patient may become unstable with signs of hypovolemia. Evaluation includes determination of the patient's hematocrit and coagulation status, gastric lavage, and consultation with a general surgeon. Endoscopy is frequently utilized to determine the source of upper gastrointestinal bleeding. Initial treatment requires placement of secure intravenous access. For the unstable patient, a central venous catheter should be placed for volume and blood administration and central venous pressure should be measured to guide fluid therapy. Blood should be typed and crossmatched for transfusion, and other preparations for a possible emergency laparotomy should be made.

Perforation of a duodenal (or gastric) ulcer is a rare occurrence after cardiac operations. The patient, if awake, experiences sudden and severe abdominal pain that often radiates to the shoulder or supraclavicular area. No bowel sounds are heard on examination, and there is rigidity with great tenderness on palpation. An upright portable chest or cross-table lateral abdominal x-ray usually shows free air underneath the diaphragm, although this finding is not always present. Management of gastrointestinal perforation requires gastric tube suction, fluid resuscitation as indicated, and antibiotic coverage. General surgical consultation should be obtained promptly, as surgical closure of the perforation (with or without a definitive peptic ulcer disease procedure) is usually required.

ACUTE CHOLECYSTITIS

Acute cholecystitis (most frequently acalculous) is a rare but often fatal complication of cardiac surgery. The diagnosis can be difficult. The patient is usually afebrile and may complain of right upper quadrant pain. A variable degree of hyperbilirubinemia and abnormal liver enzyme levels may be present although these can occur in the postoperative patient for other reasons (e.g., secondary to blood transfusions). A septic hemodynamic pattern may develop characterized by hypotension, low vascular resistance, and relatively high cardiac output. Physical examination is often difficult because the patient will frequently guard when palpated because of the nearby sternotomy incision. Abdominal ultrasonography is our usual first diagnostic test and is very helpful if an enlarged gallbladder with a thickened wall is demonstrated. Hepatobiliary scans are also useful, but they have a significant incidence of false-positive results in patients who have recently undergone major surgery. The diagnosis, however, should be pursued since untreated cholecystitis will frequently result in gangrene of the gallbladder. In one series, patients with acalculous cholecystitis after cardiac surgery had an 85% mortality rate [52]. Treatment consists of either cholecystectomy or, when indicated, cholecystostomy.

NECROTIZING ENTEROCOLITIS

Necrotizing enterocolitis is an ischemic lesion of the bowel wall affecting premature infants. Early feeding of hyperosmolar formulas and the presence of a patent ductus arteriosus or sepsis are risk factors for the development of this problem. Although the cause is uncertain, low arterial flow probably plays a role. Typically, the baby develops bilious vomiting, abdominal distention, abdominal pain, or manifestations of sepsis. The diagnosis is suspected when there is blood in the stools associated with a decrease in the patient's platelet count. Confirmation of the diagnosis is obtained when air is seen within the bowel wall on x-ray examination. Treatment consists of antibiotics, hyperalimentation, nasogastric suction, and correction of the hemodynamic problem if possible. Laparotomy is carried out when there are signs of peritonitis or free abdominal air.

ACUTE HEPATIC FAILURE

Acute hepatic failure most often accompanies prolonged low cardiac output in adult patients receiving maximum supportive therapy such as catecholamines, intraaortic balloon pumping, and dialysis. It occurs rarely in children, usually those who have had a Fontan-Kreutzer procedure [62]. Along with profound jaundice, hypoglycemia and coagulopathies may develop. Management consists mainly in general measures to support the circulation and provide nutrition and in close monitoring of blood chemical constituents. Vitamin K and fresh frozen plasma should be administered if bleeding occurs. There is evidence that amrinone (Inocor) may contribute to hepatic failure, and, thus, it should be discontinued if it is being administered. Intralipid, likewise, should not be administered as a part of the hyperalimentation formula, since this agent may contribute to hepatic insufficiency.

Gastrointestinal complications are uncommon after heart surgery; this fact probably contributes to the delay in their diagnosis and to the high overall mortality from these postoperative events. Laparotomy may be required and is best performed early rather than after the development of shock due to sepsis or bleeding. Patients who have recently undergone heart surgery often have a better cardiac status, even early after surgery, than before their operation because of the cardiac repair performed (revascularization, valve replacement, etc.). Thus, potentially lifesaving exploration of the abdomen should not be postponed because of the patient's recent heart surgery. The cardiac surgeon should participate in the decision-making process and in the preparations for laparotomy (e.g., the management of anticoagulation, if required). Although the patient is undergoing a general surgery procedure, we routinely request the services of a cardiac anesthesiologist for the postoperative cardiac surgery patient.

Neurologic Complications

STROKE

Perioperative strokes occur in about 6% of patients undergoing open heart surgery; they occur more commonly in patients with advanced age, severe atherosclerosis of the ascending aorta, a history of previous stroke, a history of congestive heart failure, mitral regurgitation, postoperative atrial fibrillation, a cardiopulmonary bypass pump time of more than 2 hours, and a previous myocardial infarction [63–67]. As more older patients are undergoing heart surgery, it is no surprise that perioperative stroke continues to be a significant cause of perioperative morbidity and mortality.

A perioperative stroke is the result of irreversible ischemic death of brain matter resulting in a gross neurologic deficit (such as hemiparesis) or, when more extensive, coma. Although often considered a "postoperative" complication, most strokes begin during the operative procedure. It is not until several hours after surgery, when the patient's anesthetic has worn off, that the deficit can be appreciated. Ischemia of the brain may occur secondary to global hypoperfusion due to inadequate blood flow and perfusion pressure while on cardiopulmonary bypass. In some cases, this may be exacerbated by the presence of occlusive lesions in the patient's cerebral vasculature. More commonly, however, strokes occur as the result of emboli to the cerebral circulation. Cardiopulmonary bypass perfusion probably results in some degree of microemboli in all patients and may be the cause of the relatively common neuropsychologic changes that are frequently evident early after open heart surgery. Larger emboli, however, result in clinically evident strokes.

Emboli to the brain during surgery may be composed of air, atherosclerotic debris (from the aorta), or thrombus (such as from the left atrium or ventricle). Massive air embolism can occur from a variety of intraoperative mishaps. It may be prevented to some degree by bubble sensor devices, arterial line filters, and careful de-airing of the heart before resumption of contractions. If a massive air embolism does occur during cardiopulmonary bypass, immediate treatment by Trendelenburg positioning of the patient, placement of a stab wound in the ascending aorta for air escape, and retrograde perfusion through the superior vena cava is recommended [68]. Smaller air emboli can also severely damage the brain; thus, careful de-airing of the heart is required whenever procedures on the left side of the heart are performed [69]. One form of therapy specific for the treatment of air embolism to the brain is the hyperbaric oxygen chamber. If available, this should be employed as early as possible after completion of the operation. This form of treatment has been shown to provide dramatic reversal of neurologic deficits occurring in some patients who have suffered large air emboli [70,71].

Particulate emboli, most commonly atherosclerotic debris from the ascending aorta, are more common and more devastating than gaseous emboli. Patients with atherosclerosis involving the ascending aorta (the usual site for aortic cannulation and the placement of proximal saphenous vein bypass anastomoses) are clearly at increased risk of suffering a stroke from dislodgement of debris from the aortic wall. Efforts to prevent this problem include careful inspection and gentle palpation of the aorta before cannulation and the use of alternative sites for cannulation and proximal graft anastomoses when significant atherosclerosis is present. Intraoperative B-mode or transesophageal ultrasonographic examination of the ascending aorta to identify regions of atherosclerotic plaque have been used in an effort to decrease the risk of embolization [72,73]. When atherosclerotic involvement of the ascending aorta is present, various alternatives to standard cannulation and bypass graft placement are available to avoid manipulation and clamping of the diseased ascending aorta [74–76]. Large thrombus emboli are less common. Patients with chronic atrial fibrillation and left atrial enlargement or with left ventricular aneurysms frequently have mural thrombi within the left atrium or left ventricle, and manipulation of the heart during surgery can lead to thrombus embolism and stroke. Thus, patients with left ventricular thrombi identified by preoperative ventriculography are at increased risk for perioperative stroke [77].

In the past, brain "protective" measures (such as barbiturate administration to lessen the degree of cerebral injury) were recommended when an intraoperative brain injury was suspected. Recent laboratory and clinical studies, however, do not support the use of barbiturates for patients with suspected brain injury without specific indication. The incidence of side effects (mainly hemodynamic instability) is significant, and benefit has not been demonstrated; thus, such measures are no longer utilized at our institutions [78]. Treatment of the patient who has suffered a perioperative stroke is largely supportive and expectant. As soon as it is realized that the patient is not awakening from anesthesia normally or that there is a focal neurologic deficit present, a CT scan of the head should be obtained if the patient is sufficiently stable for transport to the scanner. Although these examinations are often normal early in the course of a stroke, the scan will rule out large intracerebral hemorrhages and cerebral edema. If cerebral edema is present, treatment should be undertaken to lower the intracranial pressure. These measures include hyperventilation (to lower than PCO_2 level to 25–30 mm Hg), diuresis, fluid restriction, and, on occasion, monitoring of intracranial pressure.

Symptomatic visual deficits occur occasionally after open heart surgery [79]. Potential etiologies include occipital lobe infarction, retinal emboli, or anterior ischemic optic neuropathy. Embolism or hypoperfusion are the causes, although severe anemia during the operation and preexisting glaucoma may be contributing factors.

SEIZURES

Seizures are especially likely to develop in the newborn infant who has undergone surgery utilizing deep hypothermia and total circulatory arrest. They may have subtle manifestations such as jerking of the eyelids or unusual posturing. Seizures occur in 5 to 10% of patients who have undergone total circulatory arrest and are correlated with adverse long-term sequelae. It is important to be sure that other causes for seizure activity are not present. These include hypocalcemia, hypoglycemia, hypoxic brain injury, primary subarachnoid hemorrhage, and infection. Since extremely cyanotic neonates are often taken promptly to the operating room for urgent surgery, it may be impossible to determine whether brain damage leading to seizures occurred before, during, or after operation. Also, rapid resuscitation of these infants with hyperosmolar agents such as bicarbonate can cause intracerebral hemorrhage. Hypocalcemia and hypoglycemia are readily diagnosed and treated. Infection and hypoxic damage have a poorer prognosis. Ultrasound of the newborn infant's head can help determine the presence or absence of intracerebral hemorrhage.

Treatment of ongoing seizures is begun by the intravenous administration of diazepam (infants, 0.1–0.2 mg/kg slow IV bolus every 5–10 minutes up to a total dose of 0.4 mg/kg; adults, 5–10 mg slow IV bolus every 5–10 minutes up to a total dose of 20 mg). For longer-term control, phenytoin (Dilantin) is administered to adults (10–20 mg/kg IV loading dose). For children, phenobarbital is often added (5–10 mg/kg IV loading dose). When phenobarbital is used, the drug's depressant effects on respiratory drive must be kept in mind and serum levels should be monitored.

NEUROPSYCHOLOGIC DISTURBANCES

Alterations in mental function not associated with focal neurologic deficits are relatively common in patients after open heart surgery utilizing cardiopulmonary bypass. Such changes may include various degrees of confusion and disorientation, memory deficits, problem-solving deficits, coordination problems, or even psychosis. Clinically obvious neuropsychologic alterations occur in 10 to 15% of postoperative patients; the incidence appears to increase in older patients and in those who have prolonged periods of cardiopulmonary bypass. Sensitive neuropsychologic testing of early postoperative patients has found the detectable incidence of functional deterioration to be much higher [80]. With time (6–7 months), however, most patients recover and show little or no evidence of residual impairment [81,82]. It is generally believed that these neuropsychologic disturbances are secondary to microembolic damage occurring while the patient is on cardiopulmonary bypass. Treatment is supportive, with close observation of the patient to prevent self-injury, and cautious reassurance to the patient's family that the disturbance is usually self-limiting.

PERIPHERAL NERVE INJURY

Peripheral nerve injuries may occur during open heart surgery and are among the most frequent of the anesthesia-related complications leading to malpractice suits. By far, the most common injuries are to the upper extremity nerve supply, particularly either the brachial plexus or the ulnar nerve (at the elbow). The injury to the brachial plexus is probably due to traction caused by the median sternotomy incision, whereas the injury to the ulnar nerve is most likely from compression of the nerve at the elbow [83]. The overall incidence of such upper extremity neuropathies after a median sternotomy is around 6% [84]. Efforts to prevent these injuries have included not placing a rolled-up towel beneath the patient's midback region (as was once a common practice), opening the sternum only as wide as necessary, positioning the retractor low in the split sternum, and use of the hands-up position [85]. The usual presentation of this complication is numbness, sometimes with tingling, of the fifth finger and the medial portion of the fourth finger of the involved hand. Nerve conduction studies and electromyelography may be performed, although there is no specific treatment available [86]. Reassurance of the patient is indicated, and, for some patients, this is reinforced when it is heard also from a consulting physician. Thus, consultation with a neurologist may be useful in the management of this postoperative problem. Long-term resolution of the symptoms occurs in most patients with postoperative upper extremity neuropathy, and over 90% of them become asymptomatic within 3 months.

Another interesting, but rare, peripheral nerve complication may occur in patients who undergo cardiac surgery. Associated with coronary bypass procedures, and perhaps the "frog-leg" positioning of the legs for vein harvesting, *meralgia paresthetica* is characterized by a region of numbness and paresthesia on the anterolateral aspect of the thigh. The syndrome results from an injury to the lateral femoral cutaneous nerve. The problem resolves over time and requires no specific therapy [87].

Complications of Saphenous Vein Harvesting

Although the internal mammary artery has been demonstrated conclusively to be a superior conduit for myocardial revascularization (especially for grafts to the left anterior descending artery), it is usually necessary also to use segments of the saphenous vein for additional conduits in patients who undergo multivessel coronary artery bypass procedures. Leg wound complications occur in nearly one-fourth of patients in whom the saphenous vein is utilized. Such problems are more common in patients who are female, obese, diabetic, or anemic preoperatively [88]. The most common complications are inflammation, separation of the wound, cellulitis, lymphangitis, lymphocele, or lymph drainage from the wound, and abscess formation. Careful surgical technique and a good understanding of the anatomy of the leg's venous drainage are important ways for the surgeon to avoid such problems. For difficult patients (such as those with previous vein stripping, thrombophlebitis, or obesity), preoperative duplex ultrasound scanning with marking of the skin overlying the identified vein can provide a "map" to guide the surgeon in the operating room [89]. Postoperatively, some degree of distal leg edema is common; this usually resolves over a few months. Thus, patients are advised to keep the donor leg elevated when not ambulating. If the wound becomes infected, antibiotics are administered and open packing of the wound is performed as necessary. Although problems with the leg wound may seem trivial compared with the surgery performed directly on the heart, leg wound complications can lead to significant morbidity, patient discomfort, and prolonged hospitalization [90]. Proper vein harvesting technique and care of postoperative wound complications are important aspects of patient care in cardiac surgery.

Complications Related to Internal Mammary Artery Mobilization

One or both of the internal mammary (thoracic) arteries are utilized in over 90% of the coronary revascularization procedures performed at our institutions because of the proven long-term benefits of this conduit as compared with saphenous vein aortocoronary bypass grafts. It is remarkable that only rarely does the mobilization and distal division of this artery (which is the major blood supply to the sternum) contribute to wound or other postoperative complications.

The use of *bilateral* internal mammary arteries in *diabetic* patients, however, does increase the incidence of sternal wound infection [91], and we therefore avoid this situation whenever possible.

Postoperative respiratory insufficiency may be worsened by the effects of mammary artery mobilization (opening of the pleura and possible injury to the phrenic nerve) [92]. Additionally, the use of the internal mammary artery is associated with the delayed development of chronic serosanguineous pleural effusions, which can cause dyspnea and may require repeated thoracenteses [93,94].

Deep Venous Thrombosis and Pulmonary Embolism

Clinically apparent deep venous thrombosis (DVT) is a rather rare complication of open heart surgery, occurring in 0.7% in one adult patient series [95]. This low incidence probably is related to the use of intraoperative total heparinization for cardiopulmonary bypass and early mobilization of most patients after surgery. Patients with complicated courses requiring a prolonged period of immobility in bed after surgery are at increased risk for postoperative DVT. The diagnosis of DVT is based on physical examination (unexplained leg swelling or leg pain and presence of Homans' sign), with confirmation by impedance plethysmography or venous Doppler ultrasound mapping techniques [96]. Treatment consists of systemic heparinization (to keep the APTT 1.5 times normal), bed rest for several days with leg elevation, and institution of warfarin anticoagulation for 3 to 6 months. The goal of warfarin treatment is to maintain the PT at 1.3 to 1.5 times the control value.

Postoperative pulmonary emboli occur in about one-half of patients with clinically apparent DVT; of these, it may be more common in patients with postoperative atrial fibrillation or perioperative myocardial infarction. The diagnosis may be obvious in the patient with known DVT who acutely develops respiratory insufficiency. Although new-onset atrial fibrillation may be a clue to pulmonary embolism in patients after noncardiac surgery, this arrhythmia is so common in patients after open heart surgery that it has little diagnostic significance. In other patients, the diagnosis may not be so apparent (presumably due to smaller emboli). Unexplained hypoxemia may be the only clue to pulmonary emboli. In hypoxic patients, a ventilation-perfusion lung scan should be performed, although the accuracy of this test is diminished in the postoperative patient who commonly has atelectasis. If normal, then pulmonary embolism is highly unlikely. Patients with a "high probability" scan very likely have a pulmonary embolism. Those with "low" or "intermediate" probability scans but abnormal venous ultrasound examinations or abnormal impedance plethysmography will have a significant chance of pulmonary embolism and, if the clinical situation is consistent, should undergo pulmonary arteriography [97,98]. Treatment is initiated by systemic heparinization for 4 to 7 days and warfarin anticoagulation for 3 to 6 months although, for desperately ill patients, an emergency embolectomy may be lifesaving [99]. There is no role for thrombolytic therapy (streptokinase or tissue plasminogen activator) for DVT or pulmonary embolism in patients who have recently undergone cardiac surgery due to the high risk of serious bleeding problems. Patients with contraindications to anticoagulation or patients who experience recurrence of pulmonary emboli despite anticoagulation are candidates for placement of caval interruption devices such as the Greenfield filter [100].

References

1. Gomes MMR, McGoon DC. Bleeding patterns after open heart surgery. *J Thorac Cardiovasc Surg* 60:87, 1970.

2. Czer LSC. Mediastinal bleeding after cardiac surgery: etiologies, diagnostic considerations, and blood conservation methods. *J Cardiothorac Anesth* 3:760, 1989.

3. Walls, JT, et al. Heparin-induced thrombocytopenia in patients who undergo open heart surgery. *Surgery* 108:686, 1990.

4. Becker RC, Alpert JS. The impact of medical therapy on hemorrhagic complications following coronary artery bypass grafting. *Arch Intern Med* 150:2016, 1990.

5. Woodman RC, Harker LA. Bleeding complications associated with cardiopulmonary bypass. *Blood* 76:1680, 1990.

6. Taggart DP, Siddiqui A, Wheatley DJ. Low-dose preoperative aspirin therapy, postoperative blood loss, and transfusion requirements. *Ann Thorac Surg* 50:425, 1990.

7. Sethi GS, et al. Implications of preoperative administration of aspirin in patients undergoing coronary artery bypass grafting. *J Am Coll Cardiol* 15:15, 1990.

8. Goldman S, et al. and the Department of Veterans Affairs Cooperative Study Group. Starting aspirin therapy after operation: Effects on early graft patency. *Circulation* 84:520, 1991.

9. Hirsh J. Heparin. *N Engl J Med* 324:1565, 1991.

10. Aren C. Heparin and protamine therapy. *Semin Thorac Cardiovasc Surg* 2:364, 1990.

11. Pifarre R. et al. Management of blood loss and heparin rebound following cardiopulmonary bypass. *Semin Thromb Hemost* 15:173, 1989.

12. Michelson EL, et al. Early recognition of surgically correctable causes of excessive mediastinal bleeding after coronary artery bypass graft surgery. *Am J Surg* 139:313, 1980.

13. McKowen RL, et al. Infectious complications and cost-effectiveness of open resuscitation in the surgical intensive care unit after cardiac surgery. *Ann Thorac Surg* 40:388, 1985.

14. Hoffman WS, Tomasello DN, MacVaugh H. Control of postcardiotomy bleeding with PEEP. *Ann Thorac Surg* 34:71, 1981.

15. Goodnough LT, et al. Guidelines for transfusion therapy in patients undergoing coronary artery bypass grafting. *Ann Thorac Surg* 50:675, 1990.

16. Salzman, EW, et al. Treatment with desmopressin acetate to reduce blood loss after cardiac surgery. A double-blind randomized trial. *N Engl J Med* 314:1402, 1986.

17. Bolan CD, Alving BM. Pharmacologic agents in the management of bleeding disorders. *Transfusion* 30:541, 1990.

18. Bateman TM, et al. Cardiac causes of shock early after open heart surgery: Etiologic classification by radionuclide ventriculography. *Circulation* 71:1153, 1985.

19. Carter, AR, et al. Thoracic alterations after cardiac surgery. *AJR* 140:476, 1983.

20. Singh S, et al. Usefulness of right ventricular diastolic collapse in diagnosing cardiac tamponade and comparison to pulsus paradoxus. *Am J Cardiol* 57:652, 1986.

21. Chuttani K, et al. Relative value of clinical, echocardiographic, and hemodynamic signs in the diagnosis of cardiac tamponade following cardiac surgery. *Circulation* 82(Suppl III):III-577(abstr), 1990.

22. Kochar GS, Jacobs LE, Kotler MN. Right atrial compression in postoperative cardiac patients: Detection by transesophageal echocardiography. *J Am Coll Cardiol* 16:511, 1990.

23. Chuttani K, et al. Left ventricular diastolic collapse: An echocardiographic sign of regional cardiac tamponade. *Circulation* 83:1999, 1991.

24. Corwin HL, et al. Acute renal failure associated with cardiac operations. *J Thorac Cardiovasc Surg* 98:1107, 1989.

25. Abel RM, et al. Etiology, incidence, and prognosis of renal failure following cardiac operations. *J Thorac Cardiovasc Surg* 71:323, 1976.

26. Davis RF, et al. Acute oliguria after cardiopulmonary bypass: Renal functional improvement with low-dose dopamine infusion. *Crit Care Med* 10:852, 1982.

27. Magilligan DJ. Indications for ultrafiltration in the cardiac surgical patient. *J Thorac Cardiovasc Surg* 89:183, 1985.

28. Weinstein GS, et al. Serial changes in renal function in cardiac surgical patients. *Ann Thorac Surg* 48:72, 1989.

29. Gailiunas JRP, et al. Acute renal failure following cardiac operations. *J Thorac Cardiovasc Surg* 79:241, 1980.

30. Swartz RD. Interventional Support for Acute Renal Failure in the Critically Ill Patient. In RH Bartlett, WM Whitehouse, JG Turcotte (eds), *Life Support Systems in Intensive Care*. Chicago: Year Book, 1984. Pp. 409–429.

31. Maguire WC, Anderson, RJ. Continuous arteriovenous hemofiltration in the intensive care unit. *J Crit Care* 1:54, 1986.

32. Lange HW, Aeppli DM, Brown DC. Survival of patients with acute renal failure requiring dialysis after open heart surgery: early prognostic indicators. *Am Heart J* 113:1138, 1987.

33. Nelson RM, Dries DJ. The economic implications of infection in cardiac surgery. *Ann Thorac Surg* 42:240, 1986.

34. Miedzinski LJ, Keren G. Serious infectious complications of open-heart surgery. *Can J Surg* 30:103, 1987.

35. Miholic J, et al. Risk factors for severe bacterial infections after valve replacement and aortocoronary bypass operations: Analysis of 246 cases by logistic regression. *Ann Thorac Surg* 40:224, 1985.

36. Gaynes R, et al. Risk factors for nosocomial pneumonia after coronary artery bypass graft operations. *Ann Thorac Surg* 51:215, 1991.

37. Sarr MG, Gott VL, Townsend TR. Mediastinal infection after cardiac surgery (collective review). *Ann Thorac Surg* 38:415, 1984.

38. Loop FD, et al. Sternal wound complications after isolated coronary artery bypass grafting: early and late mortality, morbidity, and cost of care. *Ann Thorac Surg* 49:179, 1990.

39. Newman LS, et al. Suppurative mediastinitis after open heart surgery. *Chest* 94:546, 1988.

40. Grossi EA, et al. A survey of 77 major infectious complications of median sternotomy: A review of 7,949 consecutive operative procedures. *Ann Thorac Surg* 40:214, 1985.

41. LoCicero J. Prophylactic antibiotic usage in cardiothoracic surgery (American College of Chest Physician Section Report). *Chest* 98:719, 1990.

42. Doebbeling BN, et al. Cardiovascular surgery prophylaxis. A randomized controlled comparison of cefazolin and cefuroxime. *J Thorac Cardiovasc Surg* 99:981, 1990.

43. Ariano RE, Zhanel GG. Antimicrobial prophylaxis in coronary bypass surgery. A critical appraisal. *DICP* 25:478, 1991.

44. Kohman LJ, Coleman MJ, Parker FB. Bacteremia and sternal infection after coronary artery bypass grafting. *Ann Thorac Surg* 49:454, 1990.

45. Heath BJ, Bagnato VJ. Poststernotomy mediastinitis treated by omental transfer without postoperative irrigation or drainage. *J Thorac Cardiovasc Surg* 94:355, 1987.

46. Nahai F, et al. Primary treatment of the infected sternotomy wound with muscle flaps: A review of 211 consecutive cases. *Plast Reconstr Surg* 84:434, 1989.

47. Spencer FC, Grossi EA. Mediastinitis after cardiac operations (key references). *Ann Thorac Surg* 49:506, 1990.

48. Mathisen DJ. Surgical techniques for chest wall reconstruction (key references). *Ann Thorac Surg* 49:164, 1990.

49. Pairolero PC, Arnold PG. Management of recalcitrant median sternotomy wounds. *J Thorac Cardiovasc Surg* 88:357, 1984.

50. Jeevanandam V, et al. Single-stage management of sternal wound infections. *J Thorac Cardiovasc Surg* 99:256, 1990.

51. Norwood S, et al. Catheter-related infections and associated septicemia. *Chest* 99:968, 1991.

52. Krasna MJ, et al. Gastrointestinal complications after cardiac surgery. *Surgery* 104:773, 1988.

53. Ohri SK, et al. Intraabdominal complications after cardiopulmonary bypass. *Ann Thorac Surg* 52:826, 1991.

54. Leitman MI, Paull DDE, Barie PS. Intra-abdominal complications of cardiopulmonary bypass operations. *Surg Gynecol Obstet* 165:251, 1987.

55. Arahna GV, et al. The reasons for gastrointestinal consultation after cardiac surgery. *Ann Surg* 50:301, 1984.

56. Missavage AE, et al. Hyperamylasemia after cardiopulmonary bypass. *Am Surg* 50:297, 1984.

57. Svensson LG, Decker G, Kinsley RB. A prospective study of hyperamylasemia and pancreatitis after cardiopulmonary bypass. *Ann Thorac Surg* 39:409, 1985.

58. Fernandez-del Castillo C, et al. Risk factors for pancreatic cellular injury after cardiopulmonary bypass. *N Engl J Med* 325:382, 1991.

59. Rattner DW, et al. Hyperamylasemia after cardiac surgery. Incidence, significance, and management. *Ann Surg* 209:279, 1989.

60. Haas GS, et al. Acute pancreatitis after cardiopulmonary bypass. *Am J Surg* 149:508, 1985.

61. Baciewicz AM, Baciewicz FA. Effect of cimetidine and ranitidine on cardiovascular drugs. *Am Heart J* 118:114, 1989.

62. Jenkins JG, et al. Acute hepatic failure following cardiac operation in children. *J Thorac Cardiovasc Surg* 84:865, 1982.

63. Smith PL. Brain injury and protection. *Semin Thorac Cardiovasc Surg* 2:381, 1990.

64. Breuer AC, et al. Central nervous system complications of coronary artery bypass graft surgery. *Stroke* 14:682, 1983.

65. Gardner TJ, et al. Stroke following coronary artery bypass grafting: a ten-year study. *Ann Thorac Surg* 40:574, 1985.

66. Reed GL, et al. Stroke following coronary artery bypass surgery. *N Engl J Med* 319:1246, 1988.

67. Taylor GJ, et al. Usefulness of atrial fibrillation as a predictor of stroke isolated coronary artery bypass grafting. *Am J Cardiol* 60:905, 1987.

68. Mills NL, Ochsner JL. Massive air embolism during cardiopulmonary bypass. *J Thorac Cardiovasc Surg* 80:708, 1980.

69. Grotta JC. Current medical and surgical therapy for cerebrovascular disease. *N Engl J Med* 317:1505, 1987.

70. Utley JR, Stephens DB. Air Embolism During Cardiopulmonary Bypass. In JR Utley (ed), *Pathophysiology and Techniques of Cardiopulmonary Bypass*. Vol II. Baltimore: Williams & Wilkins, 1983. Pp. 78–100.

71. Pierce EC. Specific therapy for arterial air embolism. *Ann Thorac Surg* 29:300, 1980.

72. Marshall WG, et al. Intraoperative ultrasonic imaging of the ascending aorta. *Ann Thorac Surg* 48:339, 1989.

73. Katz ES, et al. Protruding aortic atheromas predict stroke in elderly patients undergoing cardiopulmonary bypass. Experience with intraoperative transesophageal echocardiography. *J Am Coll Cardiol* 20:70, 1992.

74. Landymore RW, et al. Prevention of neurological injury during myocardial revascularization in patients with calcific degenerative aortic disease. *Ann Thorac Surg* 41:293, 1986.

75. Holland DL, Hieb RE. Revascularization without embolization: Coronary bypass in the presence of calcified aorta. *Ann Thorac Surg* 40:308, 1985.

76. Peigh PS, et al. Coronary bypass grafting with totally calcified or acutely dissected ascending aorta. *Ann Thorac Surg* 51:102, 1991.

77. Breuer AC, et al. Left ventricular thrombi seen by ventriculography are a significant risk factor for stroke in open-heart surgery. *Ann Neurol* 10:103(abstr), 1981.

78. Rogers MC, Kirsch JR. Current concepts in brain resuscitation. *JAMA* 261:3143, 1989.

79. Shahian DM, Speert PK. Symptomatic visual deficits after open heart surgery. *Ann Thorac Surg* 48:275, 1989.

80. Shaw PJ, Bates D, Cartlidge NEF. Early intellectual dysfunction following coronary bypass surgery. *Q J Med* 58:59, 1986.

81. Townes BD, et al. Neurobehavioral outcomes in cardiac operations. *J Thorac Cardiovasc Surg* 98:774, 1989.

82. Shaw PJ, Bates D, Cartlidge NEF. Long-term intellectual dysfunction following coronary bypass surgery. *Q J Med* 62:259, 1987.

83. Graham JG, Pye IF, McQueen INF. Brachial plexus injury after median sternotomy. *J Neurol Neurosurg Psychiatry* 44:621, 1981.

84. Morin JE, et al. Upper extremity neuropathies following median sternotomy. *Ann Thorac Surg* 34:181, 1982.

85. Tomlinson DL, et al. Protecting the brachial plexus during median sternotomy. *J Thorac Cardiovasc Surg* 94:297, 1987.

86. Dawson DM, Krarup C. Perioperative nerve lesions. *Arch Neurol* 46:1355, 1989.

87. Parsonnet V, et al. Meralgia paresthetica after coronary bypass surgery. *J Thorac Cardiovasc Surg* 101:219, 1991.

88. Utley JR, et al. Preoperative correlates of impaired wound healing after saphenous vein excision. *J Thorac Cardiovasc Surg* 98:147, 1989.

89. Lemmer JH Jr, et al. Preoperative saphenous vein mapping for coronary artery bypass. *J Cardiac Surg* 3:237, 1988.

90. DeLaria GA, et al. Leg wound complications associated with coronary revascularization. *J Thorac Cardiovasc Surg* 81:403, 1981.

91. Kouchoukos NT, et al. Risks of bilateral internal mammary artery bypass grafting. *Ann Thorac Surg* 49:210, 1990.

92. Shapira N, et al. Determinants of pulmonary function in patients undergoing coronary bypass operations. *Ann Thorac Surg* 50:268, 1990.

93. Kolleff MH. Chronic pleural effusion following coronary artery revascularization with the internal mammary artery. *Chest* 97:750, 1990.

94. Scott, PP, Schonfeld SA, Reitz BA. Late post coronary artery bypass hemothorax: Description of a new entity. *Chest* 94:40S(abstr), 1988.

95. DeLaria GA, Hunter JA. Deep venous thrombosis: Implications after open heart surgery. *Chest* 99:284, 1992.

96. Polak JF. Doppler ultrasound of the deep leg veins. *Chest* 99:165S, 1991.

97. Mohr DN, et al. Recent advances in the management of venous thromboembolism. *Mayo Clin Proc* 63:281, 1988.

98. Goldharber SZ. Recent advances in the diagnosis and lytic therapy of pulmonary embolism. *Chest* 4:173S, 1991.

99. Putnam JB, et al. Embolectomy for acute pulmonary artery occlusion following Fontan procedure. *Ann Thorac Surg* 45:335, 1988.

100. Jones TK, Barnes RW, Greenfield LJ. Greenfield vena cava filter: Rationale and current indications. *Ann Thorac Surg* 42:S48, 1986.

Late Postoperative Management

Cardiac Rehabilitation

For most patients, the goal of undertaking cardiac surgery is to permit their return to as normal a lifestyle as possible including employment when appropriate. Cardiac rehabilitation has assumed greater importance in the modern era where patients with more advanced disease are undergoing cardiac surgery, and where the disability that must be overcome after some operations (e.g., cardiac transplantation for severe heart failure) is considerable. The recent trend in blood conservation and, consequently, the greater degree of postoperative anemia that is tolerated only further complicate the rehabilitative process.

A well-organized program for cardiac rehabilitation addresses both the physical and emotional needs of the postoperative patient and begins with instruction in the preoperative period [1]. An important element in cardiac rehabilitation is instilling in the patients a positive attitude beginning with the assumption that rehabilitation to an active lifestyle is the norm. The basic principle of cardiac rehabilitation is to offer the patients graded exercise in a supervised environment up to the limit of their cardiac function. With continued conditioning, many of these patients, particularly those with heart failure that has been improved or corrected, should experience considerable improvement in exercise capacity over their preoperative status. However, this may require a considerable effort over a period of time; a well-organized cardiac rehabilitation program should recognize and develop that goal.

Ambulation is initiated as early as possible in the hospital after surgery. This is medically indicated after surgery to decrease the amount of "deconditioning" and lack of mobility that occur with bedrest, to optimize pulmonary toilet and minimize atelectasis, and to decrease venous stasis in the lower extremities, consequently lowering the risk of phlebitis. The program of ambulation varies from hospital to hospital, but, in general, it should progress to supervised stair-climbing or exercise on a stationary bicycle before discharge. Both from physical and emotional perspectives, the inpatient ambulation and rehabilitation program should introduce and prepare the patient for the outpatient program. Since there is an increasing emphasis on shortening the length of the hospital stay, generating a positive attitude toward rehabilitation and de-emphasizing cardiac illness may be important factors in reducing the number of postoperative in-hospital days. Similarly, this approach should help increase the likelihood that previously employed patients will return to their jobs [2].

In patients who have undergone surgery because of coronary artery disease, an exercise stress test may be useful to provide objective evidence that ischemia has been relieved so that patients may pursue a more aggressive outpatient rehabilitative process with greater confidence. This is particularly necessary for those patients who, after initial rehabilitation, will begin heavier forms of exercise such as jogging or those patients who had silent ischemia before surgery, and for those patients with particularly severe distal coronary arterial disease. In some series, positive postoperative studies were noted in up to 10% of patients [3] and would influence the decision to restart antiischemic medications, to recatheterize, or to limit exercise. The stress test is performed approximately 2 or 3 months after surgery when patients are freely ambulatory and can perform the test to their comfortable limit of fatigue. This wait is particularly important in the modern era where blood conservation may result in a lower hematocrit at the time of discharge.

Graft Patency After Coronary Bypass Grafting

It is now recognized that coronary bypass grafting is palliative and that atherosclerosis in the native coronary arteries may progress. Approximately 10% of saphenous vein bypass grafts will be occluded at the end of the first postoperative year; hence, for patients who have received more than one saphenous vein graft, the likelihood of having at least one occluded graft increases. Graft occlusion is a complex subject, but factors that influence short-term graft patency include the technical quality of proximal and distal anastomoses, size and quality of the coronary artery, injury to the saphenous vein before implantation, and low-flow rates at the time of surgery (<40 ml/min). Long-term patency is influenced by intimal hyperplasia and recurrent atherosclerosis. By 5 years after coronary bypass grafting, approximately 25% of saphenous vein grafts are occluded, and, by 10 years, 40–50% are occluded [4,5].

In the past decade, there has been increasing attention focused on means to enhance graft patency. These efforts have concentrated in two areas: anticoagulation and atherosclerosis risk factor modification. Antiplatelet drugs can enhance graft patency and, in particular, aspirin has been demonstrated to improve graft patency rates. It was originally believed that antiplatelet therapy with both aspirin and dipyridamole administered perioperatively and postoperatively was necessary to enhance early graft patency [6]. However, patient compliance with dipyridamole, which must be taken 3 times a day and has potential gastrointestinal side effects, was often poor. More recent studies have confirmed that aspirin alone achieves the same salutary effect on early graft patency [7]. Aspirin therapy, however, must be instituted as early as possible after surgery, ideally on the day of operation [3,8]; in fact, it appears to be most effective if given within 6 hours of surgery. Aspirin can be administered by rectal suppository (325 mg) after patients are rewarmed in the intensive care unit postoperatively, as long as the patient is not bleeding. When extubated, enteric-coated aspirin (325 mg qd) is instituted. While no data is available documenting aspirin's beneficial effects on graft patency beyond 1 year, it is our practice to continue aspirin therapy indefinitely in part because of its effectiveness in decreasing the rate of future myocardial infarction [9].

With the recognition that recurrent atherosclerosis can occur both in the native circulation as well as in bypass grafts, there is now an increasing emphasis on atherosclerosis risk factor modification. This has intensified in recent years because of advances in the control of lipid metabolism. The risk factors known to accelerate atherosclerosis that can be controlled or modified include smoking, obesity, hyperlipidemia, and hypertension. The importance of risk factors must be emphasized repeatedly and must be a prominent part of the cardiac rehabilitation process. All patients with coronary artery disease are advised to have their lipid profiles (total cholesterol, triglycerides, high-density lipoprotein cholesterol, low-density lipoprotein cholesterol) checked at approximately 3 months after hospital discharge. Based on present American Heart Association recommendations, patients with elevated cholesterol (≥ 200 mg/dl), elevated triglycerides (≥ 150 mg/dl), or inadequate high-density lipoprotein levels (≤ 35 mg/dl) should have further follow-up and counseling. The initial treatment of all hyperlipidemias includes weight loss, dietary modification with respect to dietary fat intake, and aerobic exercise. In general, patients with an abnormal lipid profile on further postoperative follow-up despite these measures should be referred for further evaluation and treatment.

Endocarditis After Cardiac Surgery

Bacterial endocarditis is a potential risk in any patient who has undergone cardiac surgery [10]. In a prior era, patients were stratified into three risk categories, and prophylaxis was recommended depending on what procedure was being undertaken. More recently, it has become apparent that in certain situations — such as more than 6 months after an uncomplicated atrial septal defect repair, ligation of a patent ductus, or closure of a ventricular septal defect — the risk of subsequent endocarditis is very low, and, accordingly, prophylaxis is not indicated. In contrast, patients with prosthetic valves are at significant risk, as well as patients with previous endocarditis. Dental procedures, particularly those involving the gums (including professional cleaning), and certain surgical and endoscopic procedures carry the highest incidence of associated bacteremia. Accordingly, patients undergoing these and related procedures should receive antibiotic prophylaxis [11] which has been shown to be effective [12]. Shown in Appendix 1 are the current American Heart Association guidelines for which patients are at risk for bacterial endocarditis and the recommendations for antibiotic prophylaxis. Patients who are at risk and who sustain open injuries must be monitored more carefully for potential wound infections; the threshold to treat suspected early cellulitis should be much lower than that for patients who are not at risk for endocarditis.

A number of years ago, *prosthetic valve endocarditis* was a highly lethal disease. However, with contemporary antibiotics and an aggressive surgical approach to antibiotic-refractory endocarditis, the current potential for cure is significantly greater [13,14]. Any patient with a prosthetic valve who is febrile without an easily identifiable source must be considered as possibly having bacterial endocarditis [15,16]. These patients should undergo multiple blood cultures, ideally during the onset of a fever spike. Six to eight cultures should be obtained before antibiotic therapy is instituted for presumed endocarditis. In addition, details from the physical examination are useful to help make the diagnosis by providing evidence of new paravalvular leaks or evidence of metastatic infection. The treatment plan depends on the features of the presentation. Patients with fever and positive blood cultures without evidence of hemodynamic deterioration are initially treated with high-dose antibiotic therapy, selected on the basis of culture data and optimized according to blood levels and quantitative bactericidal studies. If patients defervesce on antibiotic therapy and if there is no evidence of prosthetic valve dysfunction, metastatic infection, or emboli, treatment is continued for 6 weeks. Then antibiotics are discontinued, and patients are observed and recultured for any evidence of recurrent fever. In some instances, particularly with extremely virulent organisms such as *Staphylococcus* species, a medical cure is not achieved [17]; erosion of the cardiac tissues is more common, resulting in paravalvular leaks, valve dysfunction due to vegetations, or erosion and detachment of a recently placed intracardiac patch. In some instances, such as infection with *Staphylococcus aureus,* destruction of the aortic annulus may occur. This may be heralded by conduction system abnormalities or development of an aortic-to-right atrial fistula. A finding of cardiac erosion during antibiotic therapy is an ominous sign and indicates the need for reoperation as early as possible. The occurrence of emboli despite antibiotic therapy is another indication for surgery. In virtually all instances of fungal endocarditis, early reoperation is necessary along with perioperative and postoperative treatment with antifungal agents.

In patients with prosthetic valve endocarditis receiving warfarin anticoagulation, we generally convert to heparin anticoagulation while the patient is hospitalized so that, if urgent operation is needed, the risk of bleeding is minimized. Stroke is a significant risk in patients with prosthetic valve endocarditis and it is not prevented by anticoagulation [18]. The need for cardiac catheterization in patients with prosthetic valve endocarditis has become more controversial with the advent of high-resolution echocardiography. Traditionally, cardiac catheterization was required to define annular anatomy, particularly where an annular abscess was suspected, and coronary artery anatomy, particularly in instances of aortic valve endocarditis where cardiac erosion may be an issue. However, with contemporary echocardiography, and in particular transesophageal echocardiography, it is now more frequently possible to delineate the anatomy less invasively [19]. If there is any question as to the involvement of the annulus or coronary arteries, or if an annular abscess is suspected but the diagnosis is not certain, cardiac catheterization with aortography or ventriculography (or both) is necessary. Because of the risk of creating emboli from endocarditis vegetations, care must be taken in selecting the route of cardiac catheterization. In some instances, particularly in patients who have undergone multiple valve replacement, transseptal or transthoracic ventriculography may be necessary.

Late Postoperative Issues Following Cardiac Valve Surgery

DETERIORATION OF BIOLOGIC VALVES

It is widely recognized that glutaraldehyde-fixed porcine bioprosthetic valves (e.g., Carpentier-Edwards or Hancock valves) offer patients the advantage of a low thromboembolic rate without the need for systemic anticoagulation [20]. However, these prostheses are subject to failure due to tissue calcification or fracture resulting in valve stenosis or, more commonly, regurgitation. Valve failure may occur as a gradual process over a few years or it may occur in a subacute or acute fashion. Although primary failure of tissue valves can occur early, the rate of failure generally begins to increase about 5 years after implantation [20]. Younger patients, particularly those less than 40 years of age, suffer deterioration of porcine bioprosthetic valves more rapidly, and, in children, porcine valve survival can be quite short (2–3 years) [21,22]. Current evidence suggests that older adults (>70 years of age) will less frequently experience calcification and degeneration of porcine valves in the aortic position, but porcine valves in the mitral position may deteriorate prematurely in patients over a wide range of ages including very elderly patients [23]. It is our current practice to consider implanting porcine aortic prostheses in patients more than 70 years of age. In selected cases where older patients are particularly vigorous and are considered to have substantial longevity, we would consider implanting a mechanical aortic valve. We usually use mechanical valves in the mitral position even in older patients. However, in older patients who are in sinus rhythm who are thought to have limited longevity, we would consider implanting a porcine valve in the mitral position. In patients in whom there is a contraindication to long-term warfarin anticoagulation, we invariably use porcine aortic and mitral prostheses.

DETERIORATION OF MECHANICAL VALVES

Over the past decade, low-profile mechanical valves incorporating pyrolytic carbon components have become the most commonly used mechanical valve prostheses in the United States. The present generation of valves offers patients thromboembolic rates less than those observed in prior decades with earlier mechanical prostheses [24]; contemporary valves also have excellent flow characteristics, even in smaller sizes.

For a given annulus diameter, mechanical valves provide less obstruction to flow than do porcine prostheses. Patients who underwent valve replacement in the 1960s and 1970s will have earlier-generation prostheses. These may be more subject to late stenosis — usually by pannus ingrowth. Early generation caged-ball (Starr-Edwards) valves may become regurgitant due to deterioration of the Silastic ball. Some Bjork-Shiley valves have undergone strut fracture with disk embolization and acute, catastrophic valve incompetence; this is especially likely to occur in convexoconcave 60° [25] and convexoconcave 70° [26] mitral valves in sizes greater than 27 mm. Because these types of valves are not currently being implanted, such complications are not as common, but they must be kept in mind in patients who present in heart failure or shock with evidence of acute prosthetic dysfunction.

PARAVALVULAR LEAKS

In prior decades, paravalvular leaks were recognized with some frequency, estimated at 14% for valves placed in the aortic position and at 9% for valves placed in the mitral position [27]. However, with improved surgical techniques (including the use of pledget-reinforced sutures) and with the decreasing frequency of patients undergoing valve surgery for advanced rheumatic heart disease (with associated annular calcification), the incidence of paravalvular leaks has been reduced to less than 1%. The use of transesophageal echocardiography as part of intraoperative monitoring and assessment offers the prospect of reducing this further by detection before decannulation of paravalvular leaks that may be a result of technical errors.

Occasionally, paravalvular leaks, particularly around mitral prostheses, may be silent. Trauma to the red blood cells can result in hemolytic anemia; this may be the clue that a paravalvular leak is present. Patients with persistent anemia after valve replacement should be evaluated by echocardiography for paravalvular leaks. Parvalvular leaks are usually repaired when there is significant anemia or hemodynamic compromise. At reoperation, some of these leaks can be repaired simply by placing additional sutures without explanting the valve.

THROMBOEMBOLISM

Thromboembolic complications of prosthetic valves occurred with a frequency approaching 5% per year with early generation caged-ball and tilting-disk valves. Contemporary, low-profile valves have a lower rate of thromboembolic complications of approximately 1 to 2% per year, even when implanted in the mitral position [24]. However, as with all other mechanical prosthetic valves, these require long-term anticoagulation with sodium warfarin.

Anticoagulation treatment for patients with prosthetic valves begins as soon as patients are able to take medications orally. It is undesirable for postoperative patients to exceed their prothrombin time (PT) goal, and, accordingly, we do not use a loading dose of warfarin. Instead, if the patient's maintenance dose is known from prior warfarin therapy, this is initiated postoperatively. For patients who are receiving warfarin for the first time, we generally start with a dose of 2.5 to 5.0 mg per day and follow the PT daily during the early postoperative period. The lower initial dose is used in patients who have had elevated right-sided filling pressures, any evidence of hepatic dysfunction, or long-standing cardiac cachexia. The dose is then increased by 2.5 mg every day or every other day until the PT begins to rise. In prior years, it was thought that a PT ratio of approximately 2.0 × control was needed for adequate anticoagulation, particularly with some tilting disk valves in the mitral position. However, recent studies have shown, particularly with contemporary prostheses, that a PT ratio of 1.5 × control is adequate to prevent thromboembolic complications [28,29]. This lower PT ratio obviates some of the potential bleeding complications of warfarin therapy. After discharge, the PT is checked weekly until a stable level is demonstrated, at which time the interval between determinations may be lengthened. With continued patient recovery and, in particular, improvement in postoperative nutrition, the dose may be increased gradually above the amount needed in the early postoperative period.

There are many pharmacologic agents that potentially interfere with warfarin anticoagulation (and alter PT) either by depressing or accelerating hepatic metabolism or by enhancing or interfering with warfarin-protein binding [30]; patients must be aware of these (Table 6-1). Patients should also be aware that dietary intake of vitamin K may affect the PT; they should be urged to be as consistent as possible in their dietary habits. In some patients, drugs that may interact with warfarin must be added to the patient's regimen. When this occurs after hospital discharge, the frequency of PT determination should be increased until PT stability is demonstrated. In patients with prosthetic valves in whom there is documented thromboembolism despite adequate anticoagulation with warfarin, it is sometimes necessary to add a platelet-inhibiting drug. Dipyridamole (100 mg tid) is the preferred second agent, since there is less gastrointestinal bleeding with dipyridamole than with aspirin and a lower risk of delayed tamponade. In patients who have mechanical prosthetic valves implanted and in whom severe contraindications to warfarin therapy appear later in life, there is some experience with the use of aspirin (325 mg bid) and dipyridamole (100 mg tid) in combination instead of warfarin for valves in the aortic position [31]; however, this alternative anticoagulation therapy is only recommended for these very exceptional circumstances.

For patients who have received porcine mitral valves, temporary warfarin anticoagulation is recommended for the first 3 months after surgery [32]. In these instances, the incidence of early thromboembolic complications is significant enough to warrant the risk of anticoagulation. Many of these patients will be in chronic atrial fibrillation, in which case warfarin anticoagulation should be continued indefinitely [33]. In instances where bioprosthetic valves are implanted only in the aortic position, temporary warfarin anticoagulation is controversial. We usually employ warfarin in these patients for 6 to 8 weeks unless there is a contraindication to anticoagulation. In patients who have had intracardiac surgery (e.g., adult atrial septal defect), if there is a background of intermittent or permanent atrial fibrillation, some surgeons employ warfarin therapy for 3 to 6 months after surgery. Patients are then evaluated by 24-hour Holter monitor; if there is no evidence of atrial irritability, warfarin is stopped.

Pericarditis and Delayed Pericardial Tamponade

Delayed postoperative pericardial effusions can occur in any patient who has undergone cardiac surgery [34–37], whether the pericardium was left open or closed and even if the pleural spaces were entered during sternotomy. The boundaries of the pericardial space

Table 6-1. Factors that may alter PT by interacting with warfarin

PROLONGS PROTHROMBIN TIME

Endogenous factors

Cancer
Collagen disease
Congestive heart failure
Diarrhea
Elevated temperature
Hepatic disorders — infectious hepatitis, jaundice
Hyperthyroidism
Poor nutritional state
Steatorrhea
Vitamin K deficiency

Exogenous factors

Alcohol
Allopurinol
Aminosalicylic acid
Amiodarone HCl
Anabolic steroids
Anesthetics, inhalation
Antibiotics
Bromelains
Chenodiol
Chloral hydrate
Chlorpropamide
Chymotrypsin
Cimetidine
Clofibrate
Coumadin overdosage
Dextran
Dextrothyroxine
Diazoxide
Diflunisal
Diuretics
Disulfiram
Ethacrynic acid
Fenoprofen
Fluoroquinolone antibiotics
Glucagon
Hepatotoxic drugs
Ibuprofen
Indomethacin
Influenza virus vaccine
Lovastatin
Mefenamic acid
Methyldopa
Methylphenidate
Metronidazole
Miconazole
Monoamine oxidase inhibitors
Nalidixic acid
Naproxen
Narcotics, prolonged use
Pentoxifylline
Phenylbutazone
Phenytoin
Propafenone
Pyrazolones
Quinidine
Quinine
Ranitidine
Salicylates
Sulfinpyrazone
Sulfonamides, long-acting
Sulindac
Tamoxifen
Thyroid drugs
Tolbutamide
Trimethoprim/sulfamethoxazole

DECREASES PROTHROMBIN TIME

Endogenous factors

Edema
Hereditary coumarin resistance
Hyperlipemia
Hypothyroidism

Exogenous factors

Adrenocortical steroids
Alcohol
Aminoglutethimide
Antacids
Antihistamines
Barbiturates
Carbamazepine
Chloral hydrate
Chlordiazepoxide
Cholestyramine
Coumadin underdosage
Diuretics
Ethchlorvynol
Glutethimide
Griseofulvin
Haloperidol
Meprobamate
Nafcillin
Oral contraceptives
Paraldehyde
Primidone
Ranitidine
Rifampin
Sucralfate
Trazodone
Vitamin C
Vitamin K–containing foods

will seal in the first 1 to 2 weeks after surgery; thus, despite what appears to be adequate drainage at the time of operation, the pericardial space can once again become "closed." Serous or serosanguineous effusions can occur from pericarditis. Sometimes, the presence of evolving pericarditis may be suggested while patients are in-hospital by the presence of a pericardial rub, fever, or pain after surgery. We generally treat such patients in-hospital after heart surgery with a nonsteroidal antiinflammatory agent such as indomethacin (25 mg tid for 5 days). However, pericarditis and effusions may still occur in the weeks after surgery in up to 1% of patients; so when patients are seen in follow-up, the surgeon conducting the postoperative examination must look for historical or physical exam evidence of a significant pericardial effusion. Patients will often have nonspecific complaints such as malaise, slow progress, lack of energy, or sometimes nausea. Heart sounds may be muffled on examination. The neck veins may be distended, and significant paradox may be present when the blood pressure is determined. The QRS voltage of the ECG may be diminished if the effusion is large enough. If there are any signs or symptoms to suggest the presence of a pericardial effusion, or if the clinical index of suspicion is high, echocardiography is necessary.

In some patients, particularly those taking warfarin anticoagulation, bleeding into the pericardial space can occur [38]. In such instances, the pericardial effusion can progress rapidly to tamponade necessitating urgent hospitalization. Most pericardial effusions and delayed tamponade may be managed by percutaneous drainage with pericardial catheters, antiinflammatory treatment (with aspirin or indomethacin), and adjustment of the PT (in patients with hemorrhagic effusions). In very unusual cases, delayed pericardial tamponade may be the result of chylous effusions [39]. These are managed by prolonged drainage, institution of a low-fat or no-fat diet, or, if needed, intravenous hyperalimentation.

In the rare case of recurrent effusions refractory to medical therapy and repeated percutaneous drainage, creation of a pericardial window may be indicated. Once patients are discharged from the hospital after treatment of delayed pericardial effusions, follow-up should include repeat echocardiographic examinations to ensure that the effusions have not recurred and that later constriction is not a complication of the effusions [40]. Children who have had certain operations (such as the Fontan-Kreutzer, atrial switch, or Gore-tex central shunt procedures) are especially prone to this complication. Echocardiography is the initial diagnostic procedure.

Arrhythmias and Cardioversion

Postoperative atrial fibrillation is most likely to occur in patients with enlarged atria, such as those who have had surgery for mitral or tricuspid valve disease, or in adult patients who have had surgery for atrial septal defects. In patients in whom fibrillation was not present preoperatively or was only of short duration (<6–12 months), pharmacologic or direct current (DC) cardioversion should be attempted before discharge from the hospital. If this is unsuccessful, then it should be attempted again 3 to 4 months after surgery. Warfarin anticoagulation should be instituted first to avoid clot formation in the atrium. The process of conversion from atrial fibrillation to sinus rhythm may dislodge a clot, particularly from the atrial appendage, and place the patient at risk for stroke. Patients will usually be already on digoxin; quinidine or procainamide may be added in an attempt to "chemically" cardiovert the rhythm. However, if this does not restore normal sinus rhythm, patients should undergo DC cardioversion.

Patients are generally admitted to the hospital for a single day for elective cardioversion. Digoxin and quinidine levels should be checked before admission to ensure that the patient has an adequate quinidine level and does not have an excessive digoxin level. Elective cardioversion is generally performed during deep sedation with a short-acting agent such as midazolam or sodium thiopental (Pentothal) administered by an anesthesiologist who then also can monitor the airway. Synchronized DC cardioversion is attempted with 50 joules, which may be increased to 100 or 200 joules if needed. Patients whose atrial fibrillation was only for a short time are usually converted with this amount of energy. Digoxin and quinidine therapy is then maintained for at least an additional month. If no atrial irritability is present at that time, quinidine is discontinued, followed by digoxin. We generally maintain warfarin anticoagulation until the stability of the patient's atrial rhythm is demonstrated on Holter monitoring 2 to 3 months later.

Transfusion-Acquired Disease

In recent years improved, sensitive screening tests for hepatitis and human immunodeficiency virus (HIV) infection have decreased the frequency with which these diseases are transmitted in blood transfusions. In addition, over the past decade, there has been a trend in our specialty toward blood conservation and toleration of greater degrees of postoperative anemia, further reducing the risk of virus transmission. While these approaches have reduced the incidence of viral disease transmission to cardiac surgery patients, such transmitted infections still remain a significant source of later morbidity and mortality [41].

HEPATITIS

Hepatitis may be transmitted readily through blood products. Antibody/antigen screening has significantly reduced the risk of hepatitis B. However, non-A, non-B hepatitis (now known as hepatitis C) is still a serious problem [41] that is associated with a significant incidence of late sequelae [42]. Hepatitis should be suspected in patients who develop jaundice after heart surgery and in patients complaining of malaise or loss of appetite. In these circumstances, liver function studies and serial serology studies should be obtained. Patients receiving warfarin anticoagulation may require a decrease in dose due to impaired hepatic metabolism. The frequency of PT determinations must be increased accordingly until liver function recovers.

HIV DISEASE

Acquired immunodeficiency syndrome (AIDS) transmission is one of the most feared complications of blood transfusion and has previously occurred in patients undergoing heart surgery [43]. Although the implementation of HIV testing has decreased the incidence of transfusion-associated AIDS, reports of HIV transmission and non–HIV-related AIDS syndrome by blood that tested seronegative reaffirm that the problem of AIDS transmission by transfusion has not been solved [44]. The risk is currently estimated to be approximately 1 in 150,000; this has served as a significant impetus for the development of blood conservation programs and autologous and directed-donor blood donation programs.

CYTOMEGALOVIRUS

Cytomegalovirus (CMV) infection usually presents 3 to 4 weeks after exposure through blood products. It produces a picture of fever and severe malaise that can last 2 to 3 weeks. It frequently results in abnormal liver function due to CMV hepatic involvement [45]. Recent evidence suggests that CMV infection may occur more commonly as a result of reactivation of previously acquired CMV, rather than de novo infection [46]. In most patients, it produces mild morbidity. However, in pregnant women, premature babies, and organ transplant recipients, it can produce significant complications. In such patients, the risk may be reduced by administration of blood products through filters which remove leukocytes [47].

References

1. Cupples SA. Effects of timing and reinforcement of postoperative education on knowledge and recovery of patients having coronary bypass graft surgery. *Heart Lung* 20:654, 1991.

2. Liddle HV, Jensen R, Clayton PD. The rehabilitation of coronary surgical patients. *Ann Thorac Surg* 34:374, 1981.

3. Fuster V, Chesebro JH. Role of platelets and platelet inhibition in aortocoronary artery vein graft disease. *Circulation* 73:227, 1986.

4. Lawrie GM, Morris GC Jr, Earle N. Long-term results of coronary bypass surgery: Analysis of 1698 patients followed 15 to 20 years. *Ann Surg* 213:377, 1991.

5. FitzGibbon GM, et al. Coronary bypass graft patency: Angiographic study of 1179 vein grafts early, one year, and five years after operation. *J Thorac Cardiovasc Surg* 91:773, 1986.

6. Chesebro JH, et al. A platelet-inhibitor-drug trial in coronary-artery bypass operations. *N Engl J Med* 307:73, 1982.

7. Goldman S, et al. Saphenous vein graft patency 1 year after coronary bypass surgery and effects of antiplatelet therapy. Results of a Veterans Administration Cooperative Study. *Circulation* 80:1190, 1989.

8. Chesebro JH. Effect of dipyridamole and aspirin on vein graft patency after coronary bypass operations. *Thromb Res Suppl* 12:5, 1990.

9. Steering Committee of the Physicians' Health Study Research Group. Final report on the aspirin component of the ongoing Physicians' Health Study. *N Engl J Med* 321:129, 1989.

10. Kaplan EL, et al. A collaborative study of infective endocarditis in the 1980s. Emphasis on infections in patients who have undergone cardiovascular surgery. *Circulation* 59:327, 1979.

11. Dajani AS, et al. Prevention of bacterial endocarditis. Recommendations by the American Heart Association *JAMA* 264:2919, 1990.

12. Imperiale TF, Horwitz RI. Does prophylaxis prevent postdental infective endocarditis. *Am J Med* 88:131, 1990.

13. Calderwood SB, et al. Prosthetic valve endocarditis: Analysis of factors affecting outcome of therapy. *J Thorac Cardiovasac Surg* 92:776, 1986.

14. Karchmer AW. Prosthetic valve endocarditis: A continuing challenge for infection control. *J Hosp Infect* 18(Suppl A):355, 1991.

15. Heimberger TS, Duma RJ. Infection of prosthetic heart valves and cardiac pacemakers. *Infect Dis Clin North Am* 3:221, 1989.

16. Masur H, Johnson WD Jr. Prosthetic valve endocarditis. *J Thorac Cardiovasc Surg* 80:31, 1980.

17. Tornos P, et al. Late prosthetic endocarditis: Immediate and long-term prognosis. *Chest* 101:37, 1992.

18. Davenport J, Hart RG. Prosthetic valve endocarditis 1976–1987: antibiotics, anticoagulation, and stroke. *Stroke* 21:993, 1990.

19. Daniel WG, et al. Improvement in the diagnosis of abscesses associated with endocarditis by transesophageal echocardiography. *N Engl J Med* 324:795, 1991.

20. Burdon TA, et al. Durability of porcine valves at fifteen years in a representative North American population. *J Thorac Cardiovasc Surg* 103:231, 1992.

21. Dunn JM. Porcine valve durability in children. *Ann Thorac Surg* 32:357, 1981.

22. Fiddler GI, et al. Calcification of glutaraldehyde-preserved porcine and bovine xenograft valves in young children. *Ann Thorac Surg* 35:257, 1983.

23. Akins CW, et al. Late results with Carpentier-Edwards porcine bioprosthesis. *Circulation* 82(Suppl IV):IV-65, 1990.

24. Antunes MJ. Clinical performance of St. Jude and Medtronic-Hall prostheses: a randomized comparative study. *Ann Thorac Surg* 50:743, 1990.

25. van der Graf Y, et al. Risk of strut fracture of Bjork-Shiley valves. *Lancet* 339:257, 1992.

26. Ericsson A, et al. Strut fracture with Björk-Shiley 70° convexo-concave valve: An international multi-institutional follow-up study. *Eur J Cardiothorac Surg* 6:339, 1992.

27. Kastor JA, et al. Paravalvular leaks and hemolytic anemia following insertion of Starr-Edwards aortic and mitral valves. *J Thorac Cardiovasc Surg* 56:279, 1968.

28. Kopf GS, et al. Long-term performance of the St. Jude Medical valve: low incidence of thromboembolism and hemorrhagic complications with modest doses of warfarin. *Circulation* 76(Suppl III):III-132, 1987.

29. Butchart EG, et al. Low risk of thrombosis and serious embolic events despite low-intensity anticoagulation. *Circulation* 78(Suppl I):I-66, 1988.

30. Hirsh J. Oral anticoagulant drugs. *N Engl J Med* 324:1865, 1991.

31. Hartz RS, et al. Comparative study of warfarin versus antiplatelet therapy in patients with a St. Jude Medical valve in the aortic position. *J Thorac Cardiovasc Surg* 92:84, 1986.

32. Hill JD, et al. Risk-benefit analysis of warfarin therapy in Hancock mitral valve replacement. *J Thorac Cardiovasc Surg* 83:718, 1982.

33. The Boston area anticoagulation trial for atrial fibrillation investigators. The effect of low-dose warfarin on the risk of stroke in patients with nonrheumatic atrial fibrillation. *N Engl J Med* 323:1505, 1990.

34. Khan AH. The postcardiac injury syndrome. *Clin Cardiol* 15:67, 1992.

35. Miller RH, et al. The epidemiology of the postpericardiotomy syndrome: A common complication of cardiac surgery. *Am Heart J* 116:1323, 1988.

36. Ikaheimo MJ, et al. Pericardial effusion after cardiac surgery: incidence, relation to the type of surgery, antithrombotic therapy, and early coronary bypass graft patency. *Am Heart J* 116:97, 1988.

37. Borkon AM, et al. Diagnosis and management of postoperative pericardial effusions and late cardiac tamponade following open-heart surgery. *Ann Thorac Surg* 31:512, 1981.

38. Ofori-Krakye SK, et al. Late cardiac tamponade after open heart surgery: Incidence, role of anticoagulants in its pathogenesis and its relationship to postpericardiotomy syndrome. *Circulation* 63:1323, 1981.

39. Thomas CS Jr, McGoon DC. Isolated massive chylopericardium following cardiopulmonary bypass. *J Thorac Cardiovasc Surg* 61:945, 1971.

40. Killian DM, et al. Constrictive pericarditis after cardiac surgery. *Am Heart J* 118:563, 1989.

41. Bove JR. Transfusion-associated hepatitis and AIDS. What is the risk? *N Engl J Med* 317:242, 1987.

42. DiBisceglie AM, et al. Long-term clinical and histopathologic follow-up of chronic posttransfusion hepatitis. *Hepatology* 14:969, 1991.

43. Schiff M, et al. Acquired immunodeficiency syndrome, a complication of cardiothoracic surgery. *J Thorac Cardiovasc Surg* 97:126, 1989.

44. Ward JW, et al. Transmission of human immunodeficiency virus (HIV) by blood transfusions screened as negative for HIV antibody. *N Engl J Med* 318:473, 1988.

45. Adler SP. Transfusion-associated cytomegalovirus infection. *Rev Infect Dis* 5:977, 1983.
46. Adler SP, Baggett J, McVoy M. Transfusion associated cytomegalovirus infection in seropositive cardiac surgery patients. *Lancet* 2(8458):743, 1985.
47. Sayers MH, et al. Reducing the risk for transfusion-transmitted cytomegalovirus infection. *Ann Intern Med* 116:55, 1992.

Complete Atrioventricular Canal

Complete atrioventricular canal is accurately defined by echocardiography in most cases. Preoperative catheterization may be useful in evaluating the degree of the patient's pulmonary hypertension and atrioventricular valve regurgitation. The size of the two ventricles must be assessed to ascertain that they are "balanced." Postoperative care can be challenging because of the young age of the patient and because pulmonary hypertension is frequently present in the postoperative period. Infants are especially prone to having spells of pulmonary vascular hypertensive crises postoperatively and this must be planned for. This aspect of complete atrioventricular canal postoperative management is aided greatly by having a pulmonary artery catheter placed at the time of surgery, not only for the measurement of pulmonary artery pressure but also to permit blood sampling to measure pulmonary artery saturation and, hence, detect any residual shunts. Atrioventricular valve function is sometimes an issue after correction; proper postoperative monitoring of atrial pressures is useful for assessing the mitral and tricuspid valves. In the past decade, the trend has been to operate on infants with complete atrioventricular canal earlier in life, typically at 3 to 6 months of age.

Tetralogy of Fallot

Tetralogy of Fallot requires complete cineangiography to define the anatomy of the ventricles and outflow tracts, ventricular septal defect, pulmonary arteries, and coronary arteries. Whether primary complete repair or a shunting procedure should be performed in neonates with tetralogy is a subject of debate and varies from center to center. In many centers initial palliation by shunting may be done if coronary anomalies are present (e.g., left anterior descending artery crossing the right ventricular outflow tract) or if there are other significant concomitant illnesses (e.g., tracheoesophageal fistula). In these instances, systemic-to-pulmonary shunting may be performed as an initial step.

In the immediate postoperative period, the patency of systemic-to-pulmonary shunts is enhanced by maintaining adequate blood volume and arterial pressure. After complete repair, postoperative care requires particular attention to the function of the right ventricle, which usually has been incised to permit relief of outflow tract obstruction. Particularly when transannular outflow tract reconstruction has been performed, these patients sometimes experience several days of low cardiac output during which they must be ventilated, carefully monitored, and supported with catecholamines. In a prior era, some of these patients experienced severe low output after correction due to failure of the right ventricle. More recently, particularly when corrections have been carried out early in the first year of life, this potential problem can be managed by leaving open a patent foramen ovale. Thus, if right heart failure occurs after surgery, elevated right atrial pressure produces a right-to-left shunt at the atrial level. The result is some systemic desaturation with maintenance of good systemic ventricular output. As right ventricular function recovers during the first 3 to 5 days after surgery, this shunt diminishes with decreased right atrial pressure.

Postoperative management of tetralogy patients is facilitated by having a catheter introduced into the pulmonary artery across the right ventricular (RV) outflow tract. This permits blood sampling from the pulmonary artery to detect residual shunts and, at the time of line removal, pressure monitoring permits the detection of any residual RV outflow tract gradient.

Pulmonary Atresia with Ventricular Septal Defect

Pulmonary atresia with ventricular septal defect may be considered a very severe form of tetralogy. Cardiac catheterization is essential in defining the ventricular anatomy and the size and location of the pulmonary arteries. When bronchial collaterals do not provide adequate pulmonary blood flow in the neonatal period, the patient is begun on prostaglandin E_1 (PGE_1) infusion to open the ductus arteriosus. Operation early in life consists of a shunt, with complete correction delayed until the child is much larger. In instances where a main pulmonary artery (PA) is present, initial palliation may also include a pulmonic valvotomy, an outflow tract patch, or an RV-to-PA conduit. Right ventricular outflow tract flow into the pulmonary arteries can promote arterial growth and provides vascular access if percutaneous pulmonary artery dilation is later required. In some instances, postoperative care can be more complex because of the multiple sources of pulmonary blood flow.

Pulmonary Atresia with Intact Ventricular Septum

Pulmonary atresia with intact ventricular septum differs from pulmonary atresia with ventricular septal defect in that the right ventricle is almost always very hypoplastic. Prostaglandin E_1 again is useful in the newborn to stabilize the patient by increasing pulmonary blood flow. If the anatomy is suitable, valvotomy is performed both to improve pulmonary perfusion and hopefully to stimulate right ventricular growth. A systemic-to-pulmonary shunt procedure is often required as well. Critical pulmonic stenosis is usually associated with a more nearly normal right ventricle and the response to percutaneous or surgical valvotomy is generally better. For both of these conditions, pulmonary vascular resistance postoperatively must be kept as low as possible using oxygen, vasodilators, and optimal ventilatory management.

Transposition of the Great Arteries

Transposition of the great arteries is the most common cause of cyanosis presenting in the neonatal period. As soon as the diagnosis is suspected, PGE_1 is begun to improve mixing across the ductus. Echocardiography is then performed to confirm the diagnosis; this may be followed by cardiac catheterization to allow further palliation with a Rashkind balloon septostomy, identification of associated lesions, and assessment of the coronary anatomy. In most institutions, an arterial switch operation is carried out within the first 2 weeks of life, unless some feature of the anatomy favors delay to an older age, at which time the type of correction is individualized.

Coarctation of the Aorta

Coarctation of the aorta varies in its presentation from profound congestive failure and peripheral hypoperfusion in neonates to asymptomatic hypertension in older children. In the newborn, PGE_1

may palliate severe coarctation until operation is performed because it opens the ductus and restores distal aortic perfusion from the pulmonary artery. Echocardiography is usually adequate to detect the presence of the coarctation and any associated intracardiac defects, but catheterization may be necessary to depict accurately the anatomy of the coarctation. Surgical correction may be postponed for a few days in newborns if the PGE_1 is effective in restoring peripheral perfusion; this allows a semielective operation to be done on a stable patient. In older children, operation is done electively, usually to treat hypertension.

Patent Ductus Arteriosus

Patent ductus arteriosus is encountered commonly in premature infants with respiratory distress syndrome. Echocardiography establishes the diagnosis and excludes other significant intracardiac conditions, such as an aortopulmonary window. In the newborn, indomethacin may be used to attempt closure of the ductus nonoperatively. Operation is usually performed for difficulty in weaning from the ventilator or for severe congestive heart failure. In children, operation should be performed electively because of the long-term risk of endocarditis, as well as the risk of developing pulmonary vascular obstructive disease with a large patent ductus.

Aortic Stenosis

Aortic stenosis, depending on its severity, may cause symptoms at any age. Severe stenosis in infancy produces profound congestive failure and acidosis and requires emergency intervention. This extreme form is best managed with prompt echocardiographic diagnosis, followed by a brief period of medical stabilization with ventilation and vasopressor support before percutaneous or operative valvotomy. Milder forms of stenosis may be followed until symptoms occur or until the patient develops a sufficiently severe gradient that makes sudden death a risk.

Univentricular Heart

Univentricular heart encompasses a wide variety of anatomic configurations that share the common feature of having a single functional ventricular chamber. The associated defects and resultant physiology determine the clinical effects, degree of cyanosis, and approach to patient management. Usually, an initial palliative operation is required to increase or decrease pulmonary blood flow with the aim of eventually carrying out a Fontan-Kreutzer type procedure to place the pulmonary and systemic circulations in series.

Tricuspid Atresia

Tricuspid atresia is a type of univentricular cardiac lesion characterized by the absence of the tricuspid valve and thus by the absence of the normal connection between the right atrium and right ventricle. The right ventricle is invariably hypoplastic. Associated defects determine the physiologic consequences of tricuspid atresia. Pulmonary blood flow may be increased, decreased, or normal depending on associated anatomic features; the degree of cyanosis is similarly variable. Most neonates have diminished pulmonary blood flow and require treatment with PGE_1 and systemic-to-pulmonary artery shunting. Eventually, a Fontan-Kreutzer operation is performed.

Hypoplastic Left Heart Syndrome

Hypoplastic left heart syndrome results in univentricular physiology based on an anatomic right ventricle, associated with unimpeded pulmonary blood flow and systemic blood flow that is ductus dependent. Consequently, on ductal closure, these infants can present with profound circulatory collapse and severe systemic acidosis. Initial management consists of intubation, PGE_1 to open the ductus arteriosus, inotropic support, bicarbonate administration to correct acidosis, and ventilatory management to limit pulmonary blood flow. With appropriate management, these very ill neonates can be stabilized for several days or even weeks. They may be treated by either the Norwood procedure or transplantation. The preferred approach remains a matter of controversy.

Truncus Arteriosus

Truncus arteriosus is an uncommon defect that presents in the neonatal period with congestive failure caused by excessive pulmonary blood flow. Cardiac catheterization is required to define the pulmonary anatomy, ventricular relations, and ventricular septal defect. Total correction is generally performed in early infancy. If operation is delayed, pulmonary vascular obstructive disease is likely to develop. Postoperative management may be challenging due to pulmonary hypertension.

Total Anomalous Pulmonary Venous Connection

Total anomalous pulmonary venous connection is another uncommon condition that usually presents in the first 6 weeks of life. The severity of the patient's symptoms is directly related to the degree of pulmonary venous obstruction, with severely obstructed pulmonary veins resulting in patient presentation in the newborn period. Operation is performed urgently in all cases, as there are few temporizing measures. Prostaglandin E_1 is avoided because restoration of ductal patency can worsen pulmonary congestion in the presence of obstructed pulmonary veins. The most critical element of postoperative care is management of the lungs, because of the potential effects of pulmonary venous obstruction and resulting pulmonary hypertension and lung injury. Invariably, several days of ventilation are required after surgery.

Preoperative Preparation

It is essential that all possible steps are taken to ensure that patients arrive in the operating room in optimal condition. The need for truly emergent operation has become rare because of improvements in diagnosis and management, especially the contributions of PGE_1 and effective resuscitation, which allow stabilization of most of the anomalies that cause severe collapse in newborns (see Chap. 1).

Laboratory studies usually include blood gases, electrolytes, glucose, calcium, and hematocrit. A specimen for blood crossmatching is obtained as well. Typically, a chest x-ray, ECG, and echocardiogram are performed as part of the initial diagnostic investigation.

Critically ill neonates are likely to develop profound metabolic acidosis as an early indicator of poor cardiac output. This should be corrected with bicarbonate infusion as the ductus is being opened with PGE_1. Respiratory acidosis should be treated with mechanical ventilation to lower the patient's PCO_2. Intubation may also be necesssary if apnea develops as a side effect of PGE_1.

All babies, particularly premature infants, have difficulty with thermal autoregulation; thus, they are at risk for hypothermia. This can further aggravate hypoperfusion. Radiant warming devices with temperature control servomechanisms permit maintenance of normal body temperature without impeding access to the patient.

Catecholamine support may be required along with transfusions if the patient is hypovolemic or cyanotic and anemic. With these management principles, it is rare nowadays for emergency operations to be performed and overall results have improved dramatically.

DUCTUS-DEPENDENT LESIONS

A considerable number of congenital heart defects that used to require urgent operative treatment in the neonatal period are now palliated by opening the ductus arteriosus and maintaining its patency with PGE_1 [3] (Table 7-1). This may be useful in patients with inadequate pulmonary blood flow (e.g., those with pulmonary or tricuspid atresia or tetralogy), inadequate systemic blood flow (e.g., those with coarctation, critical aortic stenosis, or hypoplastic left heart syndrome), or transposition of the great arteries, as well as in other, less common conditions. Prostaglandin E_1 permits time to improve the patient's hypoxia and acidosis. The patient may then come to the operating room with a lesser degree of urgency and in better condition to withstand a major operation. Prostaglandin E_1 is administered intravenously at 0.01 to 0.10 µg/kg/min. The lowest effective dose is used to prevent side effects, which include hypotension, seizures, fever, and apnea.

Table 7-1. Lesions palliated by PGE_1 infusion

Lesions with inadequate pulmonary blood flow
   Tetralogy of Fallot
   Pulmonary atresia
   Tricuspid atresia

Lesions with inadequate systemic blood flow
   Coarctation
   Interrupted aortic arch
   Critical aortic stenosis
   Hypoplastic left heart syndrome

Lesions with inadequate mixing
   Transposition of the great arteries

Key: PGE_1 = Prostaglandin E_1.

Operative Considerations

MONITORING LINES

Adequate intravenous access must be assured to permit safe initiation of the operation; additional transthoracic lines for postoperative use are easily placed during the procedure. Conventional percutaneous insertion of peripheral lines is usually possible, but cutdowns may be required as well, particularly in neonates. Scalp vein catheters are precarious and should not be relied on for any critical medication or fluid infusion.

There are a number of commercially available products that facilitate insertion of central venous lines. We commonly employ a 5 Fr. double-lumen catheter (Cook Critical Care, Bloomington, IN) inserted via the internal or external jugular vein after the patient is anesthetized. Using the Seldinger technique, this catheter can be inserted easily by experienced users and has few complications.

Peripheral arterial cannulation is generally accomplished by percutaneous insertion into the radial artery, although cutdown is sometimes required, particularly in the neonate [4]. A 22-gauge catheter is adequate for small children and infants and can be maintained for several days with proper nursing care. Percutaneous insertion may be facilitated by the use of a straight, flexible guidewire (0.015 in.). Alternatively, if this produces a poor arterial pressure tracing or if blood withdrawal is difficult, a short 22-gauge catheter may be exchanged over a guidewire to a 2.5 Fr. catheter inserted 3 to 4 cm into the radial artery. This will usually yield better blood withdrawal and improve the phasic arterial pressure tracing. Femoral artery cannulation may be used as an alternative and likewise has few complications [5,6]; meticulous attention must be directed to maintaining the sterility of the insertion site.

Patients undergoing uneventful operation for relatively simple defects generally require no additional catheters beyond those inserted preoperatively. At the conclusion of the more complex operative procedures, we often use a variety of transthoracic lines that permit more accurate hemodynamic monitoring and provide additional access for administration of volume and drugs. A right atrial catheter can be inserted easily via a venous cannulation site or by separate puncture. This line is secured by one or more pursestring sutures and brought out to the surface by a separate stab wound. Similarly, a left atrial catheter may be placed through a pursestring suture in the right superior pulmonary vein. Meticulous line care is required to minimize the risk of air embolization from left atrial catheters.

We have made extensive use of pulmonary artery catheters with oximetric capability, particularly in patients with complex heart defects and severe pulmonary hypertension. This catheter is placed through a pledgeted pursestring suture in the RV outflow tract and positioned in the main pulmonary artery. All transthoracic lines of this type must be removed before withdrawal of the patient's mediastinal drainage tubes, lest excessive bleeding from the heart lead to tamponade; this should not be done unless blood is available for transfusion and coagulation values are adequate. The complication rate from these lines is far less than 1% [7] and justifies their use in appropriate patients.

Umbilical artery catheters are often helpful in the pre- and postoperative management of neonates [8]. Often, the umbilical vessels can provide access for cardiac catheterization, and, at the conclusion of catheterization, umbilical artery and vein catheters may be inserted for subsequent intra- and postoperative use (Fig. 7-1). Multiple-lumen catheters may also be used via umbilical access [9]. Proper positioning of these lines, preferably below the level of the renal arteries, should be radiologically confirmed. It is desirable to remove umbilical artery lines as soon as possible because they have been implicated in the development of necrotizing enterocolitis and arterial thrombosis [10], particularly in premature infants. We generally remove them after patients are extubated. Usually, patients are not fed until umbilical artery lines are removed, although this practice varies from institution to institution. Similarly, *umbilical venous lines* may lead to portal vein thrombosis [11] and should be removed within a few days after insertion. Umbilical lines are removed by first discontinuing heparinized saline infusion. Beginning with the umbilical venous line, these lines are slowly withdrawn until a small amount of bleeding is noted around each catheter. The catheter is then advanced back in 1 to 2 mm. After approximately 15–20 minutes they may be completely withdrawn, as the umbilical vessels will have clotted.

Postoperative Care

Summarized in Appendix 3 are medications, dosages, and management principles commonly encountered in the postoperative intensive care of neonates, infants, and children.

ASSESSMENT OF CARDIOVASCULAR STATUS

The evaluation of the small child or infant after cardiac surgery is a demanding task requiring the utmost vigilance and attention to subtle changes [12].

Physical Examination

Because babies are capable of major alterations in their clinical status in a short period of time and because cardiac output cannot be measured directly as in adult patients, the importance of the physical examination is clearly apparent.

One of the most important indicators of tissue perfusion in the infant is the distribution of skin temperature. Often, a distinct gradation in skin temperature from abdominal wall, to thigh, to calf, and to foot can be detected as the patient's cardiac output varies. The presence and volume of the peripheral pulses are a good index of cardiac output; inspection of the skin color and capillary refill of the nailbeds is also worthwhile. Particularly in neonates, central fever with a cool periphery is an ominous sign of low cardiac output that requires prompt attention [13].

Examination of the chest and lung fields gives information regarding the adequacy of ventilation and can be an early warning of

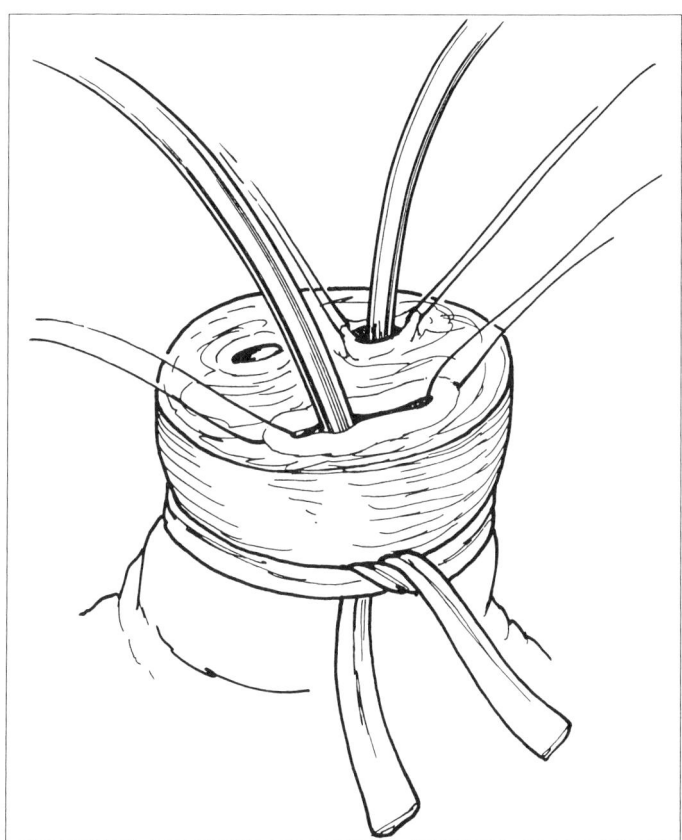

Fig. 7-1. Insertion of umbilical artery and vein catheters for neonatal monitoring and fluid and drug infusion. After a sterile prep and draping, the umbilicus is amputated to within 5–8 mm of the skin line. Two umbilical arteries and an umbilical vein (larger vessel) can be identified in the cross section. Silk traction sutures (3-0 or 4-0) are placed through the edges of the cut vessels as shown and gentle upward countertraction is exerted. An artery and the vein are then catheterized with a commercially available umbilical vessel catheter. The amount of each catheter one should insert to result in the catheter tip being at the level of the diaphragm can be estimated from the following formulas:

Artery: Inserted length (cm) = 8.5 + (1.6 × shoulder-umbilical length [cm])
Vein: Inserted length (cm) = 5.0 + (0.6 × shoulder-umbilical length [cm])

Shoulder-umbilical length is measured on a perpendicular line from the baby's shoulder to a transverse line drawn through the umbilicus. The traction sutures can be tied around each catheter to secure the insertion. To complete the procedure, umbilical tape is tied around the base of the umbilicus at the skin line to ensure a good seal around each catheter. (From P Dunn. Localization of the umbilical catheter by post-mortem measurement. *Arch Dis Child* 41:69, 1966. Adapted from *The Harriet Lane Handbook.* Chicago: Year Book Medical Publishers, 1984.)

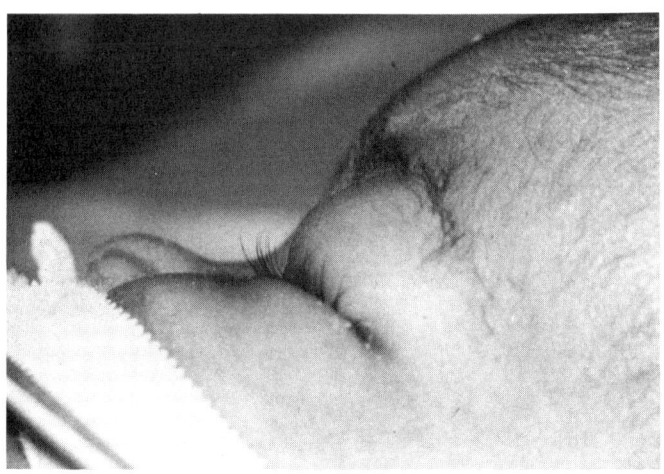

Fig. 7-2. Puffiness of the eyelid — a sign of generalized edema in the neonate and infant.

impending difficulty. When the patient is mechanically ventilated, chest excursion should be smooth and symmetric. Because the calculated ventilation tidal volume based on the patient's body weight may be misleading, we prefer to rely on a visual assessment of chest expansion to confirm the adequacy of the ventilatory volume. After extubation, the infant's breathing pattern should remain smooth and there should be no nasal flaring, intercostal retraction, or use of accessory muscles.

Hepatomegaly is a common sign of congestive failure. The liver edge is easily palpated in most children, and it will rise and fall in response to treatment. Peripheral edema is common after cardiopulmonary bypass and does not always signify failure; however, it is an important indicator of total body fluid and generally signifies a need for diuresis. Children typically exhibit a great deal of edema in the soft tissues of the upper back (the so-called flat back sign) or the face (Fig. 7-2), often to a degree not seen in the extremities. Palpating the tension of the cranial fontanelles, which are not fused in neonates, provides another method of assessing volume status.

Auscultation of the heart in the young patient is difficult because of the rapid heart and respiratory rates. Nevertheless, surgeons caring for such patients should familiarize themselves with each patient's particular auscultatory findings to permit identification of changes in heart sounds that may indicate a physiologically important alteration. A new or changing murmur, presence or resolution of a gallop, or appearance of a friction rub should be noted and compared with previous examinations.

Mixed Venous Saturation

Mixed venous oxygen saturation ($S\bar{v}O_2$) varies with the patient's oxygen consumption, hemoglobin concentration, arterial oxygen saturation, and cardiac output. If the first three factors are constant, changes in $S\bar{v}O_2$ can be followed as a rough indicator of cardiac output. In appropriate patients, we use an indwelling pulmonary artery catheter that makes colorimetric measurement of $S\bar{v}O_2$ for continuous on-line determination of this variable. The catheter must be calibrated frequently by laboratory measurements of carefully obtained pulmonary artery blood sample to ensure accuracy. We have found it most helpful to rely on fluctuations of $S\bar{v}O_2$ over time, rather than on an isolated value, as the most valuable indicator of cardiac performance [14]. In general, patients with good cardiac output maintain an $S\bar{v}O_2$ above 60%.

TREATMENT OF LOW OUTPUT

Hypovolemia occurs commonly after operations for congenital heart defects; bleeding, blood sampling, vasodilation from rewarming, and diuresis all contribute to this. Appropriate infusions of blood, colloid, and crystalloid are administered to correct volume deficits and maintain approximate oxygen carrying capacity. Left atrial or pulmonary artery catheters are useful in assessing the need for and results of volume replacement.

Volume loading can produce deleterious effects, however, and this adverse response to excessive fluid administration is most likely in infants and with more complex cardiac defects [15]. As a general rule, infants and young children do not respond favorably to high levels of preload as do adults; we rarely push the central venous pressure above 10 mm Hg or the left atrial pressure above 15 mm Hg, relying more on catecholamine administration to improve cardiac output.

The general use of pharmacologic agents in the treatment of low cardiac output is discussed in Chapter 3. Isoproterenol infusions provide both inotropic support and afterload reduction, although they may be of limited use in the already tachycardic patient. Dobutamine and moderate-dose dopamine are also useful in stimulating the myocardium without causing vasoconstriction. Amrinone is especially useful in pediatric patients because it reduces pulmonary vascular resistance, which is often a problem in these patients. Epinephrine is used in low doses when the above agents produce unsatisfactory results. Often, nitroglycerin, nitroprusside, or PGE_1 is added for afterload reduction. The target systolic arterial blood pressure, of course, is age-related, ranging from 50 to 60 mm Hg in the neonate to 100 mm Hg in the young child (see Table 3-1).

TAMPONADE PHYSIOLOGY

Cardiac tamponade represents a life-threatening complication in children as it does in adults. The volume of fluid required to produce tamponade in children is, of course, much smaller; therefore, the surgeon must have a lower theshold for reopening the sternum when this occurs. The difficulty lies in making the diagnosis of tamponade, particularly in the absence of intracardiac pressure measurements, which often facilitate the diagnosis in adult patients. Tamponade must be suspected in any child who demonstrates diminished tissue perfusion and elevated venous pressure in the postoperative period without an identifiable cause. The index of suspicion must be particularly high when these findings occur in an otherwise stable child following removal of intracardiac monitoring lines. Tamponade may be heralded by mediastinal drainage tubes that suddenly stop draining or by temporary pacing wires that falter. Echocardiography may be unreliable in excluding this diagnosis in children. Sometimes a few chest compressions in an infant will initiate evacuation of a very recent ("fresh") tamponade. However, if this is not immediately successful, prompt sternal reopening is mandatory, either in the operating room or, if needed, in the intensive care unit. Sometimes, exploration is necessary to rule out tamponade even when the clinical signs are very soft.

Infants are especially prone to develop tamponade physiology because of cardiac compression in the absence of mediastinal blood clots. A small amount of cardiac edema, swelling of the mediastinal tissues, or elevation of the diaphragm from ascites can produce this syndrome. Leaving the sternum open for a few days after surgery may prove lifesaving [16]. Also, we sometimes leave a drain in the peritoneal cavity of infants to drain ascites fluid and help avoid elevation of the diaphragm. Some have advocated continuous fluid removal early after surgery in critically ill infants as a means of alleviating the consequences of edema. This may be achieved by continuous ultrafiltration [17] or early peritoneal dialysis [18]. Late tamponade due to pericardial effusion can occur following operations for congenital heart disease and, in some patients, can be life threatening [19,20]. Prior to hospital discharge and at the first postoperative office visit, the neck veins should be examined and the patient should be checked for possible pulsus paradoxus.

RESIDUAL LESIONS

Residual lesions include those anatomic abnormalities that are not repaired at operation because of technical difficulty, unacceptable risk, or incomplete diagnosis and those that are deliberately left uncorrected for physiologic reasons. Typical examples include atrial or ventricular septal defects that are incompetely closed due to technical error, resulting in excessive pulmonary blood flow. Other residua include a persistent gradient across a coarctation repair or persistent valvular stenosis after aortic or pulmonary valvotomy. Knowledge of residual lesions obtained by postoperative monitoring or echocardiography can guide the timing of late postoperative restudy [21].

Treatment of residual lesions must be individualized according to the patient's symptoms, physical findings, and results of invasive and noninvasive studies. Residual lesions must be considered after operation if the patient has a worse-than-expected clinical course. If a patient is not progressing after surgery as expected, the adequacy of repair and the presence of residual lesions must be determined. Echocardiography is an essential first step in this process. If necessary, cardiac catheterization may be required. If a poor clinical course leads to restudy and a significant, unexpected residual lesion is found, immediate reoperation is often the best course to ensure a good short- and long-term outcome.

As mentioned above, sometimes defects are deliberately left unrepaired. An example is the atrial septal defect that is left open to allow right-to-left shunting when right ventricular function is impaired [22] or in some patients after the Fontan-Kreutzer procedure [23]. Leaving residual right-to-left shunts in such situations has decreased the morbidity and mortality from low output due to right-sided failure sometimes observed following these types of operations.

PULMONARY MANAGEMENT

Pulmonary care in the young patient usually begins in the operating room with intubation. Although practices vary from institution to institution, at the University of Iowa we prefer initial intubation via the oral route using an appropriately sized uncuffed tube (Table 7-2). Cuffed endotracheal tubes are used only in older patients (>10 years) secondary to the increased risk of subglottic stenosis in younger children. The subglottic region is the narrowest portion of the airway in young children, whereas the larynx is the narrowest portion in older children and adults. The endotracheal tube is of the appropriate size if it maintains a good seal up to 25 to 30 cm H_2O airway pressure, but "leaks" at higher airway pressures. An uncuffed endotracheal tube that does not "leak" at higher airway pressures may be too large and should be changed. In the occasional patient who will be extubated the day of operation, the orotracheal tube is left in place at the end of the procedure. For most patients, who will require mechanical ventilation for at least 12 to 24 hours, we prefer to remove the orotracheal tube at the end of the operation and replace it with a nasotracheal tube. A new, clean tube is always inserted in infants before transfer to the intensive care unit. The nasal tube provides better opportunity for secure fixation and aids in oral hygiene. Orotracheal tubes are also subject to inadvertent removal (Fig. 7-3). We obtain a postoperative chest film in the operating room prior to transfer of the patient to the intensive care unit. This confirms proper positioning of the tube in the trachea, proper positioning of intracardiac monitoring lines, and may demonstrate a need for additional chest tubes (Fig. 7-4).

Table 7-2. Endotracheal tube (ETT) size and intubation guidelines

Age	Internal diameter (mm)[a]
Premature infant[b]	2.5–3.0[c]
Term infant[b]	3.0–3.5
3 mo–1 yr	4.0
1–2 yr	4.5
2–15 yr	$\frac{16 + \text{age (years)}}{4}$

[a]If no leak is present at airway pressures >30 cm H_2O, change to the next smaller tube.
[b]The head should not be extended for placement of the ETT in newborns due to anatomic differences compared to older patients.
[c]Most premature neonates can accept a 3.0 ETT. 2.5 ETTs have increased airway resistance and are difficult to suction adequately.
Source: Adapted from *The Harriet Lane Handbook.* Chicago: Year Book Medical Publishers, 1984.

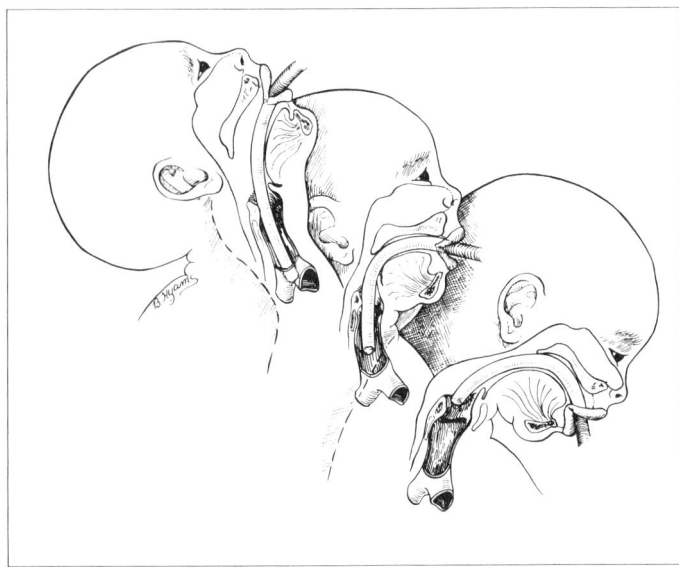

Fig. 7-3. Effect of head motion on the position of an orotracheal tube in a neonate or infant. As the neck is extended the orolaryngeal distance is shortened, and the distal end of the tube is pushed to the carina or into a (usually right) bronchus. This distance is lengthened as the neck is flexed; the tube may be pulled completely out of the trachea because the laryngotracheal distance is so short. (From BB Roe, *Perioperative Management in Cardiac Surgery*. Boston: Little, Brown, 1981. P. 14.)

At the Massachusetts General Hospital, we prefer initial intubation via the nasal route. Before intubation, 1 or 2 drops of ½% phenylephrine is placed into the selected nostril to produce mucosal vasoconstriction and, hence, reduce the risk of bleeding during heparinization. The tube is not changed at the end of the procedure. Edema can make nasal reintubation at the end of the operation more difficult, particularly in neonates following repair of complex lesions.

The connections between the endotracheal tube and the ventilator must be flexible enough to permit motion of the patient's head without moving the tube within the trachea. Failure to make this provision may lead to unplanned tube removal or trauma to the airway. It is essential that patients requiring mechanical ventilation be provided with sufficient analgesia and sedation to preclude violent movements. Particularly in patients with postoperative pulmonary hypertension, high-dose sedation with narcotics such as fentanyl (at least 10 µg/kg/hr) or morphine (0.1 mg/kg/hr) combined with pharmacologic paralysis (pancuronium 0.1 mg/kg/hr) is usually necessary for the appropriate ventilatory control of the pulmonary circulation.

The postoperative care of children (particularly neonates) following cardiac surgery involves very close attention to respiratory care and ventilatory management [24,25]. Atelectasis should be prevented

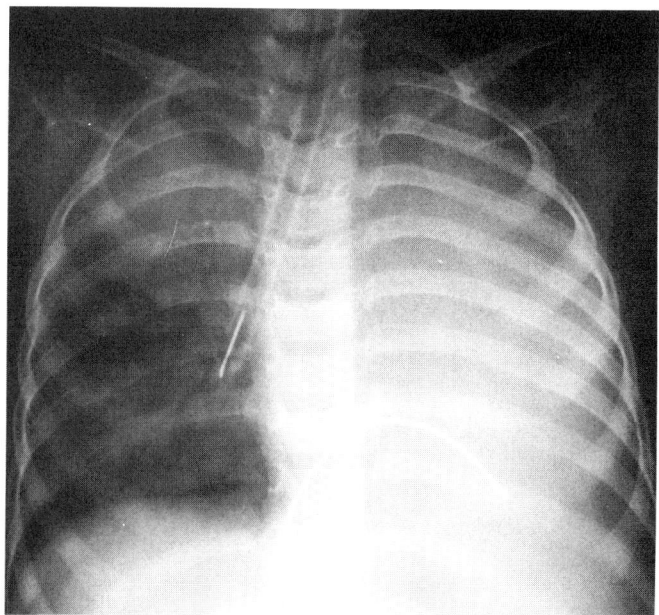

Fig. 7-4. Chest x-ray from an infant showing right bronchial intubation leading to total left lung and right upper lobe atelectasis.

by assuring adequate tidal volume and providing appropriate chest physiotherapy. Endotracheal suctioning is important, but it must be used with great caution in the hemodynamically precarious patient. Particularly in the patient with pulmonary hypertension, vigorous airway suction can produce hypoxia, pulmonary vascular spasm, and cardiovascular collapse [26]; premedication with additional narcotic plus manual hyperventilation with 100% oxygen may be needed before suctioning is performed. Tubes that may be obstructed should be removed immediately and replaced; suctioning may not succeed in removing a mucous plug or clot that is acting as a ball-valve on the tip of the tube.

Formerly, the only mechanical ventilators used for pediatric patients were of the pressure-cycled type. These ventilators deliver gas until a given pressure is reached, followed by an expiratory phase. In most neonates after cardiopulmonary bypass, inspiratory pressures of at least 20 to 25 cm H_2O are commonly required. Positive end-expiratory pressure (PEEP) of 3 to 5 cm H_2O is used to prevent alveolar collapse and to improve functional residual capacity. The ventilatory rate typically is 15 to 20 per minute. We generally employ the intermittent mandatory ventilation mode because this allows the patient to establish his or her own breathing pattern and assists in weaning. The inspiratory:expiratory ratio (I:E) is usually 1:2 (Fig. 7-5).

Volume-cycled ventilators use a similar ventilatory rate, PEEP, and I:E ratio. The tidal volume is about 15 to 20 ml/kg, slightly more

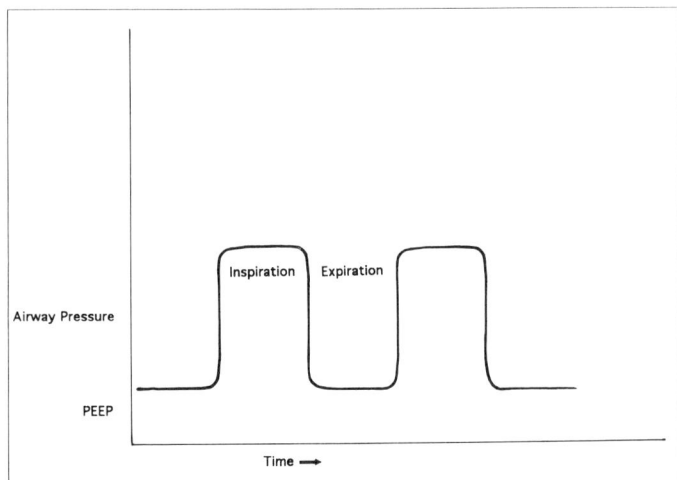

Fig. 7-5. Airway pressure as a function of time with a pressure-cycled ventilator. The inspiratory phase and expiratory phase are noted.
Key: PEEP = positive end-expiratory pressure.

than that used in adults. The inspiratory pressures must be monitored and limits set to guard against barotrauma. High-frequency jet ventilation, although not in common use in postoperative cardiac infants, may be of value in selected cases of severe pulmonary failure, acute respiratory distress syndrome, refractory pulmonary hypertension, or after a Fontan-Kreutzer procedure [27].

The fractional inspired oxygen (FIO_2) is reduced as rapidly as possible to prevent complications such as retrolental fibroplasia. It is more important to individualize this in pediatric patients than in adults because of the unique physiologic requirements imposed by some of their cardiac anomalies.

Pulmonary Hypertension

Pulmonary hypertension is typically encountered in patients with large left-to-right shunts and in those with left-sided obstructive lesions, such as mitral stenosis, cor triatriatum, and obstructed total anomalous pulmonary venous return. If left untreated, the pulmonary vascular resistance (PVR) may rise to systemic levels or higher and become irreversible (Eisenmenger syndrome). These patients are inoperable. One of the tasks of preoperative catheterization is to separate those patients with fixed elevation of PVR from those in whom the PVR falls to operable levels in response to oxygen or vasodilator drugs or both. Some of these latter, borderline-operable patients will thus be operated on and demand great attention postoperatively.

The most important component of the treatment of postoperative pulmonary hypertension is proper ventilatory management. The FIO_2 is kept high, and hypercarbia and acidosis are avoided. The patient should receive adequate sedation and paralysis to prevent

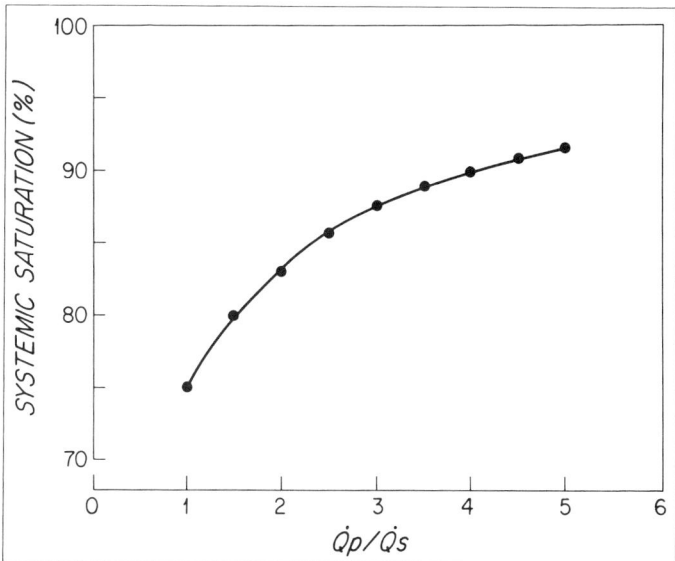

Fig. 7-6. Illustration of systemic saturation achieved as a function of the pulmonary-to-systemic flow ratio ($\dot{Q}_p/\dot{Q}_s$). Note that 100% saturation is approached asymptotically.

voluntary resistance to ventilation. These measures are often sufficient to maintain maximum pulmonary vasodilatation. Vigorous hand ventilation of the patient with 100% oxygen often alleviates those episodes of pulmonary vascular spasm that appear periodically and may be lifesaving.

Vasodilators such as nitroglycerin and nitroprusside or PGE_1 may be used. Amrinone is another valuable agent for lowering pulmonary artery resistance, and its modest inotropic effect may provide additional benefits. Dopamine may worsen the situation. Isoproterenol is useful if the heart rate is not excessive. Recently, inhaled nitric oxide has been used with good results; it appears to be a truly selective, potent pulmonary vasodilator [28].

Parallel Circulations and Control of the Pulmonary Circulation

One of the most challenging problems for postoperative management in congenital heart surgery is the care of patients with parallel circulations. Parallel circulations are encountered after palliation of any single ventricle lesion, such as after the Norwood operation for hypoplastic left heart syndrome or after creation of a systemic-to-pulmonary shunt in complex lesions that include pulmonary atresia. In these patients, the systemic saturation achieved depends on the relative amounts of pulmonary and systemic blood flow, which is expressed as the ratio $\dot{Q}_p/\dot{Q}_s$. Figure 7-6 shows an example of the systemic saturation achieved as a function of $\dot{Q}_p/\dot{Q}_s$, assuming a completely mixed circulation such as that encountered in single ventricle physiology and, for the purposes of illustration, assuming a systemic venous saturation of 50%. Note that 100% saturation is approached asymptotically so that very high ratios of $\dot{Q}_p/\dot{Q}_s$ are required to achieve high levels of systemic saturation. It is important to note that increasing saturation is obtained not only by increasing pulmonary blood flow but also by decreasing systemic flow. This has particularly important implications in the management of the neonate. In utero, there is very little pulmonary blood flow. As a result, a fetus with single ventricle physiology needs only to pump to the systemic circulation plus the blood flow to the placenta. The neonatal single ventricle has therefore not accommodated to pumping large volume loads such as may be the case in parallel circulations. Furthermore, there is evidence to suggest that single ventricles with right ventricular morphology may be less efficient than single ventricles with left ventricular morphology; the former situation is encountered in the hypoplastic left heart syndrome. In neonates with single ventricles, a higher systemic saturation may signify not only increasing $\dot{Q}_p$ but also decreasing $\dot{Q}_s$. Thus, neonates with single ventricle physiology are capable of being well saturated while having a consequent low output state and acidosis. In essence, whatever blood flow goes through the lungs does not go through the systemic circulation and vice versa.

The essence of managing neonates with parallel circulations is the control of pulmonary blood flow so as to maintain adequate systemic perfusion while having adequate saturation for oxygen transport. With time, the neonatal single ventricle can adapt to increasing volume load to easily meet the demands of the systemic circulation and can provide substantial amounts of pulmonary blood flow. However, early after operations such as the Norwood procedure for hypoplastic left heart syndrome, it may be particularly challenging to maintain adequate systemic perfusion. This issue is further complicated because it is desirable to maintain systemic output and pressure to help maintain shunt patency early after creation of a surgically placed systemic-to-pulmonary shunt.

To date, no single pharmacologic agent has been found to provide either highly selective vasoconstriction or highly selective vasodilation of only the pulmonary or only the systemic circulation. (Inhaled nitric oxide, currently under investigation, may be the first such agent available in the future [28].) Rather, the systemic and pulmonary circulations must be "balanced" in these neonates by careful postoperative ventilatory management.

There are three key ventilatory parameters that have important effects on the pulmonary circulation (Table 7-3):

1. **FiO$_2$.** The pulmonary circulation (particularly in neonates) will respond to increasing concentrations of inspired oxygen by vasodilation; conversely, decreasing FiO$_2$ down to room air will result in some pulmonary vasoconstriction. In extreme circumstances, FiO$_2$ may be decreasaed to 0.17 to 0.18% to achieve control of excessive pulmonary blood flow.
2. **pH.** Respiratory alkalosis and hypocarbia may produce pulmonary vasodilation [29] and, conversely, normal pH and normocarbia may produce some increase in PVR.
3. **Airway pressure.** By direct mechanical effect, increasing air-

Table 7-3. Control of pulmonary blood flow

Factors that increase $\dot{Q}_p$	Factors that decrease $\dot{Q}_p$
↑ FiO_2	↓ FiO_2
Alkalosis; Hypocarbia	Acidosis; Normo- or mild hypercarbia
Mean airway pressure	Mean airway pressure
↓ PEEP	↑ PEEP
↓ I:E ratio	↑ I:E ratio
↓ tidal volume	↑ tidal volume

Key: $\dot{Q}_p$ = pulmonary blood flow; FiO_2 = fractional inspired oxygen; PEEP = positive end-expiratory pressure; I:E ratio = inspiratory:expiratory ratio.

way pressure also opposes pulmonary blood flow. The airway pressure can be varied in two ways. First, PEEP can be added or removed to increase or decrease correspondingly the mean airway pressure. Second, pulmonary blood flow may also be decreased by increasing the relative amount of time the ventilator spends in inspiration versus expiration (I:E ratio). A similar effect (increasing the mean airway pressure and hence decreasing pulmonary blood flow) can be achieved by using very large tidal volumes (20–25 ml/kg); however, inspired $FiCO_2$ (1–4%) must be added to normalize PCO_2 [30].

To illustrate, after the Norwood procedure for first stage palliation of hypoplastic left heart syndrome, it frequently is necessary to limit pulmonary blood flow [30]. The single ventricle with right ventricular morphology requires time to accommodate pumping to parallel circulations, and, in these neonates, excessive systemic saturation is common and is usually accompanied by poor systemic perfusion and acidosis. Thus, these infants are frequently ventilated immediately after surgery with room air. The ventilatory rate and tidal volume are adjusted and CO_2 sometimes added so that normocarbia results and hyperventilation is avoided. Positive end-expiratory pressure may be added up to 5 to 7 cm H_2O, and a relatively long inspiratory time is selected so that the I:E ratio is 1:2 to 1:3. Cardiac performance is then maximized by ensuring optimal filling pressures and by using inotropic agents. In general, achieving precise control of ventilatory parameters early after surgery usually requires continuous narcotic sedation and phamacologic paralysis. Oxygen-carrying capacity is optimized by raising the hematocrit to about 50%.

In contrast, patients who have undergone a Fontan-Kreutzer procedure must have pulmonary vascular resistance minimized [31,32]. These patients are ventilated after surgery with little or no PEEP and with short inspiratory times; atelectasis may be minimized by the use of intermittent ventilatory sighs or by intermittent hand ventilation. Hypoxia is assiduously avoided. In-series circulations after a Fontan-Kreutzer procedure function best with spontaneous ventilation and, accordingly, efforts should be made to extubate these patients as early as possible after operation.

Extubation of the postoperative patient requires hemodynamic stability, freedom from severe edema, smooth respiratory motion of the chest wall with spontaneous breathing, and acceptable blood gases. Most patients are extubated after a short period of time with an intermittent mandatory ventilation rate of 4–5 per minute. We do not think infants should have the additional stress of a continuous positive airway pressure (CPAP) trial, because this requires great effort as the baby attempts to overcome the combined resistance of CPAP and a small-caliber endotracheal tube. The administration of dexamethasone (0.5 mg/kg IV) several hours before and after tube removal in infants assists in reducing airway edema and may help to prevent reintubation. Racemic epinephrine inhalation by nebulizer (2.25%, 1 ml in 5 ml of saline) also helps control postextubation stridor due to upper airway edema. Airway edema and consequent obstruction may be a problem following prolonged intubation or in babies who have been very active prior to extubation and more likely to have tube-related airway trauma. In addition to airway edema, phrenic nerve injury and the resulting diaphragmatic paralysis also may result in acute respiratory failure following extubation.

Tracheostomy may be required in some infants who cannot be separated from the ventilator after several weeks. It often seems that tracheostomy, by providing a shorter airway pathway and permitting easier suctioning for removal of secretions, permits weaning from the ventilator in a short time. Meticulous surgical technique is required for this procedure; the proper size tube should be inserted and secured in place to avoid trauma to the skin and trachea, and injury to the cricoid cartilage must be avoided to prevent subglottic stenosis. No one except the responsible surgical team should attempt removal or repositioning of the tube for the first 5 to 7 days; after that time, the tube can be removed easily for cleaning and reinserted.

Fluids, Electrolytes, and Nutrition

ROUTINE FLUID AND ELECTROLYTE MANAGEMENT

Postoperatively, intelligent fluid administration requires careful consideration of the patient's cardiac output, systemic and pulmonary pressures, filling pressures, urine output, and blood loss. In the immediate postoperative period, our initial plan of volume replacement dictates infusion of red blood cells and plasma equal in volume to that lost via mediastinal drainage and blood sampling on an hour-by-hour basis. The volume expander chosen is dictated by the desired hematocrit: normal or less than normal in acyanotic patients and elevated in cyanotic patients.

Usual full maintenance fluid requirements in a child are 100 ml/kg/day for the first 10 kg of body weight, plus 50 ml/kg/day for the second 10 kg of body weight, plus 20 ml/kg/day for weight over 20 kg. After cardiopulmonary bypass, this calculated volume is reduced by one-half because of the tendency for these patients to retain large volumes of excess water. Dextrose, 5% in water ($\pm$ 0.2 normal saline), with 20 mEq/liter of potassium chloride added on day 2, is generally used for maintenance fluids.

Further alterations in volume and composition of intravenously administered fluids depend on the clinical situation and measurements of hematocrit, electrolytes, and blood gases. It must be recalled that hyponatremia is almost always dilutional and requires fluid restriction, although small infants may require some sodium administration. Fluid restriction may be difficult because of the large number of intravenous lines that are at risk of occlusion if flow rates are low. Syringe infusion pumps with digital control are the most reliable devices for precise administration of small volumes of fluid as well as critical medications. For most arterial and central venous lines, at least 1.5 to 2.0 ml/hr is required to maintain patency. Arterial lines should receive saline or one-half normal saline without dextrose; other lines should receive 5% or 10% dextrose. Heparin should be added (1 U/ml).

NUTRITIONAL MANAGEMENT

The typical child who undergoes uneventful open heart operation should be able to begin clear liquids by mouth a short time (6 hr) after the endotracheal tube is removed. If liquids are well tolerated, a regular diet for age may be resumed later that day. Postoperative ileus is unusual in most cardiac patients, and there is no reason to withhold nourishment. One exception to this rule is the patient undergoing repair of coarctation. Most neonates may begin sugar solution after extubation, with a rapid progression to breast milk or formula.

The critically ill infant poses a more difficult problem in nutritional management; a need for prolonged ventilation makes normal feeding impossible. We prefer to use the patient's gastrointestinal tract as a route for alimentation whenever possible. Feedings are started via an orogastric tube with 5% dextrose or balanced electrolyte solution (e.g., Pedialyte) with frequent residuals measured to guard against gastric dilatation. Formula may then be initiated at increasing volumes and concentrations until the infant is receiving 120 to 180 kcal/kg/day. If additional volume must be administered to reach this nutritional intake, diuretics may be needed. Diarrhea or stools positive for reducing substances (e.g., on Clinitest) require discontinuation of the feedings, followed by resumption at a slightly lower rate or concentration. Intolerances to formula mandate formula changes.

Intravenous hyperalimentation may be needed if the gastrointestinal tract is not usable. Central administration is preferable, since higher solute concentrations can be given with less volume. Lipids are added to increase the calorie intake.

Glucose

Glucose homeostasis is frequently deranged in infants with severe congenital heart defects. This derangement may be most severe when circulatory arrest is employed [33]. Hyperglycemia is particularly common in the postoperative period and may lead to osmotic diuresis, dehydration, and increase in serum osmolarity, which may lead to cerebral hemorrhage. Plasma glucose values below 200 mg/dl need not be treated beyond reducing the rate or concentration of dextrose-containing intravenous solutions. Glucose levels above

300 mg/dl require the intravenous administration of regular insulin, 0.1 to 0.2 U/kg, every 6 to 12 hours until glucose levels stabilize. Standing orders for "sliding scale" insulin should never be used in infants because of the risk of dangerous hypoglycemia. Hypoglycemia must be prevented by frequent monitoring of glucose levels in patients receiving insulin, and administration of dextrose infusions if the levels fall below 100 mg/dl [34]. The small glycogen stores and limited capacity for gluconeogenesis in neonates make hypoglycemia the greater danger. Neonates may not manifest any clinical evidence of hypoglycemia until serum glucose levels fall below 30 mg/dl, at which point the patient is at risk for cerebral insult. This is completely preventable in most cases by (1) using maintenance solutions containing 10% dextrose, (2) estimating blood glucose frequently using bedside test strips [35], and (3) confirming test-strip values with measurements of blood glucose levels by the laboratory. When plasma glucose levels fall below 50 mg/dl despite these precautions, the patient should receive small dextrose-containing fluid boluses through a secure central venous catheter, and the concentration of dextrose in the maintenance solutions should be increased to 10% or more [36].

Calcium

Hypocalcemia most commonly occurs in neonates and may cause irritability, seizures, and abnormalities of cardiac rhythm. Measurement of ionized, not total, calcium is easily accomplished and is the best guide to calcium replacement (normal ionized calcium level = 1–2 mmol/liter). Replacement may be particularly necessary when blood products have been administered. Calcium supplementation should be provided as a 10% calcium gluconate infusion that is infused slowly 1 to 2 ml/kg at a time through a central venous line exclusively [37]. Particularly in neonates, hypocalcemia may be recurrent, especially if the DiGeorge syndrome is present; in this circumstance, it can be added to the maintenance solutions (calcium gluconate, 2 g/liter).

Hypomagnesemia may coexist very rarely with hypocalcemia and should be suspected when symptomatic hypocalcemia does not respond to calcium infusion alone [38]. Although laboratory measurement of serum magnesium levels is, at best, an uncertain indicator of total body magnesium, levels below 1.4 mEq/liter are abnormal. Tetany unresponsive to calcium is treated with 0.2 ml of 50% magnesium sulfate administered intramuscularly every 4 hours.

Potassium

Hypokalemia is most commonly due to urinary losses and administration of bicarbonate ion. Unlike adult cardiac patients who are often very sensitive to hypokalemia, children rarely develop ventricular irritability because of moderately low serum potassium levels. Unless the potassium falls below 3.0 mEq/liter, additional potassium supplementation is usually unnecessary. Enteral administration of potassium is preferred to intravenous administration if the gastrointestinal route is available and the deficit is modest. Intravenously administered potassium chloride requires a central venous catheter and should be given slowly at a dose of 0.1 to 0.2

mEq/kg over 20 to 30 minutes, followed by redetermination of the potassium level.

More dangerous is significant hyperkalemia, which most commonly occurs due to renal failure and metabolic acidosis. Elevated serum potassium levels lead to progressive electrical instability of the heart and eventually to cardiac arrest. Hyperkalemia may be palliated temporarily by the administration of calcium, bicarbonate, or glucose and insulin. These measures, however, only shift the potassium to the intracellular space. Removal of potassium is best accomplished with vigorous diuresis, if possible, or the use of ion-exchange resins (e.g., sodium polystyrene sulfonate [Kayexalate]) as enemas. Kayexalate is prepared as a slurry (1 g/ml of sorbitol solution) and administered through an indwelling rectal tube. Dialysis is not an efficient method of potassium removal but may be used to stabilize the serum concentration while other measures take effect.

Special Problems

COAGULATION DISORDERS AND TRANSFUSION

Younger patients are at greater risk than adults for excessive peripheral edema after cadiopulmonary bypass. Since extreme anemia and dilution of serum oncotic pressure encourage edema formation, we usually use a blood prime in our bypass circuit in infants and small children.

Patients with congenital heart defects are more likely than most individuals to have abnormal preoperative coagulation tests [39]. This is particularly evident in cyanotic patients. In most respects, replacement of blood products in the pediatric patient undergoing cardiac operation follows the same principles used for adults. Some cardiac surgeons believe that there is a beneficial effect of transfusing fresh whole blood in achieving hemostasis immediately after open heart operations, and that this benefit surpasses that of component therapy. There is some objective evidence to support this belief [40], but it is often impractical in practice due to the time required to perform screening serologic tests. It is useful to remove as much free water as possible by hemofiltration while on bypass to "make room" for fresh frozen plasma and platelet transfusions in these patients.

PARADOXICAL HYPERTENSION AFTER COARCTATION REPAIR

Despite technically adequate surgical correction of aortic coarctation, severe hypertension in the early postoperative period occurs in 37 to 63% of patients [41,42]. Proposed mechanisms of this hypertension include elevated sympathetic activity [43,44] and elevated renin [45]. It is interesting to note that paradoxical hypertension does not occur after balloon dilatation of aortic coarctation [46]. Postoperative hypertension is less of a problem following neonatal coarctation repair.

Preoperative treatment with beta blockers effectively prevents this paradoxical hypertension [47]. The patient begins propranolol (1.50

mg/kg/day PO) 2 weeks before operation, receives 0.05 mg/kg/hr IV during the immediate postoperative period, and returns to the oral regimen for the remaining postoperative week.

When hypertension does occur after coarctation repair, we prefer to treat it as we would other forms of systemic hypertension — with nitroprusside infusion beginning at 0.5 µg/kg/min and increasing as needed in addition to intravenous beta blockade. Alternatively, if hypertension is not easily controlled, intravenous esmolol [48] or labetalol [49] can be used. We use propranolol when oral intake has begun for additional blood pressure control and to assist in weaning nitroprusside. Particularly in older patients, persistent hypertension may be a significant problem. In these patients, high-dose beta blockade combined with potent antihypertensives such as angiotensin-converting enzyme inhibitors may be needed.

Blood pressure control in these hypertensive patients is important to prevent the complication of *mesenteric arteritis,* which commonly followed coarctation repair in past years. In these patients, who were generally older than the patients operated on now, hypertension occurred "paradoxically" after several days. Mesenteric arteritis may result in intestinal necrosis. For this reason, we do not permit oral intake after coarctation repair until the abdomen is soft and bowel sounds are vigorous.

TEMPERATURE REGULATION

Neonates cannot regulate their body temperature because of their relatively large surface area, limited subcutaneous fat, and inability to generate heat by shivering. Use of radiant warming devices prevents hypothermia in these patients while permitting access for necessary care (Fig. 7-7). Automatic radiant heaters incorporate skin temperature probes to regulate warming by using skin temperature in a servomechanism feedback system. Either elevation or depression of body temperature may be a sign of infection.

PROFOUND HYPOTHERMIA AND CIRCULATORY ARREST

Infants less than 5 kg in weight may benefit from operation using profound hypothermia and circulatory arrest. This technique has been applied in a wide variety of congenital heart defects [50] and permits operating in a bloodless field without the obstruction that perfusion cannulas may create in the smaller patient. Some surgeons are concerned that this technique may lead to cerebral injury and developmental delay, perhaps to a very subtle degree [51]. Detailed psychometric testing has failed to demonstrate any such deleterious effect in some studies [52]. However, more recent studies have suggested that subtle changes may occur in cognitive function, and that these changes may be related to excessively short periods of core cooling on bypass before circulatory arrest is effected [53]. A very small number of children may develop more profound neurologic sequelae such as choreoathetosis which can be manifest up to 1 week after operation [54]. While choreoathetosis is usually associated with the use of deep hypothermia and circulatory arrest, it has been reported in patients not subjected to circulatory arrest [55].

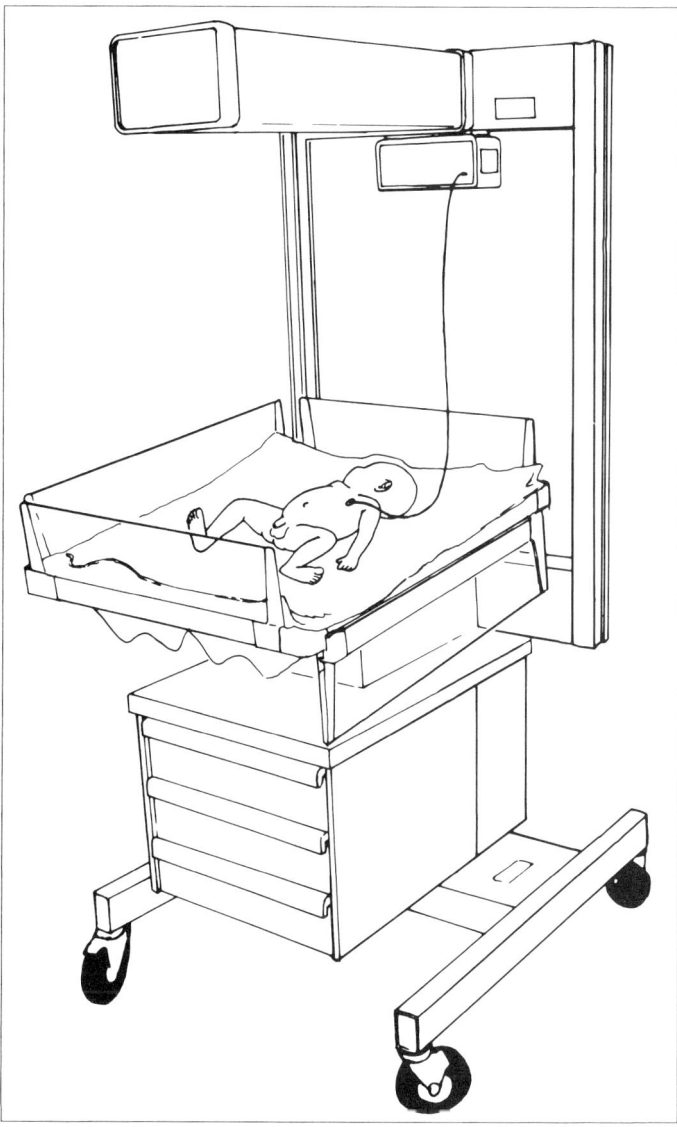

Fig. 7-7. An example of equipment designed to maintain a neonate's or infant's temperature while allowing 360-access to the baby. Overhead radiant heating is servocontrolled by skin temperature probe. The unit also incorporates fluorescent and ultraviolet lighting for hyperbilirubinemia overhead. The patient can be cared for and transported in the same bed, as it has wheels and a self-contained oxygen supply.

Control of blood glucose levels and pH during reperfusion may be of particular importance in avoiding cerebral injury [56]. Red cell sludging is avoided by hemodilution and early heparinization during cooling. Profound hypothermia results in coagulation abnormalities that may cause excessive postoperative bleeding. In most cases, meticulous hemostasis and liberal use of fresh whole blood or fresh frozen plasma and platelet concentrates are able to overcome this problem.

CENTRAL NERVOUS SYSTEM COMPLICATIONS

Infants are at high risk for seizures after cardiac operations because of electrolyte imbalance, osmotic shifts, anoxic cerebral insult, and air or thrombotic emboli through persistent shunts. Seizures most commonly occur after the use of deep hypothermic arrest. Seizure activity in babies may vary from obvious tonic-clonic motions to subtle eye, tongue, or mouth movement. In the neonate or infant who is mechanically ventilated and in those with adjunct pharmacologic paralysis, seizures may be masked and may be manifested only by tachycardia, hypertension, mydriasis, or bronchorrhea; the sudden appearance of any of these signs should raise suspicion of seizure activity in the paralyzed patient. In all cases, vigorous treatment is indicated to prevent the cerebral consequences of unchecked seizures. Initial control may be obtained with diazepam (0.1 mg/kg IV). Phenobarbital, the preferred maintenance agent, should be given intravenously in two loading doses of 10 mg/kg each, followed by a maintenance dose of 5 mg/kg/day divided into bid doses. Phenytoin (20 mg/kg IV loading dose and 5 mg/kg/day divided bid) is an alternative maintenance agent [57]. Hyperventilation and steroids are also used for treatment of this condition.

CT scanning or ultrasound examination of the brain may be needed to exclude the possibility of intraventricular hemorrhage. Sudden changes in serum osmolarity may predispose the infant to this problem. Therefore the solute load should not exceed 5 to 6 mOsm/kg/hr.

RENAL FAILURE

We generally strive to maintain a urine output of approximately 1 ml/kg/hr in children after cardiac operations. Oliguria combined with rising blood urea nitrogen and creatinine levels indicates renal failure. Renal failure in the neonatal period usually results from prerenal causes: low cardiac output, sepsis, and hypovolemia. Postrenal factors, such as obstructive uropathy, must also be considered and excluded with ultrasound. Correction of the underlying cause will correct the renal dysfunction in most cases. Peritoneal dialysis is indicated for severe volume overload or persistent metabolic acidosis. Some surgeons advocate early aggressive peritoneal dialysis in infants to prevent the edema formation and fluid and electrolyte problems common in these patients [18].

SEPSIS

Bacterial sepsis is unfortunately common in the newborn period and may further complicate the care of the patient with congenital heart defects. *Streptococcus* species are probably the most common cause of neonatal sepsis, followed by the common hospital-acquired pathogens such as *Staphylococcus* and *Pseudomonas*. Rising or falling temperature, lethargy, pallor, mottling, decreasing platelet count, hemodynamic instability, and poor feeding are typical manifestations of sepsis. The nonspecificity of these signs and the frequency with which they occur in cardiac patients without sepsis are testimony to the difficulty in prompt diagnosis of sepsis. Laboratory studies may reveal elevated or depressed white count, thrombocytopenia, hyperglycemia, and acidosis [58].

The surgeon must maintain a high index of suspicion regarding the presence of infection, even during the first postoperative night and particularly in the postoperative patient with multiple indwelling lines and foreign material within the heart. Avoidance of septic complications is achieved by minimizing the number of invasive devices and the length of time they are used, meticulous nursing procedures, and prophylactic changing of lines that must be in place for a prolonged time. When infection is suspected, vigorous attempts should be made to identify the source with blood, urine, and sputum cultures; chest radiographs; and possibly CT scans. Meningitis must also be considered, and cerebrospinal fluid cultures should be obtained.

After cultures have been obtained, the routine antibiotic regimen is changed and broad spectrum antibiotics may be instituted — usually a penicillin or vancomycin and an aminoglycoside. More specific coverage may be determined by the culture results. Doses of antibiotics may require modification according to the patient's renal function, which may be abnormal because of the immaturity of the nephron and renal injury related to the underlying illness or operative complications.

PROSTHETIC VALVES IN CHILDREN

Most surgeons make great efforts to avoid implantation of prosthetic heart valves in children with congenital defects. Poor valve longevity in pediatric patients often requires accepting a less-than-ideal reconstructive operation in preference to valve replacement. Recent experience with homograft valves and pulmonary autograft valves in the aortic position is promising, but the long-term results of these techniques will not be known for some time [59,63].

The accelerated calcification of bioprostheses is well known [60] and few such valves are used today. Mechanical valves are occasionally required despite the need for anticoagulation, which may be difficult to manage in growing children. Although some surgeons have reported early success in utilizing mechanical valves in pediatric patients without warfarin, longer follow-up revealed an excessive rate of thromboembolic complications [61]. It is well established that warfarin must be used in children who have mechanical prosthetic valves, despite the potential problems of noncompliance or bleeding complications [62]. Therefore, we have continued to use warfarin anticoagulation as we would for adult patients with mechanical valves.

Postoperative Investigations

ECHOCARDIOGRAPHY

Echocardiography, because of the detailed anatomic information it can provide and its noninvasive nature, is a nearly ideal technique for postoperative investigation of patients with congenital heart defects. We have found echocardiography to be most useful in assessing ventricular function and determining the presence of significant blood and fluid collections. Injections of saline-containing microbubbles provide an echocardiographic contrast medium to demonstrate the presence of transseptal shunts. Color flow Doppler is a recent important addition because it facilitates shunt detection and the estimation of valve regurgitation and stenosis.

CATHETERIZATION

Occasional postoperative patients following congenital heart surgery may not have sufficiently clear findings based on echocardiography and other noninvasive studies. Cardiac catheterization is helpful in evaluating residual murmurs, excluding residual shunts, and following correction of obstructive anomalies. Catheterization is never undertaken lightly in the early postoperative setting because the morbidity of the procedure is often increased. Furthermore, the technical demands of catheterization are often greater in neonates and infants because in most cases a preoperative catheterization has been performed and vascular access may be difficult to obtain. We have found early postoperative catheterization to be helpful in managing selected patients whose recovery is not going as well as expected after major operations. In addition, we use postoperative catheterization liberally for the late reevaluation of patients, particularly after arterial switch procedures, transplants, repair of tetralogy of Fallot and pulmonary atresia, and Fontan-Kreutzer procedures.

References

1. Marino B, et al. Pediatric cardiac surgery guided by echocardiography. Established indications and new trends. *Scand J Thorac Cardiovasc Surg* 24:197, 1990.

2. Krabill KA, et al. Echocardiographic versus cardiac catheterization diagnosis of infants with congenital heart disease requiring cardiac surgery. *Am J Cardiol* 60:351, 1987.

3. Freed MD, et al. Prostaglandin E_1 in infants with ductus arteriosus–dependent congenital heart disease. *Circulation* 64:899, 1981.

4. Sellden H, et al. Radial arterial catheter in children and neonates: a prospective study. *Crit Care Med* 15:1106, 1987.

5. Graves PW, et al. Femoral artery cannulation for monitoring in critically ill children: prospective study. *Crit Care Med* 18:1363, 1990.

6. Glenski JA, Beynen FM, Brady J. A prospective evaluation of femoral artery monitoring in pediatric patients. *Anesthesiology* 66:227, 1987.

7. Gold JP, et al. Transthoracic intracardiac monitoring lines in pediatric surgical patients: a ten-year experience. *Ann Thorac Surg* 42:185, 1986.

8. Butt WW, Whyte H. Blood pressure monitoring in neonates: comparison of umbilical and peripheral artery catheter measurements. *J Pediatr* 105:630, 1984.

9. Pinheiro JM, Fisher MA. Use of a triple-lumen catheter for umbilical venous access in the neonate. *J Pediatr* 120:624, 1992.

10. Marsh JL, et al. Serious complications after umbilical artery catheterization for neonatal monitoring. *Arch Surg* 110:1203, 1975.

11. Wigger HJ, Bransilver BR, Blanc WA. Thrombosis due to catheterization in infants and children. *J Pediatr* 76:1, 1970.

12. Talner NS, Lister G. Perioperative care of the infant with congenital heart disease. *Cardiol Clin* 7:419, 1989.

13. Kirklin JK, et al. Intracardiac surgery in infants under age 3 months: predictors of postoperative in-hospital cardiac death. *Am J Cardiol* 48:507, 1981.

14. Schranz D, et al. Continuous monitoring of mixed venous oxygen saturation in infants after cardiac surgery. *Intensive Care Med* 15:288, 1989.

15. Burrows FA, et al. Myocardial performance after repair of congenital cardiac defects in infants and children: Response to volume loading. *J Thorac Cardiovasc Surg* 96:548, 1988.

16. Ziemer G, et al. Staged chest closure in pediatric cardiac surgery patients preventing typical and atypical cardiac tamponade. *Eur J Cardiothorac Surg* 6:91, 1992.

17. Zobel G, et al. Continuous extracorporeal fluid removal in children with low cardiac output after cardiac operations. *J Thorac Cardiovasc Surg* 101:593, 1991.

18. Mee RBB. Invited letter concerning: Dialysis after cardiopulmonary bypass in neonates and infants. *J Thorac Cardiovasc Surg* 103:1021, 1992.

19. Kron IL, Rheuban K, Nolan SP. Late cardiac tamponade in children: A lethal complication. *Ann Surg* 199:173, 1984.

20. Beland MJ, et al. Pericardial effusion after cardiac surgery in children and effects of aspirin for prevention. *Am J Cardiol* 65:1238, 1990.

21. Lang P, et al. Early assessment of hemodynamic status after repair of tetralogy of Fallot: a comparison of 24-hour (intensive care unit) and 1-year postoperative data in 98 patients. *Am J Cardiol* 50:795, 1982.

22. DiDonato RM, et al. Neonatal repair of tetralogy of Fallot with and without pulmonary atresia. *J Thorac Cardiovasc Surg* 101:126, 1991.

23. Laks H, et al. Partial Fontan: advantages of an adjustable interatrial communication. *Ann Thorac Surg* 52:1084, 1991.

24. Lulu JA, Myrer ML. Mechanical ventilation considerations in com-

plex congenital heart disease. *Crit Care Nurs Clin North Am* 3:609, 1991.
25. Craig J. The postoperative cardiac infant: physiologic basis for neonatal nursing interventions. *J Perinat Neonat Nurs* 5:60, 1991.
26. Hopkins RA, et al. Pulmonary hypertensive crisis following surgery for congenital heart defects in young children. *Eur J Cardiothorac Surg* 5:628, 1991.
27. Meliones JN, et al. High-frequency jet ventilation improves cardiac function after the Fontan procedure. *Circulation* 84(Suppl III):III-364, 1991.
28. Frostell C, et al. Inhaled nitric oxide: A selective pulmonary vasodilator reversing hypoxic pulmonary vasoconstriction. *Circulation* 83:2038, 1991.
29. Morray JP, Lynn AM, Mansfield PB. Effect of pH and pCO_2 on pulmonary and systemic hemodynamics after surgery in children with congestive heart disease and pulmonary hypertension. *J Pediatr* 113:474, 1988.
30. Jobes DR, et al. Carbon dioxide prevents pulmonary overcirculation in hypoplastic left heart syndrome. *Ann Thorac Surg* 54:150, 1992.
31. O'Brien P, Elixson EM. The child following the Fontan procedure: nursing strategies. *AACN Clin Issues Crit Care Nurs* 1:46, 1990.
32. Fyman PN, et al. Anesthetic management of patients undergoing Fontan procedure. *Anesth Analg* 65:516, 1986.
33. Benzing G III, et al. Glucose and insulin changes in infants and children undergoing hypothermic open-heart surgery. *Am J Cardiol* 52:133, 1983.
34. Pildes RS. Neonatal hyperglycemia. *J Pediatr* 109:905, 1986.
35. Worth RC, et al. A comparative study of blood glucose test strips. *Diabetes Care* 4:407, 1981.
36. LaFranchi S. Hypoglycemia of infancy and childhood. *Pediatr Clin North Am* 34:961, 1987.
37. Tsang RC, Steichen JJ, Chan GM. Neonatal hypocalcemia: Mechanism of occurrence and management. *Crit Care Med* 5:56, 1977.
38. Noe DA. Neonatal hypocalcemia and related conditions. *Clin Lab Med* 1:227, 1981.
39. Colon-Otero G, et al. Preoperative evaluation of hemostasis in patients with congenital heart disease. *Mayo Clin Proc* 62:379, 1987.
40. Mohr R, et al. The hemostatic effect of transfusing fresh whole blood versus platelet concentrates after cardiac operations. *J Thorac Cardiovasc Surg* 96:530, 1988.
41. Fox S, Pierce WS, Waldhausen JA. Pathogenesis of paradoxical hypertension after coarctation repair. *Ann Thorac Surg* 29:135, 1980.
42. Stansel HC, et al. One hundred consecutive coarctation resections followed from one to thirteen years. *J Pediatr Surg* 12:279, 1977.

43. Benedict CR, Grahame-Smith DG, Fisher A. Changes in plasma catecholamines and dopamine beta-hydroxylase after corrective surgery for coarctation of the aorta. *Circulation* 57:598, 1978.

44. Sealy WC. Paradoxical hypertension after repair of coarctation of the aorta: a review of its causes. *Ann Thorac Surg* 50:323, 1990.

45. Rocchini AP, et al. Pathogenesis of paradoxical hypertension after coarctation resection. *Circulation* 54:382, 1976.

46. Choy M, et al. Paradoxical hypertension after repair of coarctation of the aorta in children: balloon angioplasty versus surgical repair. *Circulation* 75:1186, 1987.

47. Gidding SS, et al. Therapeutic effect of propranolol on paradoxical hypertension after repair of coarctation of the aorta. *N Engl J Med* 312:1224, 1985.

48. Smerling A, Gerson WM. Esmolol for severe hypertension following repair of aortic coarctation. *Crit Care Med* 18:1288, 1990.

49. Bojar RM, Weiner B, Cleveland RJ. Intravenous labetalol for control of hypertension following repair of coarctation of the aorta. *Clin Cardiol* 11:639, 1988.

50. Bender HW Jr, et al. Reparative cardiac surgery in infants and small children: Five years experience with profound hypothermia and circulatory arrest. *Ann Surg* 190:437, 1979.

51. Ferry PC. Neurologic sequelae of open-heart surgery in children: An 'irritating question.' *Am J Dis Child* 144:369, 1990.

52. Clarkson PM, et al. Developmental progress after cardiac surgery in infancy using hypothermia and circulatory arrest. *Circulation* 62:855, 1980.

53. Bellinger DC, et al. Cognitive development of children following early repair of transposition of the great arteries using deep hypothermic circulatory arrest. *Pediatrics* 87:701, 1991.

54. Wical BS, Tomasi LG. A distinctive neurologic syndrome after induced profound hypothermia. *Pediatr Neurol* 6:202, 1990.

55. DeLeon G, et al. Choreoathetosis after deep hypothermia without circulatory arrest. *Ann Thorac Surg* 50:714, 1990.

56. Ekroth R, et al. Elective deep hypothermia with total circulatory arrest: changes in plasma creatine kinase BB, blood glucose, and clinical variables. *J Thorac Cardiovasc Surg* 97:30, 1989.

57. Painter MJ, Bergman I, Crumrine P. Neonatal seizures. *Pediatr Clin North Am* 33:91, 1986.

58. Donovan EF. Perioperative care of the surgical neonate. *Surg Clin North Am* 65:1061, 1985.

59. Elkins RC, et al. Pulmonary autograft replacement of the aortic valve: an evolution of technique. *J Cardiac Surg* 7:108, 1992.

60. Dunn JM. Porcine valve durability in children. *Ann Thorac Surg* 32:357, 1981.

61. Sade RM, et al. Valve prostheses in children: a reassessment of anticoagulation. *J Thorac Cardiovasc Surg* 95:553, 1988.

62. Stewart S, et al. The long-term risk of warfarin sodium therapy and the incidence of thromboembolism in children after prosthetic cardiac valve replacement. *J Thorac Cardiovasc Surg* 93:551, 1987.
63. Kouchoukos NT, et al. Replacement of the aortic root with a pulmonary autograft in children and young adults with aortic-valve disease. *N Engl J Med* 330:1, 1994.

Transplantation

Preoperative Considerations

Patients waiting for heart, lung, or heart-lung transplantation represent a potentially tenuous group of individuals. They are generally less than 60 years of age and are being transplanted for end-stage cardiac or pulmonary failure. Most patients are "listed" for transplantation when their symptoms are extremely limiting (e.g., NY Heart Association class IV) and when their prognosis for survival beyond 1 year with medical therapy is poor. They will generally come to transplantation on a maximized medical regimen, often including high-dose diuretics and afterload reducing agents. Many of these patients have potentially life-threatening arrhythmias. Their pretransplant management may include an automatic internal cardiac defibrillator, pacemaker, or multiple antiarrhythmic medications, including some with potentially severe side effects such as pulmonary toxicity (amiodarone). Prior heart surgery and in particular, the location of patent bypass grafts, should be noted. Lung transplant patients may be receiving steroids, antibiotics, or home oxygen. All of this information must be available for intraoperative and postoperative management. In general, much of the transplant patient's database will have been collated during the transplant evaluation process.

INFECTION

Infection is an important issue, particularly as more desperately ill patients (e.g., patients who are intubated and supported with an intraaortic balloon pump after a massive infarction) are being evaluated for urgent transplantation. Transplantation in the face of pneumonia is doomed to failure because of progressive pulmonary infection. Bacteremia at the time of transplantation carries a high risk of seeding vascular suture lines, with the subsequent development of a mycotic aneurysm and a catastrophic rupture. Hence, an important consideration in the evaluation of a potential recipient is the prevention and eradication of infection prior to the transplant procedure.

TISSUE TYPING AND CROSSMATCHING

Donor and recipient are matched according to major ABO blood groups. In addition, when there is a possibility of preformed antibodies in the recipient, the potential donor's lymphocytes must be directly crossmatched against the recipient's serum. Serum from a potential recipient is always screened against a panel of random antigens (PRA) taken from a number (around 60) of different donors. The number or percentage of common human leukocyte antigens (HLA antigens) to which the recipient has preformed antibodies is then reported. Generally, in patients with no prior exposure to foreign antigens (e.g., blood products) or prior pregnancies, there is little or no (0%) reactivity. A PRA of more than 10% is usually an indication to obtain a prospective cytotoxic crossmatch when a prospective donor is being screened to eliminate the possibility of hyperacute rejection. In heart transplantation, a "positive" match indicates that a particular donor heart is likely susceptible to hyperacute rejection due to preformed antibody and, in such situations, the donor should be declined for a given recipient [1,2]. A PRA of less than 10%, particularly on multiple determinations over 2 or 3 months, means that such a crossmatch is not essential because hyperacute rejection is highly unlikely. It is particularly important to know whether a crossmatch is needed because additional time may be required to transport donor lymph node tissue from a remote site for the crossmatch and to perform the assay; this will add considerably to the time the donor must be maintained before organ harvesting.

SIZE MATCHING CONSIDERATIONS

Traditionally, the donor and recipient are matched according to body weight to within approximately 20%. Donor hearts that are too small may have limited ability to maintain adequate cardiac output and may require prolonged inotropic support. Conversely, a heart that is functionally suitable but too large may not "fit" into the recipient's chest or may produce a high output syndrome. This is rarely the case because the recipients usually have cardiomegaly and, especially in infants, substantial size mismatches can be tolerated.

More recent data suggest that undersizing of donor hearts may not be detrimental. Cardiac donor oversizing, while common practice, may be associated with a greater risk of postoperative death and is not associated with a better outcome of orthotopic transplantation in recipients with reversible preoperative pulmonary hypertension [3].

Patients undergoing lung transplantation should have organs matched to within 20 or 25% of their chest measurements. The measurements that are obtained are the longitudinal measurement from the apex of the diaphragm to the apex of the chest and the transverse measurement from costophrenic angle to costophrenic angle. Alternatively, total lung capacities can be estimated from the donor's and recipient's heights.

There are a few important exceptions and qualifications with regard to donor and recipient size matching. First, the obese donor may have a heart smaller than that predicted on the basis of body weight alone; this must be taken into consideration when matching a cardiac donor and potential recipient. Second and more important is the issue of the recipient's pulmonary circulation. Some potential recipients, by virtue of long-standing pulmonary hypertension secondary to chronic left heart failure, may have an elevated pulmonary vascular resistance (PVR) increasing the mortality risk early after transplantation in proportion to the amount of pulmonary hypertension [4,5], particularly if pulmonary hypertension is "fixed" and not responsive to vasodilation. Because potential donor hearts will have normal right ventricles and because the harvesting, myocardial preservation, and implantation processes will temporarily diminish right ventricular function, donor hearts may fail if suddenly required to pump against an increased PVR. In this instance, it is wise to seek donors that are at least as large or larger than the potential recipient. The risk of death is related in a continuous manner to PVR [5]. Thus, the selection of donor size with respect to such recipients must be individualized with these principles in mind.

In some patients in whom PVR exceeds 5 Wood units, cardiac transplantation can be performed, although the risk increases. It is sometimes possible to obtain significant decrements in PVR in such patients with prolonged (greater than 1 week) in-hospital vasodilatation with such agents as nitroprusside.

Conversely, patients requiring lung transplantation often have secondary right ventricular failure caused by severe pulmonary hypertension. It has been shown that this immediately improves once normal lungs are implanted, so that right heart failure is not necessarily an exclusion criterion [6]. Another problem presented by patients with end-stage lung disease is their chronic steroid dependence and severe cachexia. Before these patients can be listed for transplantation, prednisone must be tapered to less than 10 mg/day and discontinued if possible, and the patient must be started on a physical rehabilitation program including augmented caloric intake.

Donor Management

In recent years, the number of potential recipients in the United States has increased dramatically, particularly as additional centers are now offering this treatment modality and the age limits of potential transplant candidates have expanded. This demand has exacerbated the already critical donor supply and, in some instances, has made it necessary to accept either donors of more advanced age [7,8] or donors with other noncritical medical problems that previously would have precluded their use [9]. Sometimes, less-than-ideal donor hearts and lungs must be accepted for implantation in recipients who are in imminent danger of death.

Most patients who become organ donors have had either major trauma or an intracranial hemorrhage resulting in brain death [10]. Before death is declared, many of these individuals have been managed by fluid restriction and hyperosmolar therapy and often have the syndrome of inappropriate antidiuretic hormone secretion. Many have been receiving inotropic support because of hemodynamic instability created by the induced hypovolemic state. Therefore, once an individual has been declared a multiple organ donor, it is important to ensure that the blood volume is normal so that the function of the heart and lungs can be assessed accurately. If diabetes insipidus is present, as is frequently the case, substantial fluid and vasopressin administration may be required to counterbalance the losses, as well as to replete the patient's volume so that inotropic drugs can be tapered to the minimum level. For this purpose, a catheter for central venous pressure (CVP) monitoring should be inserted, if one is not already in place. Volume status should be repleted to achieve a CVP in the range of 5 to 8 mm Hg. If a lung donation will be included in the multiple-organ donation process, overhydration must be avoided; occasionally, this balance can be difficult to achieve without proper monitoring. In these circumstances, the donor hospital situation permitting, a Swan-Ganz catheter may be useful to assess left-sided filling pressures and cardiac output. This is important in order to balance the use of inotropic drugs versus volume replacement in situations where minimizing lung water is important.

In addition to the donor's cause of death, it is important to ascertain whether cardiac arrest has occurred. In general, patients who have required more than 10 minutes of CPR have probably suffered cardiac injury precluding the use of the heart for donation. In many instances, the decision to accept such a heart will require some judgment and a more detailed evaluation of cardiac function. Cardiopulmonary resuscitation does not preclude lung donation if other lung-donor criteria are met. It is also important to determine, in the trauma patient, whether closed chest trauma has occurred so that the possibility of myocardial or pulmonary contusion may be considered. Contused myocardium can undergo intramural hemorrhage when exposed to heparinized blood during cardiopulmonary bypass, resulting in a potentially significant area of wall motion abnormality or arrhythmias. Blood in the sputum or pneumothorax due to penetrating or blunt trauma to the lung is a relative contraindication to using a donor's lungs.

Certain laboratory data are important in the evaluation of the donor. First, the ECG should be relatively normal with the possible exception of sinus tachycardia; premature atrial contractions (PACs), nonspecific ST-segment or T-wave abnormalities, or even new-onset atrial fibrillation would not necessarily exclude donation. Occasionally, patients with head injuries develop subtle global abnormalities of the ST segments and T waves, unassociated with real myocardial injury. Creatine kinase (CK) determination is essential if there has been chest trauma or CPR, and it is helpful to have isoenzyme levels, since total CK may be markedly elevated from skeletal muscle sources particularly in the trauma setting. When available, echocardiography is an excellent means of evaluating the donor heart, especially in situations where weaning inotropic drug support may be difficult or the donor has received CPR. In some brain-dead patients, unusually high doses of agents such as dopamine may be required, more because of inadequate peripheral resistance than depressed cardiac function. Thus, the donor echocardiogram is useful to rule out any segmental wall motion abnormalities, as well as to assess global ventricular function. In general, we are reluctant to utilize donor hearts requiring more than 10–15 µg/kg/min of dopamine support (or the equivalent dose of some other catecholamine), particularly in older donors [11] unless echocardiography shows good biventricular function.

In donors who have been hospitalized for more than 1 week and who have had invasive CVP monitoring, it is important to ensure that there is no vegetation on the tricuspid valve. This must be ruled out by echocardiographic evaluation and inspection of the tricuspid valve at the time the heart is excised. An important concern in the pretransplant evaluation is the possibility of donor infection and the risk of transmitting this to an immunosuppressed recipient via the transplanted organ. Overall, the risk of transmitting bacterial infection from a donor source is low for heart transplants. With the exception of donor infections that have resulted in high-grade bacteremia, other donor infections, such as early pneumonia, do not pose a significant risk to the cardiac recipient [9]. The appearance of lung infiltrates on the donor chest x-ray does not necessarily exclude the donor's heart unless there is significant fever with obvious pneumonia to suggest the possibility of systemic bacteremia. Of course, these patients would be excluded as lung donors. When there is concern about infection, antibiotic therapy should be initiated in the donor based on sputum Gram-stain analysis and, if available, culture data. Sputum samples should also be obtained for transport to the bacteriology laboratory at the recipient hospital.

Other types of infectious agents, such as viruses, may be transmitted by a donor heart or lungs. Donors must be screened for human immunodeficiency virus (HIV) as well as the hepatitis antigens. Donor blood should be taken before the start of organ harvesting, and toxoplasmosis and cytomegalovirus (CMV) antibody status should be determined. When the heart from a donor who is seropositive for toxoplasmosis or CMV antibody is transplanted into a recipient who is seronegative for toxoplasmosis or CMV antibody, the risk of transmitting these infections is considerable. The risk of CMV pneumonia is highest in lung and heart-lung recipients. This information is important in postoperative management [12,13], but does not preclude donation. Posttransplant antitoxoplasmosis or anti-CMV prophylaxis (or both) is indicated for any patient at risk for primary infection with these microorganisms as discussed later in this chapter.

A thorough medical history should be recorded if it can be obtained from the donor family members, particularly for donors more than 50 years old. When the donor is at an appropriate center, cardiac catheterization must be considered when donor coronary artery disease is suspected or when the donor is over 50. In the past, such a heart would have been excluded; however, the present shortage of organs makes consideration of less optimal donor hearts necessary to accommodate the greatest number of recipients [14].

Satisfactory lungs for transplantation are difficult to obtain. In general, donors who have been intubated for more than 24 or 48 hours usually have heavily colonized airways and increased pulmonary interstitial water. In addition to fulfilling the criteria for heart donors, lung donors generally must be less than 55 years old, have normal chest x-ray appearance (immediately preharvest), a PaO_2 over 400 mm Hg on 100% oxygen, a negative Gram stain of tracheal secretions, and normal bronchoscopy (by the harvesting surgeon). Lower levels of PaO_2 may be acceptable if there is asymmetry of the lung fields and only one lung is being considered for donation; in such circumstances it may be necessary to sample selectively the pulmonary venous drainage of the lung under consideration for blood gas determination at the time of donor surgery. Ideally, there should be no history of pulmonary disease; however, a history of mild asthma or mild bronchitis in the past is only a relative contraindication to using a donor's lungs. If acceptable, the lung donor must be carefully maintained on an FIO_2 below 0.5, PEEP at 5–10 cm H_2O, peak inspiratory pressures below 20 cm H_2O, and at a tidal volume of 15 ml/kg. Optimal donor ventilation improves functional residual capacity (FRC), stimulates surfactant production by type

II pneumocytes, and results in improved function after reimplantation of the lung. Donor ventilation should be optimized before donor lungs are evaluated, so as to optimize function and obviate any atelectasis that might be present. Donor fluid administration should be minimized as much as possible while maintaining a good cardiac output and urine flow.

All heart and lung donors are treated with thyroxine (Synthroid, 3 µg/kg IV over 30 min) as soon as brain death is declared, although the efficacy of thyroid hormone replacement is controversial [15]. All donors are heparinized (3 mg/kg) immediately before organ removal.

THE DONOR OPERATION

Most cardiac and lung donations are part of a multiorgan harvest. Thus, the cardiothoracic harvesting team will have to interact with other organ harvesting teams in a coordinated effort to ensure donor stability and well-timed, optimal organ recovery. Because donor and recipient surgery must be timed appropriately to coincide, it is important at the beginning of a donor operation to ascertain the total time required for other organ harvest teams to mobilize their respective organs. The total donor operating time and transport time back to the recipient hospital must be factored against the time needed to prepare the recipient for organ implantation.

Once the sternum has been opened, the heart is inspected for gross signs of trauma, coronary plaques, and dyskinetic areas; the great vessels are mobilized and circumscribed with tapes; and a pursestring suture is placed on the ascending aorta. Once the abdominal organs have been isolated, the donor is heparinized, the abdominal aorta and vena cava are cannulated, the aorta is clamped, the inferior vena cava is transected just below the right atrium to prevent right heart distention, and a pulmonary vein is incised to prevent left heart distention. Cold cardioplegic solution (10 ml/kg) is instilled, and the heart is removed. It is packed in cold physiologic solution, surrounded with crushed ice, and transported to the recipient hospital.

Lungs may be harvested in either of two ways. The entire heart-lung block may be removed intact, with the lungs gently inflated and the trachea clamped; the individual lungs may be separated from the heart on a separate, sterile table in the donor hospital operating room. Alternatively, the heart may be excised from the donor first and removed from the surgical field before the lungs are harvested. In either technique, at the time the heart is arrested and before organ removal, 500 µg of PGE_1 IV and 6 to 10 liters of modified Euro-Collins solution (Table 8-1) or UW solution containing PGE_1 are infused at approximately 50 cm H_2O pressure over 10 to 15 minutes into the pulmonary artery. The left atrial appendage is amputated to prevent cardiac distention, rather than division of a pulmonary vein. When the heart and lungs are separated for use in different recipients, care must be exercised in dividing the pulmonary veins. A small cuff of left atrial tissue should be left with each pulmonary vein. However, enough left atrium must remain on the heart so that the recipient left atrial suture line will not encroach upon the atrioventricular groove.

Table 8-1. Modified Euro-Collins solution for donor lung preservation

Constituents per 1000 ml

Glucose	38.50 g
KH_2PO_4	2.05 g
$KHPO_4$	7.40 g
KCl	1.12 g
$NaHCO_3$	0.84 g
Final osmolality	529.00 mOsm

Recipient Preparation and Operative Management

The potential recipient is called to the hospital when the initial predonation evaluation has been completed at the donor hospital. In some instances, several hours may be needed to complete cytotoxic crossmatching; this may provide additional time for recipients to be prepared. If recipients live several hours from the transplantation center, they may need to be called to the hospital before final crossmatch information is available. Because the surgery is not elective in nature, potential recipients are rarely prepared in terms of having an empty stomach or having stopped warfarin or aspirin anticoagulation to permit normalization of the clotting system. These factors must be kept in mind for intraoperative and postoperative management.

After admission, a history and physical examination are performed to determine whether there is evidence of active infection or other problems that would contraindicate transplantation. If time allows, the patient is shaved thoroughly and then showered with an antibacterial soap (e.g., Hibiclens). A loading dose of cyclosporine (10 mg/kg PO) is administered before the patient goes to the operating room, provided renal function is adequate (creatinine <2.0 mg/dl) and azathioprine (2 mg/kg) is given orally. If the patient has been on warfarin, a vitamin K preparation (e.g., AquaMEPHYTON, 10–20 mg IV) is administered parenterally to begin the correction process. A chest x-ray is obtained; an unexplained pulmonary infiltrate would rule out transplantation. Well in advance of the anticipated starting time, the patient is brought to the operating room, and intraoperative monitoring lines are inserted: Usually, a radial arterial line is inserted, and a multiport central venous line is placed via the internal jugular route. One or two large-bore intravenous lines are also placed, particularly if there has been prior surgery. Meticulous care with sterile technique must be exercised during line placement and subsequent maintenance to decrease the risk of infection.

Anesthesia and surgery are begun as dictated by the progress of the donor operation. Because recipients have advanced heart and lung disease, anesthetic technique is important [16]; the time from the induction of anesthesia to the start of cardiopulmonary bypass is a critical period during which cardiac decompensation may occur. Under ideal circumstances, the new heart should arrive at the recipient hospital as the ascending aorta is being cannulated for car-

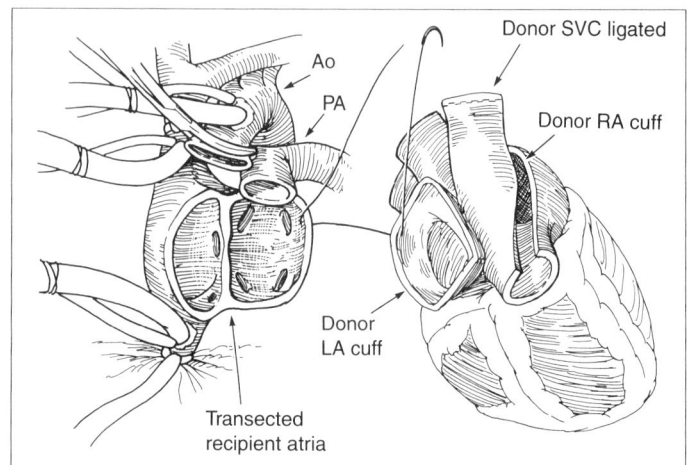

Fig. 8-1. Implantation of donor heart in recipient. Following recipient cardiectomy, the posterior portions of the left and right atria and interatrial septum remain, as well as the ends of the divided ascending aorta and main pulmonary artery. The posterior wall of the donor left atrium has been opened widely by incising between the stumps of the donor pulmonary veins. The donor right atrium has been prepared by incising from the stump of the inferior vena cava onto the free wall of the right atrium so as to avoid the region of the sinoatrial node. The left atrial suture line is completed first, beginning near the left superior pulmonary vein as shown. The right atrial suture line is completed in an analogous manner. The main pulmonary artery and the ascending aorta are then completed in an end-to-end manner.

diopulmonary bypass. The recipient heart transplant operation then proceeds in the following sequence: (1) the cardiectomy; (2) trimming of the great vessels and atrial cuffs; and (3) completion first of the atrial anastomoses, then the pulmonary artery anastomosis, and lastly the aortic anastomosis (Fig. 8-1). Alternatively, particularly when ischemic time is predicted to be long, the left-sided suture lines may be completed first, followed by cross-clamp removal, and completion of the right-sided suture lines. Careful removal of air from the heart and the ascending aorta is mandatory.

Single lung transplants are typically done through a standard thoracotomy (Fig. 8-2); double lung transplants are typically done through a bilateral transsternal thoracotomy with sequential implantation of the grafts. The need for cardiopulmonary bypass is dictated by right heart dysfunction in the presence of pulmonary artery hypertension. There should be a trial clamping of the pulmonary artery prior to removal of the native lung to assess the need for cardiopulmonary bypass at the time of donor lung implantation. Bypass, if needed, may be performed through the femoral vessels with normothermia or mild hypothermia (33–34° C.) However, for patients with severe primary pulmonary hypertension, bypass is often planned electively.

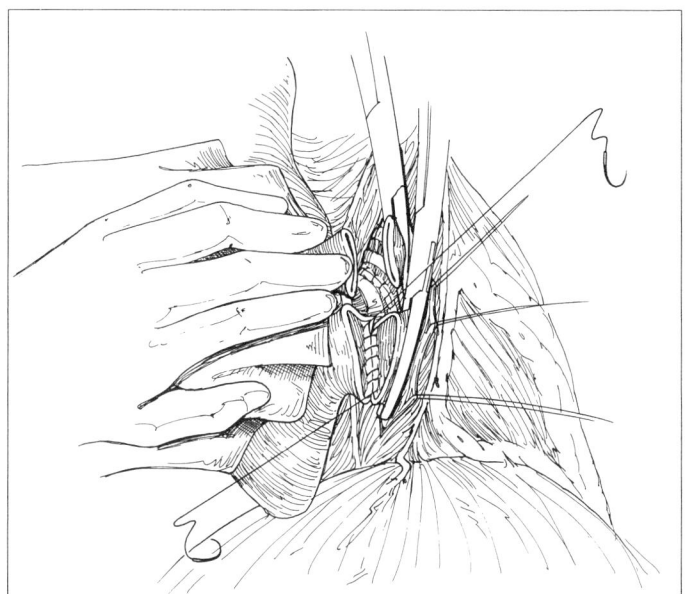

Fig. 8-2. Implantation of donor lung in recipient (right). After recipient pneumonectomy, the stumps of the bronchus and pulmonary artery and vein (clamps applied) are shown. The implantation begins with completion of the bronchial suture line. The pulmonary venous suture line is then completed, followed by the pulmonary arterial suture line. Clamps are removed, perfusion is restored, and ventilation of the transplanted lung is begun. The procedure is completed by wrapping the bronchial suture line with an omental pedicle to provide additional reinforcement and an additional source of bronchial blood supply (at MGH).

PRESERVATION OF THE DONOR HEART

Preservation of the donor heart after procurement and before restoration of its blood flow is an important issue in cardiac transplantation. The right ventricle, in particular, is very sensitive to the quality of myocardial protection. Thus, during the implant procedure, it is important to keep the heart cold until circulation can be restored. This can be achieved with the use of continuous left ventricular irrigation with ice-cold saline or with the application of iced, saline soaked sponges to the right ventricle (or both). Although practices vary from center to center, donor heart preservation may be enhanced by repeated cardioplegia infusion on arrival at the recipient hospital and during implantation. The time from procurement to removal of the aortic cross-clamp is noted so that total ischemic time may be calculated.

CHRONOTROPIC SUPPORT

Because the donor heart is denervated, it initially may require both chronotropic and inotropic support. Routinely, dopamine (3–5 µg/

kg/min) is given with isoproterenol (0.01–0.02 µg/kg/min) added, if necessary, to increase heart rate. In addition, we routinely place pairs of temporary pacing wires on the donor atrium and ventricle. If the chronotropic response to isoproterenol is inadequate (i.e., rate is less than 80 beats/min) or if temporary heart block is present, atrial (AOO) or atrioventricular sequential (DOO) pacing is begun. In patients whose conduction system has recovered and who have an adequate chronotropic effect from support medications, the pacemaker is generally left in the ventricular-demand (VVI) mode at a rate of 70 beats per minute in the event that unexpected sinus slowing or heart block occurs. In recipients whose PVR may be elevated, we place a left atrial line for monitoring left-sided filling pressures (central venous pressure may be misleading in these instances) and we often insert a Swan-Ganz catheter. Should significant right heart failure occur, pharmacologic management using right-sided infusions of PGE_1 with left-sided infusions of norepinephrine may be used as described in Chapter 4; the addition of a second left atrial line for drug infusions is useful if this intervention is needed.

When the aorta is unclamped, methylprednisolone (Solu-Medrol, 500 mg) is administered. The patient is weaned from cardiopulmonary bypass and decannulated as for other cardiac operations. Hemostasis is then secured. Patients who have been on warfarin preoperatively may require administration of 5 to 6 units of fresh frozen plasma. If excessive volume or hemodilution becomes a concern, an alternative way of managing this problem is to administer fresh frozen plasma before termination of cardiopulmonary bypass and to use hemofiltration on bypass to remove excess water volume. In the case of the recipient with a large pericardial space due to cardiomegaly who has received a smaller, normal-sized heart, accumulation of significant pericardial effusion can occur postoperatively; we generally leave one pleural space open for drainage. Some surgeons also resect the redundant pericardium. Pericardial effusion, if it occurs, generally is noted within 1 month of transplantation [17].

INOTROPIC SUPPORT

Inotropic support is generally maintained for approximately 3–4 days. This is needed, in part, because the donor heart is denervated and depends on circulating catecholamines to maintain its inotropic state. In the normal heart, CVP is usually substantially lower (by approximately 5–8 mm Hg) than left atrial pressure. This is frequently not the case after transplantation [18] for two reasons. First, the normal, donor right ventricle may have sustained some degree of ischemic injury as part of the harvest and pretransplant preservation process. Second, PVR may be elevated because of preexisting pulmonary hypertension or the effects of cardiopulmonary bypass on the lung. Consequently, in the early 24 to 48 hours after transplantation, central venous and left atrial pressures are often nearly identical. In situations where CVP exceeds left atrial pressure, some degree of right ventricular failure must be considered. As the patient awakens, this can be of particular concern because PVR often increases during emergence from anesthesia. Accordingly, it is *critical* to monitor both left and right atrial and pulmonary artery pressures continuously during the wake-up period, particularly if the recipient had any degree of pulmonary hypertension before transplantation.

An ominous sign suggesting severe right ventricular failure is a substantial increase in CVP (e.g., to over 20 mm Hg) accompanied by a *decrease* in left atrial pressure. In such circumstances, we reinstitute deep sedation and optimize inotropic drug support. Pharmacologic measures to manage right heart failure should be instituted at this time. If these measures are already in place, as is frequently the case in patients in whom right heart failure is seen on awakening, then deep sedation and paralysis are reinstituted, and further time is allowed for cardiac and pulmonary vascular recovery. After 24 to 48 additional hours, a point is usually reached where the PVR falls and right ventricular function improves sufficiently to allow the patient to be awakened and extubated. Rarely, mechanical right ventricular assist is required. Occasionally tricuspid valve regurgitation may be noted, but over the first 2 posttransplant weeks, this frequently improves as pulmonary artery pressure decreases and RV remodelling occurs [19].

Early Postoperative Considerations

Postoperatively, patients are generally placed in an intensive care unit equipped with positive-pressure isolation rooms and, in the first few days after transplantation, reverse precautions usually are observed. The transplant cubicle should be cleaned thoroughly just prior to occupancy. Recent studies have challenged whether these standard procedures are really necessary [20] provided careful handwashing and some patient isolation are practiced. Reverse-isolation precautions are decreased to using masks and handwashing when major transcutaneous lines and drains are removed — the time when prophylactic postoperative antibiotics usually are discontinued.

For the first few days after transplantation, daily chest x-rays, ECGs, and urine and sputum cultures are obtained. Bacteriologic culture and sensitivity data collected before clinical manifestations of infection may be extremely useful because infections may progress much more rapidly under conditions of immunosuppression. If the patient remains stable with clear chest x-ray and negative sputum culture, the culture frequency may be reduced 2 or 3 days after extubation.

Certain additional precautions are taken with lung transplant recipients. Because the lungs tend to undergo a "reimplantation" response, including an increase in lung water, fluid administration is kept to a minimum and diuretics and PEEP are used liberally. Postoperative ventilation management following lung transplantation can be complex and the principles vary according to the patient's underlying lung disease that led to transplantation: If a patient had primary or secondary pulmonary hypertension with systemic or suprasystemic pulmonary artery pressure prior to transplantation, we prefer to maintain deep sedation and intubation for approximately 3 days to minimize PVR in the remaining native lung, thus preventing "flooding" of the new lung with the majority of the cardiac output. All patients, regardless of their indication for lung transplantation, are weaned from an IMV mode to a pressure-support mode to decrease the work of breathing. Particularly for the patient with chronic obstructive pulmonary disease (COPD), this minimizes transpleural pressure differences and tends to prevent hyperinflation of the remaining native lung. Most COPD patients demonstrate some shift of the midline toward the graft; however, physiologic compromise is rare unless there is significant graft rejection or infection in the native lung. The bronchial anastomoses are inspected by bronchoscopy daily for the first few days and subsequently at less frequent intervals to detect breakdown, granulation formation, or stricture.

Immunosuppression, Surveillance, and Management of Rejection

ROUTINE IMMUNOSUPPRESSION

Before the 1980s and the widespread use of cyclosporine, conventional immunosuppression in transplantation was achieved with steroids and azathioprine. This regimen produced nonspecific immunosuppression and necessitated using higher doses of steroids than are used with contemporary immunosuppression. A step toward more specific immunosuppression was made when *cyclosporin A* was introduced [21]. Although its mechanism of action is not completely understood, it appears to diminish the proliferation of cytotoxic T lymphocytes. It allows the use of lower steroid doses for maintenance immunosuppression and, although cyclosporine-based regimens do not decrease the frequency of rejection, the degree and severity of rejection are much less.

MEDICATIONS USED FOR IMMUNOSUPPRESSION

Cyclosporine (Sandimmune)

Class: Fungus-derived cyclic peptide; lipophilic

Routes of administration: PO and IV

Metabolism: Primarily hepatic

Dose: Initial loading dose, 10 mg/kg PO; maintenance, 5–10 mg/kg/PO divided bid; dose titrated according to side effects and blood level determinations.

Side effects:

Dose-related and blood level-related *nephrotoxicity*. This may be potentiated by concomitant administration of other nephrotoxic drugs such as aminoglycoside antibiotics or amphotericin B
Hypertension, tremor, and neurotoxicity with decreased seizure threshold
Gingival hyperplasia and hirsutism
Hepatic toxicity
Possible increased risk of lymphoma

Blood levels: The target therapeutic range varies among institutions depending on the methodology used to determine cyclosporine concentration. When whole blood determinations are made by radioimmunoassay, the initial therapeutic range is generally 300–800 ng/ml, and when they are made by high-pressure liquid chromatography, the initial therapeutic range is 150–300 ng/ml.

Prednisone/Methylprednisolone

Class: Corticosteroid

Route of administration: PO (prednisone) or IV (methylprednisolone)

Mechanism of action: Broad suppression of the synthesis of nucleic acids and proteins in lymphocytes, resulting in lymphocyte depletion. Particularly at higher doses, all T-cell responses may be broadly suppressed. Because of a possible action to stabilize lysosomes in macrophages and neutrophils, the inflammatory response is also depressed with inhibition of bacterial killing.

Dose: Initially administered parenterally as methylprednisolone (125 mg tid) and converted to prednisone when oral intake begins. The initial prednisone dose may be high (MGH: 60–80 mg PO bid; Iowa: 70 mg PO qd) but is rapidly tapered over the first 2 weeks after transplantation. The eventual prednisone maintenance dose reached depends on the activity seen during routine surveillance biopsies, but it is generally in the range of 5–20 mg/day, given as a single dose and dependent on institutional practice. In patients with minimal tendency toward rejection for several months, we sometimes attempt to discontinue prednisone altogether at 6 months after transplantation. As mentioned previously, prednisone is often omitted for the first 2 weeks following lung transplantation.

Side effects:

Impaired wound healing and increased infection risks
Weight gain and obesity
Gastrointestinal ulceration
Glucose intolerance
Hypertension
Osteoporosis
Changes in mood

Many of these effects are dose-related, and, for this reason, efforts are made to administer prednisone in as low a dose as needed to maintain tolerance to the transplant. Although not in widespread use at the present time, some institutions are currently investigating steroid-free protocols for heart transplantation to avoid many of the undesirable steroid side effects.

We do not use maintenance steroids in newborns, and we taper the drug in older children rapidly, hoping to discontinue or at least give it on alternate days. With these precautions, children grow and develop normally and withstand the usual community-acquired infections.

Azathioprine (Imuran)

Class: Antimetabolite that results in inhibition of purine synthesis. By incorporation into nucleic acids, it slows nucleic acid synthesis and cell division. As a result, it appears to affect T-lymphocyte proliferation, thus inhibiting T-cell–mediated rejection.

Dose: 1–2 mg/kg/day given IV or PO as a single dose.

Side effects: Primarily dose-related bone marrow depression and leukopenia. Thus the WBC is monitored, and the dose is reduced if the WBC count is less than 4000/mm^3 and discontinued if it is below 2000/mm^3. Azathioprine metabolism is inhibited by allopurinol and, if given concomitantly, can result in profound bone marrow depression. Patients requiring allopurinol treatment may be treated with cyclophosphamide (CYTOXAN) instead of azathioprine.

OKT3 (ORTHOCLONE OKT3)

Class: A murine monoclonal antibody capable of neutralizing the population of lymphocytes that carry the T3 antigen–receptor complex. Because of its efficacy and specificity, OKT3 can produce profound depletion of the circulating T-cell population and thus controls the rejection process. Furthermore, there is evidence that OKT3 impairs the ability of T cells to recognize antigens, thus resulting in inactivation of T cells still present in the circulation.

Dose: 5 mg IV for 10 to 14 days in adults; occasionally, larger doses (10 mg/day) must be used to produce adequate T-cell clearance in some patients. OKT3 is produced by a mouse myeloma. Because it is a foreign protein, host antibodies against murine OKT3 can be produced, rendering the material ineffective, particularly for multiple, consecutive uses. It is unusual for this to occur during the 10 to 15 days that OKT3 is administered. However, patients who are on OKT3 therapy should have ongoing T-cell subset monitoring if available, and any increase in the T3 subset titer should raise the suspicion of antimouse antibodies. This may necessitate increasing the dose of OKT3; certainly, antimouse antibody titers must be determined before deciding whether to administer a second course of OKT3 for a subsequent rejection episode.

Side effects: Fever and chills may be experienced with the first 2 or 3 doses, and more serious side effects such as bronchospasm or pulmonary edema have been noted. Some patients also develop gastrointestinal symptoms including nausea and diarrhea. To help alleviate some of the symptoms, it is common practice to pretreat patients with acetaminophen (650 mg PO), Benadryl (50 mg PO), and cortisone (100 mg IV) before administering the first few doses of OKT3. Severe pulmonary edema can occur with OKT3 administration, so this drug should not be utilized in patients with fluid overload (by chest x-ray and body weight measurement).

Antilymphocyte Globulin (ALG)/Antithymocyte Globulin (ATG)

Class: Polyclonal, animal-derived antibodies to human lymphocytes or thymocytes.

Dose: 15 mg/kg/d (IV or IM) for 14 days

Side effects: Reactions noted in patients include: bronchospasm, fever, chills, serum sickness, and even anaphylactic shock. Like OKT3, antibodies to antilymphocyte serums can occur and may limit repeated use, but these are not usually measured.

Lymphocytes are inactivated and subsequently cleared from circulation by the reticuloendothelial system, in a manner analogous to that of OKT3, but without the specificity of the newer agent. Although ALG and ATG have been prepared in a number of different species, rabbit- and horse-derived globulins are the most commonly used preparations today.

CURRENT PROTOCOLS

Presently, cyclosporine-based regimens are standard practice in heart, heart-lung, and lung transplantation [22,23]. This practice takes the form of protocols involving two drugs (cyclosporine and prednisone) or three drugs (cyclosporine, azathioprine, and prednisone). The use of the three-drug regimen may permit lower doses of cyclosporine and steroids to be administered, thereby diminishing the potential for nephrotoxicity and infection [24]. It is our current practice to use a three-drug regimen as shown in Table 8-2 for both heart and lung recipients.

Polyclonal antiserums (equine or rabbit antilymphocyte or antithymocyte globulin) have been used for years either as induction immunotherapy or as rescue therapy in treating severe rejection episodes. While still used for treating rejection, polyclonal antibodies have been largely replaced by monoclonal antibodies. Monoclonal antibodies to human T lymphocytes were first used in renal transplantation in 1981 [25]. Monoclonal antibodies (e.g., OKT3) are able to remove circulating T lymphocytes within a very short time after administration. They have been utilized by some centers prophylactically for the first 2 weeks after heart transplantation and appear to be effective in the prevention of early rejection episodes. In heart transplantation we have reserved the use of antiserums for special circumstances, such as significant renal failure before transplantation, where it is desirable to keep the initial dose of cyclosporine low or to omit it for the first 1 or 2 weeks after transplantation. In lung transplantation, some use OKT3 for the first 10 days for prophylaxis against rejection.

As mentioned previously, immunosuppression is initiated preoperatively in heart and lung recipients by the administration of cyclosporine and azathioprine. When renal function is known to be impaired (creatinine ≥ 2.0 mg/dl) or the patient is hemodynamically unstable (e.g., intraaortic balloon pump support or high-dose dobutamine), we often omit preoperative cyclosporine in favor of OKT3 induction.

Following heart transplantation in the operating room, methylprednisolone (500 mg IV) is given when the donor heart is reperfused. When the patient reaches the intensive care unit, methylprednisolone (125 mg IV q8–12hr) is started and continued until the patient is extubated (generally for 3 doses); if prolonged intubation occurs, the dose is tapered slowly down to 30 IV qd. Prednisone is begun after extubation. The dose and tapering schedule for prednisone may vary widely (see Table 8-2).

Cyclosporine (3–4 mg/kg bid) is instilled through the nasogastric tube when the patient reaches the intensive care unit and then given orally when the patient is extubated. The cyclosporine dose is ad-

Table 8-2. Immunosuppressive drug regimen for heart and lung transplantation

Procedure	Preoperative	Intraoperative	Postoperative
Heart transplantation (Massachusetts General Hospital)	Cyclosporine 6 mg/kg PO*	Azathioprine 5 mg/kg IV Methylprednisolone 500 mg IV	Cyclosporine 6 mg/kg/d PO divided bid; dose adjusted according to blood levels Azathioprine 2 mg/kg/d PO, decreased if WBC < 4000 mm³ Methylprednisolone 125 mg IV q8hr × 48hr, then prednisone 2 mg/kg/d divided bid, tapering to 0.4 mg/kg/d by discharge; Prednisone tapered to 10 mg/d by 6–9 mo postop depending on rejection activity on surveillance biopsies
Lung transplantation (University of Iowa)	Azathioprine 5 mg/kg PO or IV Cyclosporine 10 mg/kg PO	Methylprednisolone 500 mg IV	Azathioprine 1 mg/kg/d PO or IV Cyclosporine 8–12 mg/kg/d divided bid, adjusted according to blood levels, eventually to 5–6 mg/kg/d OKT3 5 mg IV qd for 10 d Prednisone PO (or methylprednisolone IV) start on POD #8 60 mg qd, tapered weekly to 30 mg qd by POD #36 Prednisone then weaned by 2.5 mg/d per mo, down to 15 mg/d by eighth mo. Prednisone may then be converted to 15 mg qod over next 6–8 mo in clinically stable patient

*Given if renal function is normal; otherwise not given preoperatively.
Key: WBC = white blood (cell) count.

justed daily to maintain target blood levels of 200–300 ng/dl (HPLC method). Azathioprine (2 mg/kg qd) is given intravenously as a single daily dose and then orally after extubation, and the azathioprine dose is reduced if the WBC count falls below 4000/mm^3.

The early concerns expressed by surgeons about administering steroids during the first 2 weeks to patients undergoing lung and heart-lung transplantation may not be warranted. However, there exist considerable differences of opinion about this issue. Some avoid steroids for the first week following lung transplantation and depend on OKT3 prophylaxis against rejection.

REJECTION SURVEILLANCE

One of the most difficult issues in the management of transplant patients is proper surveillance for detection of allograft rejection. Unlike the transplantation of other organ systems, where more severe degrees of allograft dysfunction can be tolerated, there is a much narrower margin of safety in heart and lung transplantation. Thus, the early detection of rejection, before significant mechanical failure, electrical instability, or pulmonary failure appears, is of utmost importance.

For heart transplant recipients, standard clinical indicators such as heart size, blood pressure, heart rate, and the ECG may not suggest the diagnosis until it is substantially advanced [26]. Although recent efforts have been directed toward the development of more sophisticated techniques such as nuclear magnetic resonance imaging, the gold standard for the detection of cardiac allograft rejection remains the endomyocardial biopsy and for lung allograft rejection, transbronchial biopsy [27,28].

Endomyocardial Biopsy

Endomyocardial biopsies in cardiac transplant patients are generally performed under fluoroscopic guidance in the cardiac catheterization laboratory. They provide a simple, low-morbidity method for obtaining tissue samples (generally 4–6) of the right ventricular myocardium, usually via the internal jugular vein approach. At the time the biopsy is performed, right-sided pressures and a thermodilution cardiac output should be obtained if indicated. Endomyocardial biopsies are initially performed weekly after transplantation in adults and children until three negative biopsies are obtained. These usually are done before the patient is discharged. Subsequent biopsies are performed every 2 to 4 weeks for the next 2 months; then monthly for the first 6 months; and less frequently after the first year as individually required. Additional biopsies may be needed when the clinical status changes. It has been our policy not to perform routine biopsies in newborns unless there is a serious suspicion of rejection, and to perform routine biopsies in older infants less frequently than in adults.

Transbronchial Biopsy

The diagnosis of pulmonary rejection is even more problematic and must be distinguished from pulmonary infection. Most lungs undergo a reimplantation response manifested by increased lung water and pulmonary infiltrates during the first few days. Subsequently, pulmonary infiltrates may appear radiographically from infection or atelectasis. These cannot be distinguished from early rejection. In the past, the empiric response to antirejection therapy was used to establish this diagnosis. Nowadays, transbronchial biopsies are performed at routine intervals and are of some assistance. Routine surveillance lung biopsies are performed at 1, 3, and 6 weeks; 3, 6, 9, and 12 months; and annually thereafter. The majority of patients will develop at least one episode of rejection within the first 3 months following transplantation, prompting some alteration in this biopsy schedule. However, the diagnosis of early lung rejection is usually made on clinical criteria such as the occurrence of a subjective sense of dyspnea, a decrease in saturation, or a change in chest x-ray. Within the first 3 months following lung transplantation, FEV_1 continues to improve and the improvement continues despite an episode of rejection. Beyond 3 months, spirometry is more useful as an indicator of rejection. Chest CT scanning may be useful in discriminating between rejection and infection: Rejection presents with prominent septal lines in the lung parenchyma; infection produces more of a ground-glass appearance to the pulmonary parenchyma.

A new infiltrate in a lung transplant recipient always mandates bronchoscopy. If there is no purulence in the airways, a transbronchial biopsy is performed; if there is excessive purulence, a bronchoalveolar lavage is performed to collect material for microbiologic study and a chest CT is obtained. If the patient does not respond to antimicrobial therapy within 4 to 5 days, the patient is rebronchoscoped for transbronchial biopsy.

DIAGNOSIS AND GRADING OF ACUTE REJECTION

The primary reason for performing biopsies in the postoperative period is to detect allograft rejection. The assignment of numerical grades to the degree of rejection facilitates documentation, record keeping, and progress in the monitoring of transplant patients. We employ the grading systems presented by The Working Group of the International Society for Heart and Lung Transplantation that utilize a total of five numerical categories ranging from 0 to 4, which may have advantages over previous grading systems [29]. The details of these grading schemes are enumerated in Tables 8-3 and 8-4 [30].

The two most significant findings in cardiac biopsy evaluation are the extent of inflammatory infiltration and the degree of myocyte necrosis (grades 2–4); these findings are pivotal in deciding whether to treat for rejection. In all cases, the biopsy findings must be interpreted in the light of the clinical scenario and the previous biopsy histology. Endomyocardial biopsy is subject to sampling error because rejection may occur in a heterogeneous manner. Thus, in the patient who may have new-onset atrial or ventricular arrhythmias, low-grade fever, or fluid retention and who is found to have grade 1 rejection, a course of antirejection treatment may still be indicated. In general, however, the appearance of myocyte necrosis, irrespective of the clinical state, is an indication to treat for rejection. One important exception to this can occur in the first 10 to 21 days after transplantation. The transplanted heart will have sustained various degrees of ischemic injury during the time it was not perfused. This

Table 8-3. Classification and grading of cardiac rejection

Grade	Classification
0	No rejection
1	1A = Focal (perivascular or interstitial) infiltrate without necrosis 1B = Diffuse but sparse infiltrate without necrosis
2	One focus only with aggressive infiltration and/or focal myocyte damage
3	3A = Multifocal aggressive infiltrates and/or myocyte damage 3B = Diffuse inflammatory process with necrosis
4	Diffuse aggressive polymorphous process, ± infiltrate, ± edema, ± hemorrhage, ± vasculitis, with necrosis

Source: ME Billingham, et al. A working formulation for the standardization of nomenclature in the diagnosis of heart and lung rejection: Heart Rejection Study Group. *J Heart Transplant* 9:587, 1990. Reproduced with permission.

can result in myocyte necrosis that must be distinguished from that produced by rejection; generally, ischemic injury is not accompanied by as much interstitial infiltrate and occurs only early after transplantation. In addition, biopsy specimens can include healing biopsy sites from previous endomyocardial biopsies. These can be misleading and must be distinguished histologically from areas of potential rejection.

The grading system for pulmonary rejection quantitates the extent of mononuclear cell infiltration, pneumocyte damage, and vasculitis (see Table 8-4) [31]. Perivascular infiltration is the hallmark of early lung rejection.

THE TREATMENT OF ACUTE REJECTION

Pulse doses of steroids remain first-line therapy for the initial treatment of non–life-threatening acute rejection, usually grade 2 [32]. We treat grade 1 rejection if patients have other manifestations such as cardiac arrhythmias, or, in the case of lung transplants, a symptomatic decrease in pulmonary function. The route of administration depends on the time interval since transplantation and, to some extent, on the degree of rejection. Generally, within the first 3 months after transplantation, single daily doses of methylprednisolone are administered intravenously for 3 consecutive days. We generally use 500–1000 mg/day for heart recipients and 500 mg/day for lung recipients, although the minimum dose needed remains controversial [33,34]. This dose may be decreased in adults weighing less than 60 kg. Approximately 3 months after transplantation, patients who do not have severe degrees of rejection may be treated with pulse doses of prednisone (100 mg/day PO) for 3 days followed by a slow tapering back to the maintenance dose. In each patient, approximately 1 week after completion of steroid pulse therapy, a repeat endomyocardial or transbronchial biopsy is obtained. Biopsy may be done sooner if there are clinical manifestations of worsening rejection. If rejection improves, orally administered steroids are con-

Table 8-4. Classification and grading of pulmonary rejection

I. Acute rejection
    Grade 0 — No significant abnormality
    Grade 1 — Minimal acute rejection
        A. With evidence of bronchiolar inflammation
        B. Without evidence of bronchiolar inflammation
        C. With large airway inflammation
        D. No bronchioles to evaluate
    Grade 2 — Mild acute rejection
        A. With evidence of bronchiolar inflammation
        B. Without evidence of bronchiolar inflammation
        C. With large airway inflammation
        D. No bronchioles to evaluate
    Grade 3 — Moderate acute rejection
        A. With evidence of bronchiolar inflammation
        B. Without evidence of bronchiolar inflammation
        C. With large airway inflammation
        D. No bronchioles to evaluate
    Grade 4 — Severe acute rejection
        A. With evidence of bronchiolar inflammation
        B. Without evidence of bronchiolar inflammation
        C. With large airway inflammation
        D. No bronchioles to evaluate
II. Active airway damage without scarring
    Lymphocytic bronchitis
    Lymphocytic bronchiolitis
III. Chronic airway rejection
    Bronchiolitis obliterans — subtotal
        A. Active
        B. Inactive
    Bronchiolitis obliterans — total
        A. Active
        B. Inactive
IV. Chronic vascular rejection
V. Vasculitis

Source: SA Yousem et al. A working formulation for the standardization of nomenclature in the diagnosis of heart and lung rejection: Lung Rejection Study Group. *J Heart Transplant* 9:593, 1990. Reproduced with permission.

tinued at their maintenance level. During this period, care is taken to ensure that the cyclosporine blood level is optimized.

If rejection fails to resolve after treatment with orally administered steroids and if the patient is clinically stable, a 3-day course of intravenously administered methylprednisolone may be tried. In all instances, if patients fail to improve with parenterally administered steroids, if the initial biopsy revealed grade 4 rejection, or if there are significant clinical manifestations (e.g., failure), the next tier of therapy at our institutions is with the monoclonal antibody OKT3. In clinical studies to date, OKT3 has been shown to be highly effective for reversing allograft rejection [25,35]. OKT3 is not an option for treating early rejection if it was used for early posttransplant prophylaxis.

Some precautions must be exercised when OKT3 is administered. The starting dose is 5 mg/day given as a single intravenous bolus. OKT3 can produce pulmonary edema in a small percentage of patients; preexisting fluid overload or congestive heart failure due to rejection may predispose to this complication. Premedication is essential to prevent this complication. The efficacy of OKT3 therapy may be confirmed by peripheral T-cell monitoring, especially in patients who have received prior OKT3 therapy and may have produced antibodies to it. Unless indicated by clinical findings, patients generally undergo biopsy 5 to 10 days after completion of OKT3 therapy.

In instances where rejection is still present after OKT3 therapy, or where OKT3 has not produced adequate T-cell clearance (e.g., when there has been prior use and anti-OKT3 antibodies are present), other antilymphocyte preparations may be used [36]. Equine antithymocyte globulin (ATGAM, Upjohn) is administered intravenously in a single daily dose via a central venous catheter (15 mg/kg/day) for 14 days. As with OKT3 therapy, efficacy of treatment may be assessed by measuring T-cell subsets. A 0.1-ml subcutaneous test dose is administered before therapy is initiated and patients are premedicated with acetaminophen, diphenhydramine hydrochloride (e.g., Benadryl), and methylprednisolone, as is the practice with OKT3. In our experience, adverse patient reactions to ATGAM are less common than with OKT3. ATGAM has been intermittently unavailable due to manufacturing problems.

Alternative antilymphocyte serums have been made in other animals, generally at university laboratories. They are not widely available and may be subject to some variability in potency.

Several other agents are useful in patients who experience recurrent or recalcitrant rejection. Orally administered methotrexate has proved very helpful in our practice [37]. The dose is 5 to 10 mg/wk given as a single dose for 6 weeks. If the response is inadequate, a second course (20 mg/wk) may be given for 6 weeks. Actinomycin D and thalidomide have been reported to be useful for chronic rejection in a few cases. Phototherapy has reversed difficult rejection in a few of our patients; the mechanism of this modality is unknown [38]. An alternative mode of "salvage" therapy for unresponsive cardiac rejection is total lymphoid irradiation, which may be of value in some patients [39].

In very rare instances, progressive, ongoing rejection cannot be reversed. This results in eventual progressive heart or lung failure. When all antirejection therapies (including experimental medications) have failed, retransplantation must be considered, especially for heart transplant recipients. Particularly in instances where hemodynamic deterioration of the heart recipient is rapid and where the waiting time for a donor organ may be considerable, temporary mechanical support with an intraaortic balloon pump or ventricular assist device may be needed until a new heart becomes available. Retransplantation of the lung is associated with substantial mortality and this modality is used infrequently.

Antibiotic Prophylaxis

Because of immunosuppression, infection continues to be a significant source of morbidity and mortality in transplant patients, especially those with lung and heart-lung transplants. Early after surgery, these patients are susceptible to the usual types of bacterial infections, including wound infections, pneumonia, and urinary tract infections. The risk of infection may be increased even further when patients come to surgery with marked degrees of debility. Furthermore, if patients have been hospitalized for an extended period of time, such as for management of heart failure or for preoperative mechanical support, there may be additional risk for nosocomial infection.

Thus, routine antibiotic prophylaxis may be of particular value in the cardiac and pulmonary transplant setting. For most patients, we use a cephalosporin such as cephapirin or cefazolin, in combination with vancomycin. In patients who have been hospitalized for an extended period of time, this regimen, while providing excellent *Staphylococcus* coverage, may not be adequate, particularly against colonization by common gram-negative organisms. For these patients, coverage with advanced-generation cephalosporins may be included.

There are additional special circumstances that may warrant additional antibiotic therapy. For example, when a donor may be heavily colonized with bacteria, we retrieve a donor sputum sample at the time of organ harvesting. Microbial identification and antibiotic sensitivities can help guide the use of additional antibiotic prophylaxis or guide initial treatment of suspected postoperative infections. Lung transplant patients receiving OKT3 may also be given fungal prophylaxis with intravenous fluconazole. In cystic fibrosis patients receiving lung transplants, antifungal prophylaxis may be provided with amphotericin B until final fungal culture reports are available to rule out *Aspergillus* colonization of the recipient.

After the initial recovery following transplantation, when immunosuppression becomes well established, the risk of opportunistic infection begins to increase and is related to the *cumulative* doses of immunosuppressants utilized and especially to the amount of steroid used. Although the list of potential opportunistic etiologic agents is long, there are a few instances where prophylaxis has proved useful.

THRUSH PROPHYLAXIS

Oral thrush can be a source of extreme discomfort in transplant patients and may impair nutrition. We generally use a nystatin suspension for prophylaxis against thrush. One teaspoonful is used as an oral rinse and subsequently swallowed 3 times per day. More resistant cases usually respond to clotrimazole troches (10 mg bid).

PNEUMOCYSTIS PROPHYLAXIS

There is a 10% incidence of *Pneumocystis carinii* pneumonia in the first 6 months following organ transplantation. Because of this risk, most centers routinely administer prophylaxis for at least 6 months posttransplant. Long-term, low-dose treatment with trimethoprim-sulfamethoxazole (1 single-strength tablet daily) [40] has been shown to be highly effective in eliminating not only infections caused by *Pneumocystis carinii* but also those due to *Nocardia asteroides* and *Listeria monocytogenes*. This prophylactic regimen is begun when patients begin oral intake. For those patients unable to tolerate trimethoprim-sulfamethoxazole, monthly aerosolized pentamidine has been shown to be a useful alternative.

TOXOPLASMOSIS PROPHYLAXIS

Toxoplasmosis, a disease caused by the protozoan *Toxoplasma gondii*, can result in serious central nervous system, cardiac, and pulmonary infections in immunosuppressed hosts. *Toxoplasma gondii* is present in the environment and many individuals, when subjected to serologic testing, are often positive. Infection in cardiac transplant recipients can occur from either of two mechanisms. In patients who are seropositive at the time of transplantation, reactivation of toxoplasmosis may occur in the immunosuppressed state. Fortunately, this reactivation-type of toxoplasmosis is usually not serious and is rarely identified clinically.

Second, patients who are seronegative at the time of transplantation are at risk if they receive a heart from a seropositive donor. In these instances, *Toxoplasma* protozoa may be transmitted by the donor organ and prophylaxis is indicated [41]. For these patients, we employ a prophylactic course of treatment with pyrimethamine (50 mg PO qd) and sulfadiazine (500 mg PO qd) for 6 months. To prevent the bone marrow depression associated with these drugs, especially in patients receiving azathioprine, we administer folinic acid (1 mg PO qwk). This regimen also provides effective prophylaxis against *Pneumocystis, Nocardia,* and *Listeria;* trimethoprim-sulfamethoxazole is not needed in patients receiving this regimen of antitoxoplasmosis prophylaxis.

ANTIVIRAL PROPHYLAXIS

The most important infectious disease problem following organ transplantation is that caused by *cytomegalovirus* (CMV) [42]. The incidence and severity of CMV disease are modulated by two major factors: (1) the donor's and recipient's past experiences with the virus (with the presence of circulating anti-CMV antibody connoting both past experience and latent infection capable of being reactivated by immunosuppressive therapy) and (2) the type and intensity of immunosuppressive therapy administered. Seronegative recipients of organs from seropositive donors have at least a 50–60% incidence of clinical CMV disease, with some series reporting an even higher incidence [43]; those recipients who are CMV seropositive prior to transplantation have a 20% incidence of clinical disease. However, the administration of OKT3 or antithymocyte globulin (ATG) can double or triple the incidence of clinical disease in these individuals. Clinical CMV disease typically occurs 3 weeks to 3 months posttransplantation and consists of variable combinations of fever, leukopenia, hepatitis, pneumonia, gastrointestinal ulceration, and thrombocytopenia (with pneumonia being the most dreaded manifestation). Pulmonary involvement can be particularly devastating in lung transplant recipients. In addition, CMV has immunomodulatory effects, rendering the individual susceptible to life-threatening superinfection. Chorioretinitis may develop — either as the first manifestation of CMV infection or as a sequela of previous manifestations of the virus.

Optimal regimens for preventing CMV disease are still being defined [44–46]. One efficacious *prophylactic* regimen at present consists of a combination of hyperimmune anti-CMV globulin (150 mg/kg/wk for 2–3 weeks) plus high-dose oral acyclovir (800 mg qid for 3–4 months). *Preemptive* therapy consisting of the administration of ganciclovir (2.5–5.0 mg/kg/day IV) during a course of OKT3 or ATG provides significant protection against the added morbidity and mortality caused by the virus-promoting effects of these potent antirejection therapies [47]. When clinical CMV disease develops, the therapy of choice is intravenous ganciclovir (5 mg/kg bid) with or without weekly hyperimmune globulin for a minimum of 2–3 weeks.

The other herpes-group viruses causing difficulties in transplant recipients are *herpes simplex* (HSV), *Epstein-Barr* (EBV), and *varicella-zoster* (VZV) viruses. Localized orofacial or anogenital HSV infection is common and responds equally well to ganciclovir or the less toxic acyclovir (200 mg PO 5 times/day), with disseminated HSV disease being almost unheard of in this patient group. Although EBV can cause clinical effects similar to CMV, its most important effects in the transplant recipient have to do with its role in the pathogenesis of EBV-associated lymphoproliferative disease. How best to prevent this is still under evaluation. Finally, reactivation VZV (zoster) is common, rarely disseminates, and responds well to acyclovir (800 mg PO qid) or ganciclovir (5 mg/kg IV bid). Indeed, such therapy should be viewed as optional, since zoster rarely disseminates in the organ transplant patient. Primary VZV infection, on the other hand (occurring in VZV-seronegative recipients) is a medical emergency, requiring high-dose acyclovir (800 mg PO 4–5 times per day). Varicella-zoster virus–seronegative transplant recipients should receive varicella-zoster immune globulin prophylaxis whenever exposure to individuals with zoster or chickenpox occurs.

Long-term Follow-up

REHABILITATION

Cardiac and lung transplant recipients frequently face a more extensive postoperative rehabilitation process than patients who have had other types of cardiac surgery because of the restricted lifestyle and physical debility that patients often experience prior to transplantation. This process encompasses several aspects including (1) physical rehabilitation, (2) attention to dietary considerations, and (3) a compulsive and well-organized approach to managing the medication regimen [48].

Physical rehabilitation begins preoperatively to the extent possible and is resumed in the hospital before discharge. Patients are often exercised on a stationary bicycle at low levels of workload 7 to 10 days after the transplant; however, in patients who have been on bedrest for extensive periods before transplantation (e.g., patients on intraaortic balloon pump support), the rehabilitative process may be prolonged. An individualized program of graded physical exercise must be prescribed for each patient and must recognize the individual's pretransplant disability as well as the exercise response of the denervated transplant heart [49].

Dietary management also must be individualized; dietary instruction should begin during the preoperative evaluation period. There are several issues germane to this patient population. First, caloric intake must be monitored and controlled. Because of the changes in appetite that occur in most individuals on prednisone, weight gain (typically >20 lbs) is often a problem. Thus, monitoring fat and total calorie intake becomes important. Second, because some patients will face the risk of developing late cardiac graft atherosclerosis, monitoring the fat content and consequent lipid profile of each patient becomes essential. Third, because of the tendency of cyclosporine to increase blood pressure in most individuals, salt intake is frequently restricted. Finally, because of the immunosuppressed state, raw foodstuffs (e.g., raw fruits and vegetables) must be assiduously avoided; an exception are items that may be peeled to remove the outside skin — a potential source of infection. The entire dietary program is important and, in the face of these considerations, adequate protein intake must be maintained. Thus, as part of the rehabilitative process, these patients require substantial instruction.

Even more critical than compulsive dietary management is the patient's understanding of the medication regimen and awareness of early signs of complications and toxicity. It is essential that the physician in charge of the patient's management and the transplant coordinator know that the patient is taking his or her medications properly, particularly if there are clinical events or laboratory findings that appear to be inconsistent. For example, tremendous fluctuations in the blood cyclosporine level may signify difficulties in medication compliance or errors in taking cyclosporine.

FOLLOW-UP INVESTIGATIONS

Patients who undergo heart and lung transplantation initially require relatively frequent visits to the transplant center. In addition to endomyocardial or transbronchial biopsies and laboratory monitoring, cardiac function will be checked frequently by echocardiography and pulmonary function by spirometry. We commonly evaluate cardiac transplant patients thoroughly on an annual basis with cardiac catheterization. This includes measurement of right heart pressures, ventriculography, and coronary angiography. It is important that quantitative coronary angiography be performed because these patients may develop graft coronary artery atherosclerosis characterized by a gradual and diffuse decrease in coronary vessel diameter [50]. The time course for investigations and testing in the average heart transplant patient is summarized in Table 8-5. Lung recipients undergo periodic pulmonary function testing and bronchoscopy.

Table 8-5. Timetable for investigations following heart transplantation

Postoperative procedure	When to perform
Right heart catheterization and endomyocardial biopsy[a]	Weekly, first 4 wk Biweekly, next 8 wk Monthly, next 3 mo Every 3 mo, remainder of first yr Every 4 mo for the second yr Every 6 mo, beyond second yr
Quantitative coronary angiography	At time of hospital discharge, to establish baseline measurements[b] Annually thereafter
Cyclosporine levels, electrolytes, renal function studies	Biweekly for 6 mo Monthly, next 12 mo Every 3 mo thereafter

[a] The biopsy schedule may be altered depending on the presence and severity of detected rejection.
[b] Optional.

LONG-TERM COMPLICATIONS

Heart Transplantation

Graft atherosclerosis remains the bête noire of cardiac transplantation and is the major source of long-term morbidity and mortality. Risk factors for the development of graft atherosclerosis include CMV infection [51], particularly with a prolonged course [52]; older recipients or donors; possibly a pretransplant history of coronary artery disease [53]; and chronic mild rejection. There is some evidence that prophylactic treatment with diltiazem may slow the progression of this disease [54].

When heart failure occurs beyond the first or second year after transplantation, ischemia due to graft atherosclerosis must be considered as a potential etiology. Presumably because the donor heart is denervated, transplant recipients do not manifest angina as a symptom of ischemia; the transplant cardiologist should pursue the diagnosis of ischemic cardiomyopathy in any heart transplant recipient with late heart failure. This pursuit should include thallium scintigraphy and repeat angiography. Unfortunately, discrete lesions amenable to angioplasty or bypass are rarely the etiology. The only effective treatment for such patients may be retransplantation.

Lung Transplantation

The long-term problem for lung transplant recipients is chronic rejection, most commonly manifested as *bronchiolitis obliterans,* which occurs at a rate of approximately 2 to 5% per year and is roughly parallel in incidence to chronic rejection in other solid organs. Unfortunately, obliterative bronchiolitis appears to be truly immunologic in nature and does not, in most cases, respond to augmented immunosuppression. Retransplantation for chronic rejection in lung transplantation patients has been done with a very high mortality, and the long-term results are discouraging.

References

1. Pennock JL, et al. Cardiac transplantation in perspective for the future: survival, complications, rehabilitation, and cost. *J Thorac Cardiovasc Surg* 83:168, 1982.

2. Weil R III, et al. Hyperacute rejection of a transplanted human heart. *Transplantation* 32:71, 1981.

3. Costanzo-Nordin MR, et al. Oversizing of donor hearts: beneficial or detrimental? *J Heart Lung Transplant* 10:717, 1991.

4. Bourge RC, et al. Analysis and predictions of pulmonary vascular resistance after cardiac transplantation. *J Thorac Cardiovasc Surg* 101:432, 1991.

5. Kirklin JK, et al. Pulmonary vascular resistance and the risk of heart transplantation. *J Heart Transplant* 7:331, 1988.

6. Pasque MK, et al. Single lung transplantation for pulmonary hypertension: Technical aspects and immediate hemodynamic results. *J Thorac Cardiovasc Surg* 103:475, 1992.

7. Schuler S, et al. Extended donor age in cardiac transplantation. *Circulation* 80:III-133, 1989.

8. Mulvagh SL, et al. The older cardiac transplant donor: Relation to graft function and recipient survival longer than 6 years. *Circulation* 80(Suppl III):III-126, 1989.

9. Lammermeien DE, et al. Use of potentially infected donor hearts for cardiac transplantation. *Ann Thorac Surg* 50:222, 1990.

10. Frist WH, Fanning WJ. Donor management and matching. *Cardiol Clin* 8:55, 1990.

11. Wahlers T, et al. Donor heart-related variable and early mortality after heart transplantation. *J Heart Lung Transplant* 10:22, 1991.

12. Hakim M, et al. Toxoplasmosis in cardiac transplantation. *Br Med J* 292:1108, 1986.

13. Hakim M, et al. Significance of donor transmitted diseases in cardiac transplantation. *J Heart Transplant* 4:302, 1985.

14. Menkis AH, et al. Successful use of the "unacceptable" heart donor. *J Heart Lung Transplant* 10:28, 1991.

15. Taniguchi S, et al. Effects of hormonal supplements on the maintenance of cardiac function in potential donor patients after cerebral death. *Eur J Cardiothorac Surg* 6:96, 1992.

16. Hensley FA Jr, et al. Anesthetic management for cardiac transplantation in North America — 1986 survey. *J Cardiothorac Anesthesia* 1:429, 1987.

17. Valantine HA, et al. Increasing pericardial effusion in cardiac transplant recipients. *Circulation* 79:603, 1989.

18. Stinson EB, et al. Hemodynamic observations in the early period

after human heart transplantation. *J Thorac Cardiovasc Surg* 69:264, 1975.

19. Bhatia SJ, et al. Time course of resolution of pulmonary hypertension and right ventricular remodelling after orthotopic cardiac transplantation. *Circulation* 76:819, 1987.

20. Gamberg P, Miller JL, Lough ME. Impact of protection isolation on the incidence of infection after heart transplantation. *J Heart Transplant* 6:147, 1987.

21. Morris PJ. Cyclosporin A. *Transplantation* 32:349, 1981.

22. Bolman R III, Saffitz J. Early postoperative cases of the cardiac transplantation patient: routine considerations and immunosuppressive therapy. *Prog Cardiovasc Dis* 33:137, 1990.

23. Renlund DG, O'Connell JB, Bristow MR. Strategies of immunosuppression in cardiac transplantation. *Semin Thorac Cardiovasc Surg* 2:181, 1990.

24. Olivari MT, et al. Five year experience with triple drug immunosuppressive therapy in cardiac transplantation. *Circulation* 82(Suppl):IV-276, 1990.

25. Cosimi AB, et al. Use of monoclonal antibodies to T-cell subsets for immunologic monitoring and treatment in recipients of renal allografts. *N Engl J Med* 305:308, 1981.

26. Bolling SF, et al. Hemodynamics versus biopsy findings during cardiac transplant rejection. *Ann Thorac Surg* 51:52, 1991.

27. Billingham ME. The pathology of transplanted hearts. *Semin Thorac Cardiovasc Surg* 2:233, 1990.

28. Billingham ME. Endomyocardial biopsy diagnosis of acute rejection in cardiac allografts. *Prog Cardiovasc Dis* 33:11, 1990.

29. Nakhleh RE, et al. Correlation of endomyocardial biopsy findings with autopsy findings in human cardiac allografts. *J Heart Lung Transplant* 11(Pt I):479, 1992.

30. Billingham ME, et al. A working formulation for the standardization of nomenclature in the diagnosis of heart and lung rejection: Heart rejection study group. *J Heart Lung Transplant* 9:587, 1990.

31. Yousem SA, et al. A working formulation for the standardization of nomenclature in the diagnosis of heart and lung rejection: Lung rejection study group. *J Heart Lung Transplant* 9:593, 1990.

32. Miller LW. Treatment of cardiac allograft rejection with intravenous corticosteroids. *J Heart Transplant* 9:283, 1990.

33. Heublein B, Wahlers T, Haverich A. Pulsed steroids for treatment of cardiac rejection after transplantation. What dosage is necessary? *Circulation* 80:III-97, 1989.

34. Wahlers T, et al. Treatment of rejection after heart transplantation: what dosage of pulsed steroids is necessary? *J Heart Transplant* 9:568, 1990.

35. Macris MP, et al. Clinical experience with Muromonab-CD3 monoclonal antibody (OKT3) in heart transplantation. *J Heart Transplant* 8:281, 1989.

36. Carey JA, Frist WH. Use of polyclonal antilymphocyte preparations for prophylaxis in heart transplantation. *J Heart Transplant* 9:297, 1990.

37. Hosenpud JD, et al. Methotrexate for the treatment of patients with multiple episodes of acute cardiac allograft rejection. *J Heart Lung Transplant* 11:739, 1992.

38. Costanzo-Nordin MR, et al. Successful treatment of heart transplant rejection with photopheresis. *Transplantation* 53:808, 1992.

39. Hunt SA, et al. Total lymphoid irradiation for treatment of intractable cardiac allograft rejection. *J Heart Lung Transplant* 10:211, 1991.

40. Kramer MR, et al. Trimethoprim-sulfamethoxazole prophylaxis for *Pneumocystis carinii* infections in heart-lung and lung transplantation — how effective and for how long? *Transplantation* 53:586, 1992.

41. Wreghitt TG, et al. Toxoplasmosis in heart and heart and lung transplant recipients. *J Clin Pathol* 42:194, 1989.

42. Rubin RH. Impact of cytomegalovirus infection on organ transplant recipients. *Rev Infec Dis* 12(Suppl 7):S754, 1990.

43. Grossi P, et al. Three-year experience with human cytomegalovirus infections in heart transplant recipients. *J Heart Transplant* 9:712, 1990.

44. Snydman DR. Cytomegalovirus immunoglobulins in the prevention and treatment of cytomegalovirus disease. *Rev Infec Dis* 12(Suppl 7):S839, 1990.

45. Snydman DR, et al. Use of cytomegalovirus immune globulin to prevent cytomegalovirus disease in renal transplant recipients. *N Engl J Med* 317:1049, 1987.

46. Levinson ML, Jacobson PA. Treatment and prophylaxis of cytomegalovirus disease. *Pharmacotherapy* 12:300, 1992.

47. Duncan SR, et al. Ganciclovir prophylaxis for cytomegalovirus infections in pulmonary allograft recipients. *Am Rev Respir Dis* 146:1213, 1992.

48. Thompson JA, et al. Management and long-term follow-up of outpatient care in the cardiac transplant recipient. *Cardiovasc Clin* 20:213, 1990.

49. Kavanaugh T, et al. Cardiorespiratory responses to exercise training after orthotopic cardiac transplantation. *Circulation* 77:162, 1988.

50. Zhou GS, et al. Cardiac transplantation: clinical and laboratory correlates of accelerated coronary artery disease in the cardiac transplant patient. *Circulation* 76(Suppl I):I-56, 1987.

51. Grattan MT, et al. Cytomegalovirus infection is associated with cardiac allograft rejection and atherosclerosis. *JAMA* 261:3561, 1989.

52. Everett JP, et al. Prolonged cytomegalovirus infection with viremia

is associated with development of cardiac allograft vasculopathy. *J Heart Lung Transplant* 11:S133, 1992.

53. Sharples LD, et al. Risk factor analysis for the major hazards following heart transplantation — rejection, infection, and coronary occlusive disease. *Transplantation* 52:244, 1991.

54. Schroeder JS, et al. Accelerated graft coronary artery disease: diagnosis and prevention. *J Heart Lung Transplant* 11:S258, 1992.

Appendixes

Recommendations for Preventing Bacterial Endocarditis

Patients at risk for bacterial endocarditis*

High-risk group	Moderate-risk group	Low-risk group
Aortic or mitral valve disease	Mitral valve prolapse	Isolated atrial septal defect
Prosthetic valve or conduit	Ventricular septal defect	Pulmonary stenosis — trivial
Tetralogy of Fallot	Status post tetralogy repair	Status post complete VSD closure
Coarctation of aorta	Endocardial cushion defect	Status post complete PDA closure
Patent ductus		AV fistula, peripheral
Asplenia		

*Patients with congenital heart disease in the high-risk or moderate-risk groups should receive careful prophylaxis at times of predictable high risk of bacteremia (e.g., during dental extraction, genitourinary or gastrointestinal surgery, open heart surgery, tonsillectomy, or drainage of an abscess). Some less strict prophylaxis should be given at times of lower risk (e.g., during cardiac catheterization, bronchoscopy, normal vaginal delivery, dilatation and curettage, or nasotracheal intubation). Patients in the low-risk group appear not to require any antibiotic prophylaxis.

Antibiotic prophylaxis regimens[a]

For dental/oral/upper respiratory tract procedures

Standard Regimen in patients at risk (includes those with prosthetic heart valves and other high- and moderate-risk patients)
Amoxicillin 3.0 g PO 1 hr before procedure, then 1.5 g 6 hr after initial dose.[b, c]
For amoxicillin/penicillin-allergic patients
Erythromycin ethylsuccinate 800 mg or erythromycin stearate 1.0 g PO 2 hr before procedure, then one-half the dose 6 hours after the initial administration.[b]
OR
Clindamycin 300 mg PO 1 hr before procedure and 150 mg 6 hr after initial dose.[b]
Alternate Regimen
For patients unable to take oral medications
Ampicillin 2.0 g IV (or IM) 30 min before procedure, then ampicillin 1.0 g IV 6 hr after initial dose.[b]
For ampicillin/amoxicillin/penicillin-allergic patients unable to take oral medications
Clindamycin 300 mg IV 30 min before procedure and 150 mg IV 6 hr after initial dose.[b]

For high-risk patients who are not candidates for the standard regimen
 Ampicillin 2.0 g IV (or IM) plus gentamicin 1.5 mg/kg IV (or IM) (not to exceed 80 mg) 30 min before procedure, followed by amoxicillin 1.5 g PO 6 hr after the initial dose. Alternatively, the parenteral regimen may be repeated 8 hr after the initial dose.[b]

For amoxicillin/ampicillin/penicillin-allergic patients who are not candidates for the standard regimen
 Vancomycin 1.0 g IV administered over 1 hr, starting 1 hr before procedure. No repeat dose is necessary.[b]

For genitourinary/gastrointestinal procedures

Standard Regimen
Ampicillin 2.0 g IV (or IM) plus gentamicin 1.5 mg/kg IV (or IM) (not to exceed 80 mg) 30 min before procedure, followed by amoxicillin 1.5 g PO 6 hr after the intial dose. Alternatively, the parenteral regimen may be repeated once 8 hr after the initial dose.[b]

For amoxicillin/ampicillin/penicillin-allergic patients
 Vancomycin 1.0 g IV administered over 1 hr plus gentamicin 1.5 mg/kg IV (or IM) (not to exceed 80 mg) 1 hr before procedure. May be repeated once 8 hr after initial dose.[b]

Alternate oral regimen for low-risk patients
Amoxicillin 3.0 g PO 1 hr before procedure, then 1.5 g 6 hr after the initial dose.[b]

---

[a]**Note:** During prolonged procedures or in the case of delayed healing, it may be necessary to provide additional doses of antibiotics. For brief outpatient procedures such as uncomplicated catheterization of the bladder, 1 dose may be sufficient.

Antibiotic regimens used to prevent recurrences of acute rheumatic fever are inadequate for the prevention of bacterial endocarditis. In patients with markedly compromised renal function, it may be necessary to modify or omit the second dose of gentamicin or vancomycin. Intramuscular injections may be contraindicated in patients receiving anticoagulants.

[b]Initial pediatric doses are listed below. Follow-up oral dose should be one-half the initial dose. Total pediatric dose should not exceed total adult dose.

Amoxicillin:[c]	50 mg/kg
Ampicillin:	50 mg/kg
Clindamycin:	10 mg/kg
Erythromycin ethylsuccinate or stearate:	20 mg/kg
Gentamicin:	2.0 mg/kg
Vancomycin:	20 mg/kg

[c]The following weight ranges may also be used for the initial pediatric dose of amoxicillin:
 < 15 kg (33 lbs): 750 mg
 15–30 kg (33–66 lbs): 1500 mg
 > 30 kg (66 lbs): 3000 mg (full adult dose)

Source: Adapted from Heart Valve Surgery, and Prevention of Bacterial Endocarditis: Recommendations by the American Heart Association. *JAMA* 264:2919, 1990. Copyright 1990, American Medical Association.

Usual Dosages of Drugs Commonly Used in Adults

Combination drugs commonly used in adults

Trade name	Drugs	Oral dose
Aldactazide	Spironolactone & hydrochlorothiazide	1–2 tabs qd or bid
Ascriptin	Aspirin, magnesium hydroxide, aluminum hydroxide and calcium carbonate	1–2 tabs qd to qid
Darvocet–N 100	Propoxyphene napsylate (100 mg) & acetaminophen (650 mg)	1–2 tabs q6hr prn
Dyazide	Triamterene & hydrochlorothiazide	1–2 capsules qd-bid
Moduretic	Amiloride & hydrochlorothiazide	1–2 tabs qd
Percocet	Oxycodone hydrochloride (5.0 mg) & acetaminophen (325 mg)	1 tab q6hr prn
Percodan	Oxycodone hydrochloride (4.50 mg), oxycodone terephthalate (0.38 mg) & aspirin (325 mg)	1–2 tabs q6hr

Usual dosages of drugs commonly used in adults

Drug	Trade name	Oral	Intramuscular	Intravenous
Adenosine	Adenocard	—	—	6 mg rapid bolus
Aminocaproic acid	Amicar	—	—	May repeat with 12 mg q1–2min × 2 doses
				4–5 g load over 1 hr; then 1 g qhr × 4
Amrinone	Inocor	—	—	0.75 mg/kg bolus; then 5–10 µg/kg/min
Atenolol	Tenormin	25–100 mg/day	—	5 mg IV slowly; repeat in 10 min
Atropine sulfate	—	—	0.4–0.6 mg	0.4–2.0 mg bolus
Bretylium tosylate	Bretylol	—	—	5–10 mg/kg bolus over 10 min q6hr, or, 1–2 mg/min continuous infusion
Bumetanide	Bumex	0.5–2.0 mg qd	—	0.5–1.0 mg q2–3hr; not to exceed 10 mg/day
Calcium chloride	—	—	—	0.5–1.0 g slow bolus
Calcium gluconate	—	—	—	1–2 g slow bolus
Captopril	Capoten	12.5–100.0 mg bid-tid	—	—
Cefazolin sodium	Ancef, Kefzol	—	0.5–1.0 g q6–8hr	0.5–1.0 g q6–8hr
Cephalexin	Keflex	250–500 mg qid	—	—
Chlorothiazide	Diuril	0.5–2.0 g qd or bid	—	0.5–1.0 g qd-bid
Chlorpromazine	Thorazine	10–50 mg q6–8hr	10–50 mg q6–8hr	—

Cimetidine	Tagamet	300 mg qid	300 mg q6–8hr
Diazepam	Valium	2–10 mg q6–8hr	2–5 mg q3–6hr prn
Digoxin	Lanoxin	Load with 0.5 mg, then 0.25 mg q4–6hr for total of 1 mg; then 0.125–0.250 mg qd; follow levels	Same as oral
Diltiazem	Cardizem	30–90 mg tid-qid	For arrhythmias: 0.25 mg/kg load over 2 min; if response inadequate, may repeat in 15 min with 0.35 mg/kg. Continuous infusion at 5–10 mg/hr
Diphenhydramine hydrochloride	Benadryl	25–50 mg q4–6hr	10–50 mg q4–6hr
Dobutamine	Dobutrex	—	2.5–15.0 µg/kg/min
Dopamine	Intropin	—	2.5–15.0 µg/kg/min
Enalapril	Vasotec (several)	2.5–40 mg qd	1.25–2.50 mg IV q6hr
Epinephrine		—	1–10 µg/min
Esmolol	Brevibloc	—	Load with 500 µg/kg over 1 min then 50–200 µg/kg/min continuous infusion; may omit loading dose and begin with infusion, titrate as needed

Usual dosages of drugs commonly used in adults (continued)

Drug	Trade name	Oral	Intramuscular	Intravenous
Ethacrynic acid	Edecrin	25–200 mg qd	—	50–100 mg
Famotidine	Pepcid	20–40 mq qd-bid	—	20 mg q12hr
Flurazepam	Dalmane	15–30 mg qhs prn sleep	—	—
Furosemide	Lasix	20–80 mg q6–24hr	Same as oral	20–80 mg q6–24hr; large single bolus (up to 500 mg) may be indicated in acute renal failure
Hydralazine	Apresoline	10–50 mg qid	10–20 mg q6–8hr	10–20 mg q6–8hr
Hydrochlorothiazide	Esidrix, Hydro-DIURIL	25–100 mg bid or qd	—	—
Hydromorphone	Dilaudid	2–4 mg q4–6hr	1–2 mg q4–6hr	—
Ibuprofen	Advil, Motrin	200–400 mg q4–6hr	—	—
Isoproterenol	Isuprel	—	—	2–10 μg/min
Ketorolac	Toradol	10 mg q6hr PO prn	30–60 mg load; then 15–30 mg q6hr prn	—
Labetalol	Normodyne, Trandate	100–400 mg bid	—	10–20 mg bolus; infusion at 2 mg/min
Lidocaine	Xylocaine	—	—	50–100 mg bolus load; infusion at 1–4 mg/min

Lisinopril	Prinivil, Zestril	5–40 mg qd	—
Mannitol	—	—	12.5–100.0 g bolus or as continuous infusion
Meperidine	Demerol	50–100 mg PO q4–6hr prn	Same as oral
Methylprednisolone	Medrol (PO) Solu-Medrol (IV)	4–40 mg qd individualized	10–125 q4–6hr; up to 30 mg/kg q4–6hr; individualize; may require taper
Metolazone	Diulo, Zaroxolyn	2.5–10.0 mg daily	—
Metoprolol	Lopressor	100–400 mg daily	5 mg q2min × 3 doses (early treatment of acute myocardial infarction)
Nicardipine	Cardene	20–40 mg tid	—
Nifedipine	Adalat, Procardia (several)	10–30 mg tid-qid	—
Nitroglycerin		0.15–0.60 mg sublingual	5–300 µg/min continuous infusion
Norepinephrine	Levophed	—	0.5–30 µg/min

Usual dosages of drugs commonly used in adults (continued)

Drug	Trade name	Oral	Intramuscular	Intravenous
Oxymorphone	Numorphan	—	1.0–1.5 mg q4-6hr prn	0.2–0.5 mg q4-6hr
Pancuronium bromide	Pavulon	—	—	0.04–0.10 mg/kg initial paralyzing dose
Phenylephrine hydrochloride	Neo-Synephrine	—	—	40–200 µg/min; titrate effect
Phenytoin sodium	Dilantin	—	—	For status epilepticus: load 10–15 mg/kg slow; maintenance dose 100 mg q6-8hr
Phytonadione	AquaMEPHYTON	—	2.5–25.0 mg; repeat in 6–8 hr if required	—
Procainamide	Procan SR (PO) Pronestyl (IV, PO)	250–500 mg q3-4hr; 500–1000 mg q6-8hr (slow release)	—	Load with 500–1000 at 20–30 mg/min; maintenance dose 1–4 mg/min; follow levels
Prochlorperazine	Compazine	5–10 mg q3-4hr (up to 40 mg/day)	—	2.5–10.0 mg slow injection (over 2–5 min); up to 40 mg/day total
Quinidine gluconate	Quinaglute	324–648 mg q8-12hr	—	—
Quinidine sulfate	Quinidex Extentabs	300–600 mg q8-12hr	—	—
Ranitidine	Zantac	150 mg q12hr or 300 mg qhs	50 mg q6-8hr	50 mg q6-8hr
Sodium nitroprusside	Nipride	—	—	0.3–8.0 µg/kg/min; titrate effect

Spironolactone	Aldactone	25–50 mg PO bid	—
Sucralfate	Carafate	1 g qid	—
Theophylline	(several)	5 mg/kg load; then 1–3 mg/kg bid to tid; follow levels	5 mg/kg load; then 0.24–0.70 mg/kg/hr; follow levels
Trimethaphan	Arfonad	—	0.4–6.0 mg/min
Trimethobenzamide	Tigan	250 mg tid or qid	200 mg tid or qid
Vancomycin	Vancocin	—	1 g q12hr
Vecuronium bromide	Norcuron	—	0.08–0.10 mg/kg initial bolus; maintenance dose 0.010–0.015 mg/kg prn
Warfarin	Coumadin	Individualized; common initial dose of 5–10 mg qd for 2–3 days; follow prothrombin time	—

Usual Dosages of Drugs Commonly Used in Infants and Children

Intravenous cardiovascular medications

Pressors

Amrinone	0.75–1.50 mg/kg bolus, then 5–10 mg/kg/min
Dopamine	2–5 μg/kg/min (renal effect); 5–20 μg/kg/min (cardiac effect)
Dobutamine	5–20 μg/kg/min
Epinephrine	0.1 μg/kg/min starting dose; titrate to effect
Isoproterenol	0.1 μg/kg/min starting dose; titrate to effect, keeping HR < 200
Norepinephrine	0.1 μg/kg/min starting dose; titrate to effect
Phenylephrine	0.1 μg/kg/min starting dose; titrate to effect

Vasodilators

Nitroglycerin	1 μg/kg/min starting dose; titrate to effect
Nitroprusside	1 μg/kg/min starting dose; titrate to effect; monitor BP and cyanide level
Prostaglandin E_1 (PGE_1)	0.05–0.20 μg/kg/min starting dose; when effect noted, decrease to lowest effective dose which may be as low as 0.01 μg/kg/min

Analgesics/narcotics

Aspirin/Acetaminophen	10 mg/kg/dose PO/PG/PR q4hr
Demerol	1 mg/kg/dose IM/IV q2–4hr
Fentanyl	2–10 μg/kg/dose IV q2–3hr; 5–40 μg/kg/hr continuous IV infusion for deep sedation
Morphine	0.1 mg/kg/dose IM/IV/SC q2–4hr; 0.1 mg/kg/hr continuous IV infusion for deep sedation

Narcotic reversal

Naloxone	0.1 mg/kg/dose, repeat prn

Muscle relaxants

Atracurium	0.5 mg/kg/dose VI, repeat q20–40min prn
Pancuronium	0.1 mg/kg/dose IV, repeat q1–2hr prn or 0.1 mg/kg/min continous IV infusion
Succinylcholine	< 1 yr: 2 mg/kg dose IV; > 1 yr: 1 mg/kg/dose IV; 4 mg/kg/dose IM
Tubocurarine	0.5 mg/kg/dose IV, q2–3hr
Vecuronium	0.1 mg/kg/dose IV, repeat q20–40min prn

Muscle relaxant reversal (except succinylcholine)

Atropine	0.02 mg/kg IV
Neostigmine	0.06 mg/kg IV (always precede with atropine)

Anticonvulsants

Diazepam	0.1–0.3 mg/kg slow IV administration; contraindicated in hyperbilirubinemia
Lorazepam	0.1 mg/kg slow IV

Phenobarbital	10 mg/kg IV load × 2 (may repeat to total 40 mg/kg); maintenance 5 mg/kg/day ÷ bid; therapeutic level 20–40 μg/ml
Phenytoin	15–20 mg/kg IV (slow administration ≤ 1 mg/kg/min); maintenance 5 mg/kg/day ÷ bid; therapeutic level 10–25 μg/ml

Antihypertensives

Captopril	1 mg/kg/day PO ÷ tid
Hydralazine	0.1–0.2 mg/kg/dose IM/IV q4–6hr
Labetalol	0.25 mg/kg slow over 2 min (pt. supine). Repeat prn
Nifedipine	0.25 mg/kg SL/PO q4–6hr
Nitroprusside	1 μg/kg/min starting dose; titrate to effect; monitor BP and cyanide level
Propranolol	0.05–0.10 mg/kg/dose IV 21–3hr; 0.5–1.0 mg/kg/day PO ÷ tid-qid

Sedatives/anesthetics

Chloral hydrate	50–75 mg/kg/dose PO/PR q4–8hr
Diphenhydramine	0.25–0.50 mg/kg/dose IV q4–6hr; 5 mg/kg/day PO ÷ qid
Ketamine	1–2 mg/kg IV (useful for shock, asthma)
Lorazepam	0.1 mg/kg IV
Methohexital	1.0 mg/kg IV; 20 mg/kg PR
Midazolam	0.05 mg/kg IV
Pentobarbital	2 mg/kg/dose IV; "Barbiturate coma": load 5–10 mg/kg IV, maintenance 1–2 mg/kg/hr IV infusion
Thiopental	3–5 mg/kg IV

Diuretics

Chlorothiazide	20–30 mg/kg/day PO ÷ bid
Furosemide	1–2 mg/kg/dose PO/IM/IV
Mannitol	0.25–1.00 g/kg/dose; repeat q2–4hr
Spironolactone	2.0–3.5 mg/kg/day PO

Antibiotics (IV)	1st week of life	1–4 weeks	4+ weeks
Ampicillin	100–200 mg/kg/d ÷ q12hr	200 mg/kg/d ÷ q8hr	200–300 mg/kg/d ÷ q4–6hr
Cefotaxime	100 mg/kg/d ÷ q12hr	150 mg/kg/d ÷ q6–8hr	200 mg/kg/d ÷ q4–6hr
Cefuroxime	—	—	75–150 mg/kg/d ÷ q8hr
Clindamycin	15 mg/kg/d ÷ q12hr	15 mg/kg/d ÷ q12hr	20 mg/kg/d ÷ q8hr
Gentamicin*	5 mg/kg/d ÷ q12hr	5.0–7.5 mg/kg/d ÷ q8hr	6 mg/kg/d ÷ q8hr
Nafcillin	50 mg/kg/d ÷ q12hr	100 mg/kg/d ÷ q6–8hr	200 mg/kg/d ÷ q4–6hr
Penicillin G	100,000 U/kg/d ÷ q12hr	200,000 U/kg/d ÷ q6–8hr	200,000–300,000 U/kg/d ÷ q4–6hr
Ticarcillin	150 mg/kg/d ÷ q12hr	200–300 mg/kg/d ÷ q6–8hr	300–400 mg/kg/d ÷ q4–6hr

Tobramycin*	4 mg/kg/d ÷ q12hr	6 mg/kg/d ÷ q8hr	6 mg/kg/d ÷ q8hr
Vancomycin*	20–30 mg/kg/d ÷ q12hr	30–45 mg/kg/d ÷ q8hr	30–45 mg/kg/d ÷ q8hr

*Monitoring of blood levels required

Gastrointestinal/nutrition/metabolic

Calcium	Maintenance = 50 mg elemental Ca^{++}/kg/day
Cimetidine	5 mg/kg/dose q6hr
Glucose	5 mg/kg/min
Insulin	0.1 U/kg/hr SC/IV drip. When blood sugar reaches ≥ 300, begin infusion of D_5W
Intralipid	1 mg/kg/d; increase by 1 gm/kg/d to maximum 4 gm/kg/d
Kayexalate	1 gm/kg/dose PO; 1.5–2.0 gm/kg/dose in 20% sorbitol PR (1 g removes 1 mEq K^+)
Calories	Term neonate: 100–120 kcal/kg/d, increased following surgery
Fluids	Full-term newborn, Day 1: $D_{10}W$ @ 60 ml/kg/d; Day 2: $D_{10}W$ @ 80 ml/kg/d ± electrolytes; Day 3: $D_{10}W$ + (Na^+ 2–3 mEq/kg/d) + (K^+ 1–2 mEq/kg/d) @ 100 ml/kg/d. Decrease rate 20% if on ventilator
	Older infants and children: 4 ml/kg/hr for first 10 kg; 2 ml/kg/hr for next 10 kg; 1 ml/kg/hr for every kg over 20 kg

Resuscitation

Fluid bolus	10–20 ml/kg IV bolus (saline, Ringer's lactate, colloid)
Oxygen	100% O_2
Cardioversion	SVT/V Tach = 0.5 watt-sec/kg (synchronous), repeat at 2 watt-sec/kg
Defibrillation	V Fib/V Tach = 2 watt-sec/kg (asynchronous), repeat at 4 watt-sec/kg
Atropine	0.02 mg/kg IM/IV/ETT: min 0.1 mg, max 1.0 mg
Bicarbonate	1–23 mEq/kg IV; repeat according to blood gas determinations
Bretylium	5 mg/kg IV (repeat × 1)
Calcium	10 mg/kg elemental Ca^{++} IV slow push; 0.3 ml/kg 10% $CaCl_2$ or 1.0 ml/kg 10% calcium gluconate
Epinephrine	0.1 ml/kg (1:10,000) IV/(4 × Dose for ETT instillation)
Glucose	1 gm/kg = 4 ml/kg $D_{25}W$ IV push
Lidocaine	1 mg/kg IV bolus, then 20–50 μg/kg/min IV infusion

Key: ETT = Endotracheal tube.

Desired Serum Concentration of Drugs Commonly Used in the Care of Cardiac Surgery Patients

Drug	Effective level	Potentially toxic level
Amiodarone	1.0–2.5 µg/ml	> 2.5 µg/ml
Digoxin	0.5–2.0 ng/ml	> 2 ng/ml
Gentamicin	Peak 4–10 µg/ml; Trough <2 µg/ml	Trough > 2 µg/ml
Lidocaine	1–5 µg/ml	> 5 µg/ml
Mexiletine	0.5–2.0 µg/ml	> 2 µg/ml
Phenobarbital	15–40 µg/ml	> 40 µg/ml
Phenytoin	10–20 µg/ml	> 20 µg/ml
Procainamide	4–10 µg/ml	> 10 µg/ml
NAPA	9–19 µg/ml	—
Procainamide + NAPA	10–30 µg/ml	> 30 µg/ml
Quinidine	2–5 µg/ml	> 5 µg/ml
Theophylline	10–20 µg/ml	> 20 µg/ml
Vancomycin	Peak 35–45 µg/ml; Trough 5–10 mg/ml	Peak > 45 µg/ml

Key: NAPA = *N*-acetylated procainamide (an active metabolite).

Adjustments in Drug Dose or Dosing Interval for Cardiac Surgery Patients with Renal Impairment

Drug	Normal dose intervals	Dosage in renal failure	Significant dialysis of drug (H, hemodialysis; P, peritoneal dialysis)	Route of excretion and normal half-life (hr)	Remarks
Antibiotics					
Amphotericin B	q24hr	Reduce if severe	No (H,P)	Hepatic, renal (24)	Nephrotoxicity
Ampicillin	q3hr	Reduce if severe	Yes (H)	Renal, hepatic (1.5)	—
Carbenicillin	q3hr	Reduce if severe	Yes (H,P)	Renal, hepatic (1.5)	—
Cefazolin	q8hr	Reduce unless mild	Yes (H)	Renal (2)	—
Ceftazidime	q12hr	Reduce unless mild	Yes (H)	Renal (1.2)	—
Erythromycin	q6hr	Unchanged	?	Hepatic (1.5)	—
Gentamicin	q8hr	Reduce	Yes (H)	Renal (2.5)	Ototoxicity; nephrotoxicity
Imipenem	q6hr	Reduce unless mild	Yes (H)	Renal (1)	Can cause seizures in end-stage renal failure
Kanamycin	q8hr	Reduce	Yes (H,P)	Renal (3–4)	Ototoxicity; nephrotoxicity
Methicillin	q4hr	Reduce if severe	No (H,P)	Renal, hepatic (0.5)	—
Nitrofurantoin	q8hr	Avoid unless mild	?	Renal (0.5)	—
Oxacillin	q6hr	Reduce if severe	No (H,P)	Renal, hepatic (0.5)	—
Penicillin G	q4–6hr	Reduce if severe	No (H,P)	Renal, hepatic (0.5)	Convulsions with very high levels
Streptomycin	q12hr	Reduce	Yes (H,P)	Renal (2.5)	Ototoxicity; rare nephrotoxicity

Drug	Normal dose intervals	Dosage in renal failure	Significant dialysis of drug (H, hemodialysis; P, peritoneal dialysis)	Route of excretion and normal half-life (hr)	Remarks
Sulfisoxazole	q6hr	Reduce	Yes (P)	Renal (3–4)	—
Tetracycline	q6hr	Reduce	No (H,P)	Renal, hepatic (6–8)	May potentiate acidosis; catabolic; increases BUN
Tobramycin	q8hr	Reduce	Yes (H)	Renal (2.5)	Ototoxicity, nephrotoxicity
Vancomycin	q6hr	Reduce	No (H,P)	Renal (6)	Hypotension with rapid infusion
Antiarrhythmics					
Amiodarone	q24hr	Unchanged	No (H,P)	Hepatic (up to 120d)	—
Phenytoin	q8–12hr	Unchanged	Yes (H)	Hepatic, renal (15)	—
Lidocaine	IV drip or intermitten boluses	Unchanged	?	Hepatic	—
Mexiletine	q8hr	Reduce if severe	No (H,P)	Hepatic, renal (8–12hr)	—
Procainamide	q6hr	Reduce unless mild	Yes (H)	Renal	Suggest supplemental dose with each dialysis
Propranolol	q6hr	Probably unchanged	?	Hepatic	—

Quinidine	q6hr	Reduce unless mild	Yes (H,P)	Renal	Exacerbates GI symptoms due to uremia
Antihypertensives					
Hydralazine	q8hr	Unchanged	No (H,P)	?Nonrenal	—
Nitroprusside	IV drip	Contraindicated in severe renal failure	Yes (H,P)	Renal	Cyanide poisoning in renal failure
Cardiac glycosides					
Digitoxin	q24hr	Reduce	No (H,P)	Hepatic, renal (25% converted to digoxin) (72–144)	—
Digoxin	q24hr	Reduce	No (H,P)	Renal (nonrenal: 15%) (36)	Dose proportional to creatinine clearance
Calcium channel blockers					
Diltiazem	q8hr	Unchanged	No (H,P)	Hepatic	—
Nifedipine	q6hr	Unchanged	No (H,P)	Hepatic	—
Verapamil	q8hr	Unchanged	No (H,P)	Hepatic	—
Diuretics					
Bumetanide	q12hr	Unchanged	No (H,P)	Hepatic (1.5)	—
Ethacrynic acid	q6hr prn for diuresis	Avoid if severe	?	Hepatic	Ototoxicity
Furosemide	q6hr prn for diuresis	Unchanged	?	Hepatic	Rare ototoxicity; may use large doses to achieve effect with relative safety in renal failure
Metolazone	q12–24hr	Unchanged	No (H,P)	Hepatic	—

Drug	Normal dose intervals	Dosage in renal failure	Significant dialysis of drug (H, hemodialysis; P, peritoneal dialysis)	Route of excretion and normal half-life (hr)	Remarks
Spironolactone	q12hr	Avoid unless mild	?	Hepatic	Hyperkalemia
Thiazides	q12hr	Ineffective if severe	?	Renal	Hyperuricemia
Anticoagulants					
Heparin	q4hr or IV drip	Unchanged	?	Nonrenal	—
Warfarin	q24hr	Unchanged	?	Hepatic	—
Sedative, tranquilizing, and analgesic agents; muscle relaxants					
Acetaminophen	q4hr	Reduce	?	Renal	—
Aspirin	q4hr	Reduce unless mild	Yes (H,P)	Renal, hepatic	Platelet effects; aggravation of GI symptoms
Chloral hydrate	q4hr	Unchanged	Yes (H,P)	Hepatic	—
Chlordiazepoxide (Librium)	q8hr	Reduce if severe	No (H)	Hepatic, renal	—
Chlorpromazine (Thorazine)	q6hr	Reduce unless mild	No (H,P)	Hepatic	—
Diazepam	q6–8hr	Unchanged	No (H)	Hepatic	—
Fentanyl	Continuous	Unchanged	No (H,P)	Hepatic (3)	—
Meperidine	q4hr	Unchanged	?	Hepatic	—
Meprobamate	q6hr	Reduce unless mild	Yes (H)	Hepatic	—
Morphine	q4hr	Unchanged	?	Hepatic	—

Pancuronium	q1–2hr	Reduce	?	Renal (2)	Avoid in severe renal failure
Phenobarbital	q8–12hr	Reduce unless mild	Yes (H)	Renal	—
Secobarbital	qhs	Unchanged	No (H,P)	Hepatic	—
Sufentanil	Continuous	Unchanged	?	Hepatic (2)	—
Vecuronium	q1–2hr	Unchanged	?	Hepatic (1)	—
Immunosuppressive agents					
Azathioprine	q24hr	Reduce	Yes (H)	Renal	—
Cyclophosphamide	q24hr	Reduce	Yes (H)	Renal	—
Cyclosporine	q12hr	Unchanged	No (H,P)	Hepatic	—
Prednisone	q12–24hr	Unchanged	No	Hepatic	—
H₂-blocking agents					
Cimetidine	q12hr	Reduce	No (H,P)	Renal	—
Ranitidine	q12hr	Reduce	Yes (H)	Renal	—

Key: ? = Unknown; BUN = blood urea nitrogen; GI = gastrointestinal.
Sources: Adapted from WM Bennett, I Singer, CH Coggins. A practical guide to drug usage in adult patients with impaired renal function. *JAMA* 214:1468, 1970, and WM Bennett. Guide to drug dosage in renal failure. *Clin Pharmacokinet* 15:326, 1988.

Nomogram for Determining Body Surface Area from Height and Weight

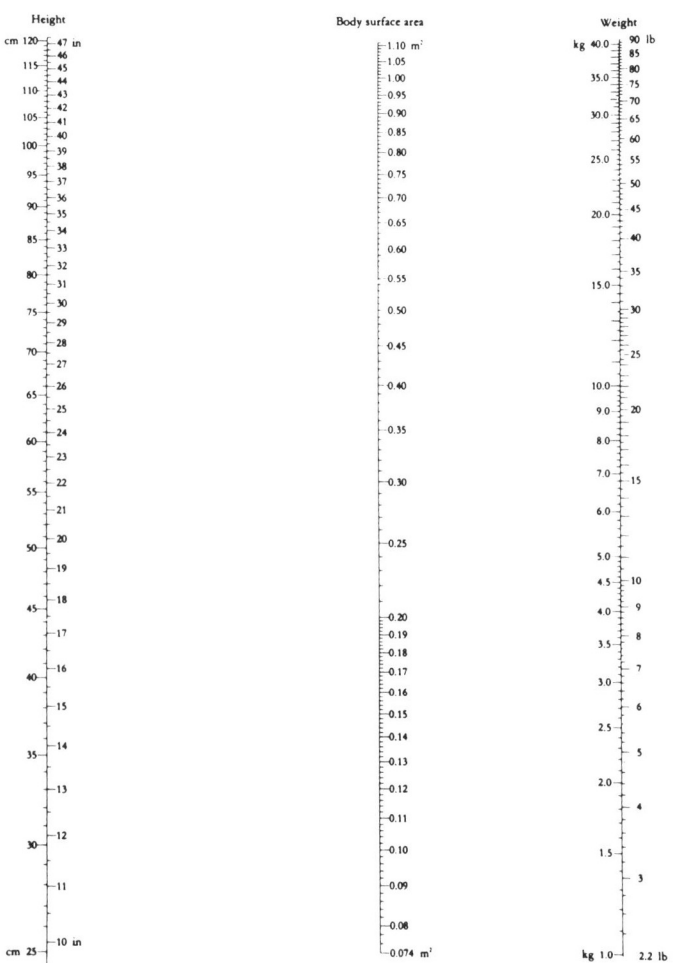

Source: From Documenta GEIGY Scientific Tables, 7th edition. Courtesy of CIBA-GEIGY Ltd., Basel, Switzerland.

Index

A-a (arterial-alveolar) gradient, 144
Abdominal fascia, closure of, 53
Acetaminophen
  pediatric dosage of, 270
  in renal failure, 278
Acid-base balance, 88–91
Acid-base nomogram, 89
Acidosis, 88–90
  in infants, 202
Acne, preoperative evaluation and, 3
Acquired immunodeficiency syndrome
  from transfusion, 193
  from transplantation, 233
Actinomycin D, for rejection of transplant, 249
Activated clotting time (ACT), 38–39, 158, 159
Activated partial thromboplastin time (APTT), 159
Acyclovir, for antiviral prophylaxis following transplantation, 252
Adalat. *See* Nifedipine
Adenosine (Adenocard)
  adult dosage of, 264
  for arrhythmias, 126
  for junctional ectopic tachycardia, 136
  with thallium scintigraphy, 8
  for wide QRS tachycardia, 129–130
Admission orders, adult, 6, 7
Adrenalin. *See* Epinephrine
Adult respiratory distress syndrome, postoperative, 76, 145–146
Advanced Cardiac Life-Support (ACLS) guidelines, 121
Advil (ibuprofen), adult dosage of, 266
Afterload, 68
  and hypotension, 71

AIDS
  from transfusion, 193
  from transplantation, 233
Air embolism, 172
Airway pressure, and pulmonary circulation, 214–215
Alarm system, 121, 144
Albumin levels, 97
Albuterol, for bronchospasm, 142–143
Aldactazide, adult dosage of, 263
Aldactone. *See* Spironolactone
ALG (antilymphocyte globulin), following transplantation, 242–243
AlitraQ, 99
Alkalosis, 90–91
Allen's test, 29, 30
Alpha-adrenergic receptors, 21, 112
Ambulation, 82, 183
Amiloride and hydrochlorothiazide (Moduretic), adult dosage of, 263
Amin-Aid, 99
Aminocaproic acid (Amicar)
  adult dosage of, 264
  for fibrinolysis, 159
Amiodarone (Cordarone)
  and postoperative ARDS, 76
  in renal failure, 276
  serum concentration of, 273
Amoxicillin, for endocarditis prophylaxis, 5, 261, 262
Amphotericin B, in renal failure, 275
Ampicillin
  for endocarditis prophylaxis, 261, 262
  pediatric dosage of, 271
  in renal failure, 275
Amrinone (Inocor)
  adult dosage of, 264
  and hepatic failure, 171
  for low cardiac output, 111, 114–115
  in children, 207

281

Amrinone (Inocor) — *Continued*
  pediatric dosage of, 270
  for pulmonary hypertension, 213
  for right ventricular failure, 120
Analgesia, postoperative, 94–95
Ancef. *See* Cefazolin sodium
Anemia
  postoperative
    blood products for, 91–92, 93
    hypotension with, 71
    low cardiac output with, 109
  preoperative, 93
Anesthesia, 36–37
  for transplantation, 235–236
Angina, unstable
  aspirin use for, 21
  heparin for, 20
  left main coronary artery disease with, 10
  nitrates for, 19
Angiography, quantitative coronary, after transplantation, 253, 254
Angioplasty, failed, preoperative management of, 13
Angiotensin-converting enzyme inhibitors, 21
Antacids, with renal failure, 165
Antibiotic prophylaxis
  for bacterial endocarditis, 261–262
  for cardiac surgery, 167
  for dental work, 6, 185, 261–262
  for transplantation, 250–252
Antibiotics
  for endocarditis, 185–186
  for sepsis in infants, 223
Anticoagulant therapy, preoperative, 20–21
Antihypertensive medications, preoperative use of, 21
Antilymphocyte globulin (ALG), following transplantation, 242–243
Antithymocyte globulin (ATGAM), for rejection following transplantation, 249
Antiviral prophylaxis, following transplantation, 251–252
Aortic cannulation, 39, 40, 41
Aortic coarctation, 199–200
  paradoxical hypertension after repair of, 219–220
Aortic dissection, from cannulation, 39, 41
Aortic regurgitation, preoperative management of acute, 11
Aortic stenosis
  in children, 200
  preoperative management of, 10–11
Aortic valvuloplasty, percutaneous, 10–11
Apresoline. *See* Hydralazine
Aprotinin, and need for blood products, 93
AquaMEPHYTON
  adult dosage of, 268
  warfarin use and, 20
ARDS (adult respiratory distress syndrome), postoperative, 76, 145–146
Arrhythmias
  and cardiac output, 108
  intraoperative, 33–36, 43–45, 46, 47
  postoperative, 124
    bradyarrhythmia, 124–129
    late, 191–192
    management strategies for, 124
    parenteral drugs for, 126–127
    tachyarrhythmias, 129–137
Arterial-alveolar (A-a) gradient, 144
Arterial blood gases, 80
  in acidosis, 88–89
  in alkalosis, 90
Arterial blood pressure, with low cardiac output, 107
Arterial monitoring line
  complications of, 29–30, 68
  insertion of
    intraoperative, 47, 50
    preoperative, 29–33, 34–35
  intraoperative, 29–33
  postoperative, 66–68
Arteriography, coronary, preoperative, 6
Ascriptin, adult dosage of, 263
Aspirin
  for graft patency, 184
  pediatric dosage of, 270
  postoperative administration of, 63, 158
  preoperative use of, 21
    and postoperative bleeding, 92, 158

products that contain, 22
  with renal failure, 165, 278
Atelectasis, postoperative, 141–142
  in children, 210–211
Atenolol (Tenormin)
  adult dosage of, 264
  preoperative use of, 19
  for prophylaxis of atrial arrhythmias, 132
ATGAM (antithymocyte globulin), for rejection following transplantion, 249
Atherosclerosis
  graft
    with coronary bypass graft, 184–185
    after transplantation, 254
  risk factor modification for, 184–185
Atracurium, pediatric dosage of, 270
Atrial fibrillation
  cardiac output with, 108
  diagnosis of, 131, 132
  factors contributing to, 131
  intraoperative, 43–44
  late postoperative, 191–192
  management of, 125, 132–135
  postoperative, 131–135
  prophylaxis for, 131–132
Atrial flutter
  characteristics of, 131
  diagnosis of, 131, 132
  factors contributing to, 131
  intraoperative, 44
  management of, 132–135
  postoperative, 125, 131–135
  prophylaxis for, 131–132
Atrial premature beats, 125
Atrial septal defect, 197
Atrioventricular canal, complete, 198
Atrioventricular interval, 108–109
Atropine sulfate
  adult dosage of, 264
  for bradycardia, 124
  pediatric dosage of, 270, 272
Augmented ventilation, 78
Auscultation
  of children, 206
  with low cardiac output, 107
  postoperative, 62

Autologous blood donations, 23–24, 92
Automatic implantable cardioverter defibrillator, 137–138
Azathioprine
  in renal failure, 279
  for transplantation, 235, 241–242, 243, 244, 245

Bacterial endocarditis, 185–186
  prophylaxis for, 261–262
Bactrim. See Trimethoprim-sulfamethoxazole
Balloon pump. See Intraaortic balloon counterpulsation
Base excess, 90
Benadryl (diphenhydramine hydrochloride)
  adult dosage of, 265
  pediatric dosage of, 271
Benzodiazepines, anesthesia with, 36
Beta-adrenergic receptors, 112
Beta-blocking agents
  for postoperative hypertension, 76
  preoperative use of, 19–20
Bicarbonate. See Sodium bicarbonate
Biologic valves
  deterioration of, 187
  warfarin anticoagulation with, 189
Bleeding, postoperative, 157–159
  cardiac tamponade from, 162–163
  factors in, 157–159
  gastrointestinal tract, 169–170
  management of, 160–162
  rate of, 157
Blood conservation
  intraoperative, 48, 92–93
  preoperative, 23–24, 92
Blood group crossmatching, for transplantation, 229–230
Blood pressure
  with low cardiac output, 107
  postoperative, 65–66, 71–76
Blood products, in perioperative period, 91–94
Blood samples, postoperative, 62
Body surface area, nomogram for determining, 280

Brachial plexus, injury to, 174–175
Bradyarrhythmias, postoperative, 124–129
Bradycardia, sinus
　intraoperative, 33–36
　postoperative, 124, 125
Bretylium tosylate (Bretylol)
　adult dosage of, 264
　for arrhythmias, 126
　pediatric dosage of, 272
　for ventricular tachycardia, 137
Brevibloc. *See* Esmolol
Bronchiolitis obliterans, following lung transplantation, 254
Bronchospasm, postoperative, 142–143
Bubble oxygenators, 39
Bumetanide (Bumex)
　adult dosage of, 264
　preoperative use of, 23
　in renal failure, 277

Cachexia
　chest closure with, 52
　postoperative management of, 97–98, 99–100
　preoperative management of, 17–18
Calcium
　for cardiac arrest, 123
　pediatric dosage of, 272
Calcium channel blockers
　for postoperative hypertension, 74–76
　preoperative use of, 19
Calcium chloride
　adult dosage of, 264
　for low cardiac output, 115
Calcium gluconate
　adult dosage of, 264
　for hyperkalemia, 86
　in infants, 218
Calcium levels
　in infants, 218
　postoperative, 87–88
Calories, pediatric requirements for, 272
Cannulation, 39, 40, 41
Captopril (Capoten)
　adult dosage of, 264
　pediatric dosage of, 271

Carafate (sucralfate)
　adult dosage of, 268
　for ulcer disease, 170
Carbenicillin, in renal failure, 275
Cardene *See* Nicardipine
Cardiac arrest, postoperative, 121–124
Cardiac catheterization
　postoperative, 108
　of children, 224
　preoperative, 6
　after transplantation, 253, 254
Cardiac index, postoperative, 68, 69
Cardiac massage, 122
Cardiac output
　arrhythmias and, 108
　evaluation of, 62, 65–66
　hypothermia and, 108
　low
　　in children, 207
　　defined, 70
　　effects of, 70–71
　　factors causing, 70, 105–106, 108–109
　　incidence of, 105
　　inotropic drug treatment of, 110–116
　　management of, 106–110
　　mechanical support for, 118–119
　　from right ventricular failure, 119–121
　　vasoactive drugs for, 116–118
　monitoring of, 67–70
　after separation from bypass, 44–45
　thermodilution, 62, 67–70
Cardiac rehabilitation, 183–184
Cardiac tamponade, 162–163
　in children, 207–208
　delayed, 189–191
Cardiogenic shock
　with acute mitral regurgitation, 11
　with depressed left ventricular function, 10
　from postinfarction ventricular septal defect, 12
Cardioplegia, 41–42
　and cardiac output, 106
Cardiopulmonary bypass
　separation from, 42–43, 44–45
　with transplantation, 236

Cardiopulmonary resuscitation (CPR), 121–122
of donor heart, 232
Cardiovascular function, postoperative evaluation and monitoring of, 65–70
in children, 204–207
Cardioversion
for atrial arrhythmias, 133
with automatic implantable cardioverter defibrillator, 137–138
of children, 272
for late postoperative arrhythmias, 191, 192
for ventricular tachycardia, 137
Cardizem. *See* Diltiazem
Carotid bruits
physical examination and, 3, 16
Carotid artery disease, preoperative management of, 16–17
Catheterization. *See* Arterial monitoring line; Cardiac catheterization
Catheter sepsis, 168–169
Cefazolin sodium (Kefzol, Ancef)
adult dosage of, 264
prophylactic use of, 167
in renal failure, 275
Cefotaxime, pediatric dosage of, 271
Ceftazidime, in renal failure, 275
Cefuroxime, pediatric dosage of, 271
Central nervous system complications, 171–174
in infants, 222
Central venous pressure, in donor heart evaluation, 231, 238–239
Cephalexin (Keflex), adult dosage of, 264
Chest percussion, 82
Chest tubes, 82–83, 146–147
Chest x-ray, postoperative, 62
Children. *See also* Infants
anesthesia for, 36
assessment of cardiovascular status in, 204–207
coagulation disorders and transfusion of, 219

diagnostic considerations for, 197–201
drug dosages for, 270–272
endocarditis prophylaxis for, 262
fluid and electrolyte management of, 216–217
low cardiac output in, 207
morphine for, 94
nutritional management of, 217–219
operative considerations for, 203–204
paradoxical hypertension after coarctation repair of, 219–220
phrenic nerve paralysis in, 143
pleural effusions in, 148
postoperative care of, 204–216
postoperative investigations of, 224
preoperative preparation of, 201–202
prosthetic valves in, 223
pulmonary management of, 209–216
residual lesions in, 208–209
tamponade in, 207–208
Chloral hydrate
pediatric dosage of, 271
postoperative use of, 94
in renal failure, 278
Chlordiazepoxide (Librium), in renal failure, 278
Chlorothiazide (Diuril)
adult dosage of, 264
pediatric dosage of, 271
Chlorpheniramine, for allergic response to protamine, 51
Chlorpromazine (Thorazine)
adult dosage of, 264
in renal failure, 278
Cholecystitis, acute, 170
Choreoathetosis, 220
Christmas disease, preoperative management of, 13
Chronic obstructive pulmonary disease (COPD)
chest closure with, 52–53
preoperative evaluation of, 9
transplantation with, 240
Chronotropic support, of donor heart, 237–238
Cigarette smoking, 77, 141

Cimetidine (Tagamet)
  adult dosage of, 265
  for allergic response to protamine, 51
  pediatric dosage of, 272
  in renal failure, 279
Circulatory arrest, profound hypothermia and, 39–41
  in infants, 220–222
Citrate, hypocalcemia from, 87
CK-MB (creatine kinase MB), in myocardial ischemia, 138–139
Cleocin. *See* Clindamycin
Clindamycin
  for endocarditis prophylaxis, 261, 262
  pediatric dosage of, 271
Closed chest massage, 122
Closure
  of chest, 52–53
  pericardial, 51–52
Clotrimazole troches, for thrush prophylaxis following transplantation, 250
Clotting factors, transfusion of, 93–94
CMV (controlled mechanical ventilation), 78
CMV infection. *See* Cytomegalovirus (CMV) infection
Coagulation disorders
  in children, 219
  postoperative bleeding due to, 158, 162
  preoperative management of, 13–14
Coagulation studies, preoperative, 6
Coarctation, of aorta, 199–200
  paradoxical hypertension after repair of, 219–220
Colloidal solutions, for volume expansion, 109
Compazine (prochlorperazine), adult dosage of, 268
Complications. *See* Postoperative complications
Congenital anomalies, 197–201
Congenital heart disease
  cyanotic, 18–19
  preoperative evaluation and, 14
Continuous positive airway pressure, 78
Controlled mechanical ventilation, 78

COPD. *See* Chronic obstructive pulmonary disease
Core cooling, 39–41
Coronary angiography, quantitative, following transplantation, 253, 254
Coronary arteriography, preoperative, 6
Coronary artery disease, left main, with unstable angina, 10
Coronary artery spasm, 140, 141
Coronary bypass grafting, graft patency after, 184–185
Coronary revascularization surgery, peripheral vascular examination for, 3
Corticosteroids. *See* Steroids
Coumadin. *See* Warfarin
CPR, 121–122
  of donor heart, 232
Creatine kinase MB (CK-MB), in myocardial ischemia, 138–139
Critical aorrtic stenosis, 10–11
Crossmatching, for transplantation, 229–230
Cryoprecipitate, for fibrinogen level, 159
Crystalloid solutions, for volume expansion, 109
Cutdown, for catheter insertion, 29, 31
Cyanotic congenital heart disease, preoperative management of, 14, 18
Cyclophosphamide, in renal failure, 279
Cyclosporine (Sandimmune)
  in renal failure, 279
  for transplantation, 235, 240–241, 243–245
  monitoring of, 254
Cytomegalovirus (CMV) infection
  transfusion-acquired, 193
  from transplantation, 233
  prophylaxis for, 251–252

Dalmane (flurazepam), adult dosage of, 266
Darvocet-N 100 (propoxyphene napsylate and acetaminophen), adult dosage of, 263
Database, for preoperative evaluation, 2–3, 4–5

DDAVP. *See* Desmopressin acetate
Decannulation, 47–48
Deep venous thrombosis, 176–177
Defibrillation
 of children, 272
 for postoperative cardiac arrest, 121
 in separation from bypass, 43
Defibrillator, automatic implantable cardioverter, 137–138
Defibrillator electrode pads, 37
Demerol. *See* Meperidine (Demerol)
Dental work, antibiotic prophylaxis for, 6, 185, 261–262
Dentition, preoperative evaluation of, 3, 6
Desmopressin acetate (DDAVP)
 and need for blood products, 93
 for postoperative bleeding, 162
Dexamethasone, for extubation of infants and children, 216
Diabetes
 internal mammary artery mobilization in, 176
 postoperative management of, 95–97
 preoperative management of, 15
Diabetes insipidus, in heart donor, 231
Diazepam (Valium)
 adult dosage of, 265
 pediatric dosage of, 270
 postoperative use of, 94
 in renal failure, 278
 for seizures, 174
Diet. *See* Nutritional management
Digitalis. *See* Digoxin; Digitoxin
Digitoxin
 preoperative use of, 19
 in renal failure, 277
Digoxin
 adult dosage of, 265
 for arrhythmias, 126
 for atrial fibrillation and flutter, 133–134
 for low cardiac output, 115–116
 preoperative use of, 19
 in renal failure, 277
 serum concentration of, 273

Dilantin. *See* Phenytoin sodium
Dilaudid (hydromorphone), adult dosage of, 266
Diltiazem (Cardizem)
 adult dosage of, 265
 for arrhythmias, 126
 for atrial fibrillation and flutter, 134
 for graft atherosclerosis following heart transplantation, 254
 for hypertension, 75
 in renal failure, 277
Diphenhydramine hydrochloride (Benadryl)
 adult dosage of, 265
 pediatric dosage of, 271
Diphenylhydantoin. *See* Phenytoin sodium
Dipyridamole
 for graft patency, 184
 with prosthetic valves, 189
 with thallium scintigraphy, 8
Directed donor program, 24
Diulo. *See* Metolazone
Diuretic therapy
 postoperative, 85, 95
  and alkalosis, 91
  and potassium level, 86
 preoperative, 21
Diuril. *See* Chlorothiazide
Dobutamine (Dobutrex)
 adult dosage of, 265
 for low cardiac output, 111, 113
  in children, 207
 pediatric dosage of, 270
 for right ventricular failure, 120
Donor heart, preservation of, 237–239
Donor management, for transplantation, 231–235
Dopamine (Intropin)
 adult dosage of, 265
 for bradycardia, 124–128
 for donor heart management, 232, 237–238
 for low cardiac output, 111, 112–113
  in children, 207
 pediatric dosage of, 270
 for renal failure, 164
Drugs. *See* Medications; *specific drug*

Ductus arteriosus
  patent, 200
  use of prostaglandin E$_1$ to reopen, 18
Ductus-dependent congenital cardiac lesions, 202
Dyazide (triamterene and hydrochlorothiazide), adult dosage of, 263

EBV (Epstein-Barr virus), with transplantation, 252
ECG
  of donor heart, 232
  in myocardial infarction, 139
  preoperative, 6
Echocardiography
  of cardiac tamponade, 163
  of donor heart, 232
  postoperative, 108
    of children, 224
  preoperative, 6, 8
Edecrin See Ethacrynic acid
Edema
  in children, 206
  postoperative management of, 83, 85
Eisenmenger syndrome, 212
Ejection fraction, 105–106
Electrical cardioversion. See Cardioversion
Electrocardiogram
  of donor heart, 232
  in myocardial infarction, 139
Electrolyte management
  postoperative, 83–88
    of infants and children, 216–217
  after transplantation, 254
Electromechanical dissociation (EMD), 123–124
Electrophysiologic testing, preoperative, 7
Elliptocytosis, hereditary, preoperative management of, 13
Emboli
  to brain, 172–173
  with prosthetic valves, 188–189
  pulmonary, 176–177
Enalapril (Vasotec)
  adult dosage of, 265
  preoperative use of, 21
Endocarditis, 185–186
  prophylaxis for, 261–262

Endomyocardial biopsy, of transplant patient, 245, 254
Endotracheal intubation, postoperative, 80, 81, 145
  of infants and children, 209–210, 211
Endotracheal suctioning, of children, 211
Enflurane, anesthesia with, 36
Ensure, 98
Ensure Plus, 98
Enteral formulas, 98–99, 100
Epinephrine (Adrenalin)
  adult dosage of, 265
  for bradycardia, 128
  for bronchospasm, 142
  for cardiac arrest, 122–123
  for extubation of infants and children, 216
  for low cardiac output, 111, 113
    in children, 207
  pediatric dosage of, 270, 272
  for ventricular tachycardia, 137
Epstein-Barr virus, with transplantation, 252
Equalization, of filling pressures, 163
Erythromycin
  for endocarditis prophylaxis, 261, 262
  in renal failure, 275
Erythropoietin, recombinant, and need for blood products, 93
Esidrix, adult dosage of, 266
Esmolol (Brevibloc)
  adult dosage of, 265
  for arrhythmias, 126
  for atrial fibrillation and flutter, 135
  for hypertension, 73, 76
  for paradoxical hypertension after coarctation repair, 220
  for sinus tachycardia, 130
Ethacrynic acid (Edecrin)
  adult dosage of, 266
  in renal failure, 277
Euro-Collins solution, modified, for donor lung preservation, 234, 235
Exercise, following transplantation, 252–253
Exercise-induced stress, with thallium scintigraphy, 8

Extubation
  of adults, 80, 82
  of infants and children, 216

Failed angioplasty, 13
Failure to thrive, 97
Famotidine (Pepcid), adult dosage of, 266
Femoral arterial catheters, 29
Fentanyl
  anesthesia with, 36
  pediatric dosage of, 270
  for postoperative sedation of children, 210
  in renal failure, 278
Ferrous sulfate, preoperative, 23, 93
Fever, preoperative evaluation and, 15–16
Fibrinogen, and postoperative bleeding, 159
Fibrinolysis, postoperative bleeding due to, 159
Filling pressures, equalization of, 163
Filling volume, adequate, 44
FiO_2 (fractional inspired oxygen)
  postoperative, 144
  and pulmonary circulation, 214, 215
Flat back sign, 206
Flecainide, for atrial arrhythmias, 135
Fluid bolus, in children, 272
Fluid management, postoperative, 83–85
  of infants and children, 216–217, 272
Flurazepam (Dalmane), adult dosage of, 266
Folinic acid, for toxoplasmosis prophylaxis, 251
Fontan procedure. *See* Fontan-Kreutzer procedure
Fontan-Kreutzer procedure
  control of pulmonary circulation after, 215
  pleural effusion with, 148
Fractional inspired oxygen (FiO_2)
  postoperative, 144
  and pulmonary circulation, 214, 215

Fresh frozen plasma
  for postoperative bleeding, 162
  in transplantation for patients taking warfarin, 20, 238
Furosemide (Lasix)
  adult dosage of, 266
  pediatric dosage of, 271
  postoperative use of, 86, 95
  preoperative use of, 21
  in renal failure, 164, 277

Gancyclovir, for antiviral prophylaxis following transplantation, 252
Gastric drainage, 33
Gastrointestinal complications, 169–171
Gastrointestinal procedures, endocarditis prophylaxis for, 262
Gastrointestinal tract bleeding, 169–170
Genitourinary procedures, endocarditis prophylaxis for, 262
Gentamicin
  pediatric dosage of, 271
  in renal failure, 275
  serum concentration of, 273
Glucose
  for diabetes, 96–97
  for hyperkalemia, 86
  pediatric dosage of, 272
Glucose homeostasis, in infants, 217–218, 222
Glucose-insulin-potassium (GIK) infusion, for low cardiac output, 116
Glucose-6-phosphate deficiency, preoperative management of, 13
Graft atherosclerosis
  with coronary bypass graft, 184–185
  after transplantation, 254
Great arteries, transposition of, 199
Guanethidine, preoperative use of, 21

Halothane, anesthesia with, 36
Heart block, 125, 128
  pulmonary artery catheter with, 33

Heart failure, postoperative, 66
Heart sounds, postoperative, 62
Heart transplantation. *See* Transplantation
Hematocrit
  in congenital heart disease, 14
  postoperative, 91–92, 93
Hematologic abnormalities, preoperative management of, 13–14
Hemodialysis, 165
Hemodynamic state, postoperative management of, 65–71
Hemofiltration, 165
Hemophilia, preoperative management of, 13
Henderson-Hasselbalch acid-base nomogram, 89
Heparin-associated thrombocytopenia, 157
Heparinization
  for deep venous thrombosis, 176
  intraoperative, 38–39
  preoperative, 20
  in renal failure, 278
  reversal of, 49–51
  of transplantation donor, 234
Heparin rebound, and postoperative bleeding, 158–159
Hepatic failure, postoperative acute, 171
Hepatic function, abnormal, preoperative management of, 16
Hepatic function studies, preoperative, 6
Hepatitis
  transfusion-acquired, 192
  from transplantation, 233
Hepatomegaly, in children, 206
Hereditary elliptocytosis, preoperative management of, 13
Hereditary spherocytosis, preoperative management of, 13
Hernia, incisional, 53
Herpes simplex virus (HSV), with transplantation, 252
History, 3
  for donor heart, 233
Homologous blood transfusions, 24
H_2 blockers, for ulcer disease, 169
Human immunodeficiency virus (HIV) infection
  transfusion-acquired, 193
  from transplantation, 233

Hydralazine (Apresoline)
  adult dosage of, 266
  pediatric dosage of, 271
  in renal failure, 277
Hydrochlorothiazide, adult dosage of, 266
Hydrocortisone, preoperative, 15
HydroDIURIL, adult dosage of, 266
Hydromorphone (Dilaudid), adult dosage of, 266
Hyperglycemia
  in diabetes, 96
  in infants, 217–218
Hyperkalemia, 86
  in children, 219
Hyperlipidemia, 185
Hypertension
  paradoxical, after coarctation repair, 219–220
  postoperative, 71–76
  in children, 210, 211, 212–213
Hypercalcemia, 87–88
  in infants, 218
Hypoglycemia, 96–97
  in infants, 218
Hypokelamia, 85–86
  in children, 218–219
Hypokalemia-induced alkalosis, 91
Hypomagnesemia, 88
  in infants, 218
Hyponatremia, 86–87
Hypoplastic left heart syndrome, 201
  parallel circulations after Norwood procedure for, 213–216
Hypotension
  drug treatment of, 111
  postoperative, 71
Hypothermia
  and cardiac output, 109
  in infants, 202, 220, 221
  myocardial, 42
  profound, 39–41
    in infants, 220–222
  topical, 42

Ibuprofen, adult dosage of, 266
Imipenem, in renal failure, 275
Immunosuppression, for transplantation, 240–245

Implantable cardioverter defibrillator, 137–138
Imuran. *See* Azathioprine
Incentive spirometer, 77, 82
Incision, 37
Incisional hernia, 53
Inderal. *See* Propranolol
Infants. *See also* Children
  arterial monitoring line for, 67
  assessment of cardiovascular status of, 204–207
  cardiac index for, 68, 69
  central nervous system complications in, 222
  coagulation disorders and transfusion of, 219
  diagnostic considerations for, 197–201
  drug dosages for, 270–272
  endotracheal tube in, 80, 81
  fluid and electrolyte management in, 85, 216–217
  hematocrit of, 92
  hypocalcemia in, 87
  hypoglycemia in, 97
  hypokalemia in, 85
  left atrial catheter for, 68
  low cardiac output in
    evaluation of, 108
    treatment of, 207
  morphine for, 94
  necrotizing enterocolitis in, 170–171
  nutritional management of, 97, 217–219
  operative considerations for, 203–204
  paradoxical hypertension after coarctation repair of, 219–220
  postoperative care of, 204–216
  postoperative examination of, 65–66
  postoperative investigations of, 224
  postoperative sedation of, 94
  preoperative preparation of, 201–202
  profound hypothermia and circulatory arrest of, 220–222
  pulmonary management of, 209–216
  renal failure in, 222
  residual lesions in, 208–209
  seizures in, 173–174, 222
  sepsis in, 222–223
  tamponade in, 207–208
  temperature regulation in, 202, 220, 221
Infection
  in heart donor, 232–233
  postoperative, 166–169
    in infants, 222–223
  post-transplant, 250–252
  preoperative management of, 15–16
  in transplant candidate, 229
Inocor. *See* Amrinone
Inotropic drugs, for low cardiac output, 110–116
Inotropic support, of donor heart, 238–239
Inspiratory pressure support, 79
Inspired oxygen concentration (FIO_2)
  postoperative, 144
  and pulmonary circulation, 214, 215
Insulin
  for diabetes, 96
  for hyperkalemia, 86
  pediatric dosage of, 218, 272
Intensive care unit flow sheet, 62, 63
Intermittent mandatory ventilation, 78
Internal jugular access, 29, 32
Internal mammary artery mobilization, complications related to, 175–176
Intraaortic balloon counterpulsation
  during cardiopulmonary bypass, 45, 46, 47
  for low cardiac output, 118–119, 120–121
  percutaneous insertion of, 45, 46
  preoperative, 21, 23
    for depressed left ventricular function, 10
    for left main coronary artery disease with unstable angina, 10
  transthoracic placement of, 45, 47
Intracardiac monitoring lines, 45–47, 49, 50
Intralipid, pediatric dosage of, 272
Intraoperative management. *See* Operative management

Intropin. *See* Dopamine
Ischemia, postoperative, 138–140
Ischemic cardiomyopathy, after transplantation, 254
Isoflurane, anesthesia with, 36
Isoproterenol (Isuprel)
  adult dosage of, 266
  for bradycardia, 124
  for donor heart, 238
  for low cardiac output, 111, 114
    in children, 207
  pediatric dosage of, 270
  for pulmonary hypertension, 213
  for right ventricular failure, 120
Isradipine, for postoperative hypertension, 75
Isuprel. *See* Isoproterenol

Jevity, 98
Junctional ectopic tachycardia, 135–136

Kanamycin, in renal failure, 275
Kayexalate
  for hyperkalemia, 86
  pediatric dosage of, 272
Keflex (cephalexin), adult dosage of, 264
Kefzol. *See* Cefazolin sodium
Ketamine
  anesthesia with, 36
  pediatric dosage of, 271
Ketorolac (Toradol), adult dosage of, 266

Labetalol
  adult dosage of, 266
  for paradoxical hypertension after coarctation repair, 220
  pediatric dosage of, 271
  for postoperative hypertension, 73, 76
Laboratory studies, preoperative, 6
Lanoxin. *See* Digoxin
Lasix. *See* Furosemide
Left atrial catheter
  following heart transplantation, 238
  intraoperative placement of, 45–47, 49, 50
  postoperative monitoring of, 68–70
Left bundle branch block, pulmonary artery catheter with, 33
Left-to-right shunt, cardiac output with, 68, 119
Left ventricular end-diastolic pressure, 67
Left ventricular filling pressure, and cardiac output, 109, 110
Left ventricular function, depressed, preoperative management of, 9–10
Levophed. *See* Norepinephrine
Librium, in renal failure, 278
Lidocaine (Xylocaine)
  adult dosage of, 266
  for arrhythmias, 126–127
  pediatric dosage of, 272
  in renal failure, 276
  in separation from bypass, 43
  serum concentration of, 273
  for ventricular tachycardia, 136, 137
  for wide QRS tachycardia, 129
Lipid profiles, 185
Lipisorb, 99
Lisinopril
  adult dosage of, 266
  preoperative use of, 23
Long-term follow-up, after transplantation, 252–254
Lopressor (metoprolol), adult dosage of, 267
Lorazepam, pediatric dosage of, 270, 271
Lung transplantation
  donor management for, 233–234
  donor operation for, 234, 235
  early postoperative considerations with, 239–240
  long-term complications after, 254
  operative management for, 236, 237
  recipient operation for, 236
  rejection of, 245–246, 247, 248
  retransplantation, 249
  size matching for, 230, 231
  transbronchial biopsy of, 245–246

Lymphoid irradiation, total, for refractory rejection following transplantation, 249

Magnesium levels, 88
  in infants, 218
Magnesium sulfate, for ventricular tachycardia, 137
Mandatory minute ventilation, 79
Mannitol
  adult dosage of, 266
  pediatric dosage of, 271
Massage, cardiac, 122
Mean left atrial pressure, 67
Mechanical support, for low cardiac output, 118–119
Mechanical valves, deterioration of, 187–188
Mechanical ventilation, 77–79
  of children, 210, 211–213
  postoperative use of, 144
  prolonged, 144
  weaning from, 80, 82
Mediastinal drainage tubes, 52, 53, 157
Mediastinitis, 166–168
  with chronic obstructive pulmonary disease, 52
Medications
  adult dosages of, 263–269
  dosages with renal impairment, 275–279
  history of, 3
  pediatric dosages of, 270–272
  preoperative, 19–21
  serum concentration of, 273
Medrol. See Methylprednisolone
Membrane oxygenators, 39
Meperidine (Demerol)
  adult dosage of, 266
  pediatric dosage of, 270
  in renal failure, 278
Meprobamate, in renal failure, 278
Meralgia paresthetica, 175
Mesenteric arteritis, 220
Metabolic acidosis, 88–90
  in infants, 202
Metabolic alkalosis, 90–91
Metabolic patterns, in postoperative period, 84
Methicillin, in renal failure, 275
Methohexital, pediatric dosage of, 271

Methotrexate, for rejection of transplant, 249
Methylprednisolone (Medrol, Solu-Medrol)
  adult dosage of, 267
  for allergic response to protamine, 51
  for rejection following transplantation, 247, 248
  for transplantation, 238, 241, 243, 244
Metocurine, with anesthesia, 36
Metolazone (Diulo, Zaroxolyn)
  adult dosage of, 267
  in renal failure, 277
Metoprolol (Lopressor), adult dosage of, 267
Mexiletine (Mexitil)
  in renal failure, 276
  serum concentration of, 273
Microbubbles, in separation from cardiopulmonary bypass, 42–43
Midazolam (Versed)
  pediatric dosage of, 271
  postoperative use of, 94
Minute ventilation, 79
Mitral regurgitation
  balloon pump with, 118–119
  preoperative management of acute, 11–12
Mixed venous oxygen saturation, in children, 206–207
Moduretic, adult dosage of, 263
Monitoring lines
  arterial, 29–33, 34–35, 47, 50
  for infants and children, 203–204, 205
  left atrial, 45–47, 49, 50
  in postoperative management, 62
Monoclonal antibodies
  for rejection following transplantation, 248–249
  for transplantation, 242, 243
Morphine
  anesthesia with, 36
  pediatric dosage of, 270
  postoperative
    for pain control, 94
    for sedation of children, 210
  in renal failure, 278
Motrin (ibuprofen), adult dosage of, 266

Murmurs
  postoperative, 62
  preoperative, vs. carotid bruit, 16
  Muscle relaxants, with anesthesia, 36–37
Myocardial hypothermia, 42
Myocardial infarction
  postoperative, 138–140
  preoperative management of recent, 12
Myocardial ischemia, postoperative, 138–140
Myocardial protection, 41–42

Nadolol, preoperative use of, 19
Nafcillin, pediatric dosage of, 271
Naloxone, pediatric dosage of, 270
Narcotics, anesthesia with, 36
Nasal prongs, 81
Nasogastric catheters
  intraoperative, 33
  postoperative, 62
Nasotracheal tube, postoperative, 80
  in infants and children, 209–210
Necrotizing enterocolitis, 170–171
Neonates. *See* Infants
Neostigmine, pediatric dosage of, 270
Neo-Synephrine. *See* Phenylephrine hydrochloride
Nepro, 99
Neurologic complications, 171–175
  in infants, 222
Neuropsychologic disturbances, 174
Newborns. *See* Infants
Nicardipine (Cardene)
  adult dosage of, 267
  for postoperative hypertension, 75, 76
Nifedipine
  adult dosage of, 267
  for coronary artery spasm, 140
  for hypertension, 73, 75, 76
  pediatric dosage of, 271
  in renal failure, 277
Nipride. *See* Nitroprusside
Nitric oxide, for pulmonary hypertension, 213

Nitrofurantoin, in renal failure, 275
Nitroglycerin
  adult dosage of, 267
  for coronary artery spasm, 140
  for hypertension, 73, 74
    in children, 213
  for low cardiac output, 117
    in children, 207
  for myocardial infarction, 140
  pediatric dosage of, 270
  preoperative use of, 19
Nitroprusside (Nipride)
  adult dosage of, 268
  for hypertension, 71–74
    in children, 213
  for low cardiac output, 117
    in children, 207
  for paradoxical hypertension after coarctation repair, 220
  pediatric dosage of, 270, 271
  in renal failure, 277
Nitrous oxide, anesthesia with, 36
Nodal rhythm, 125
Nodal tachycardia, 135–136
Norcuron. *See* Vecuronium bromide
Norepinephrine (Levophed)
  adult dosage of, 267
  for donor heart, 238
  for hypotension, 71
  for low cardiac output, 111, 113–114, 118
  pediatric dosage of, 270
Normodyne. *See* Labetalol
Norwood procedure, parallel circulation after, 213–215
Numorphan, adult dosage of, 267
Nutrient, 99
Nutritional management
  of infants and children, 217–219
  postoperative, 97–100
  with prolonged ventilatory support, 145
  after transplantation, 253
Nutrivent, 98
Nystatin suspension, for thrush prophylaxis, 250

Obese patient
  chest closure in, 52
  transplantation from, 230
  venous mapping in, 3

OKT3
  for rejection of transplant, 248–249
  for transplantation, 242, 243
Open chest massage, 122
Operative management
  anesthesia in, 36–37
  arrhythmias in, 33–36, 43–45, 46, 47
  basic monitoring in, 29–36
  closure of chest in, 52–53
  decannulation in, 47–48
  heparinization in, 38–39
  incision in, 37
  myocardial protection in, 41–42
  oxygenator in, 39
  pacing in, 33–36
  pacing wires and intracardiac lines in, 45–47, 48–51
  patient positioning and preparation in, 37–38
  perfusion techniques in, 39, 40, 41
  pericardial closure in, 51–52
  profound hypothermia and circulatory arrest in, 39–41
  for reoperations, 37–38
  reversal of heparin in, 49–51
  separation from cardiopulmonary bypass in, 42–43
  transport of patient in, 53–54
Oral surgical and dental procedures, endocarditis prophylaxis for, 261–262
Orders
  admission, 6, 7
  postoperative, 63, 64
  transfer, 63, 65
Orogastric catheters, 33
Orotracheal tube, postoperative, 80, 81
  in infants and children, 209, 210
Orthoclone OKT3
  for rejection of transplant, 248–249
  for transplantation, 242, 243
Osmolite, 98
Osmolite HN, 98
Overdrive pacing, for premature ventricular contractions, 136
Oxacillin, in renal failure, 275
Oxycodone hydrochloride and acetaminophen (Percocet), adult dosage of, 263
Oxycodone hydrochloride, oxycodone terephthalate, and aspirin (Percodan), adult dosage of, 263
Oxygen, for children, 272
Oxygenator, 37, 39
Oxygen mask, 81
Oxygen saturation monitors, transcutaneous, 33
Oxymorphone (Numorphan), adult dosage of, 267

Pacemaker
  cardioversion with, 137
  intraoperative management of, 36
Pacing
  asynchronous mode of, 128–129
  demand mode of, 128, 129
  of donor heart, 238
  failure of, 129
  generator for, 128
  intraoperative, 33–36, 44
  overdrive, 136
  postoperative
    for atrial flutter, 133
    for bradycardia, 124, 128–129
    for premature ventricular contractions, 136
  rapid atrial, 44, 133
  temporary, 128–129
Pacing wires, temporary, intraoperative placement of, 45, 48
Pain control, postoperative, 94–95
Pancreatitis, acute, 169
Pancuronium bromide (Pavulon)
  adult dosage of, 267
  with anesthesia, 36
  pediatric dosage of, 270
  postoperative use of, 94
    in children, 210
  in renal failure, 279
Panel of random antigens (PRA), 229–230
Paradoxical hypertension, after coarctation repair, 219–220
Parallel circulations, 213–216
Paravalvular leaks, 188
Parenteral nutrition, 100
Paroxysmal supraventricular tachycardia, 125

Patent ductus arteriosus, 200
Patient positioning, 37
Patient teaching, preoperative, 1–2
Pavulon. See Pancuronium bromide
Pediatric patients. See Children; Infants
PEEP. See Positive end-expiratory pressure
Penicillin G
 pediatric dosage of, 271
 in renal failure, 275
Pentamidine, for pneumocystis prophylaxis, 251
Pentobarbital, pediatric dosage of, 271
Pepcid (famotidine), adult dosage of, 266
Perative, 99
Percocet, adult dosage of, 263
Percodan, adult dosage of, 263
Percutaneous aortic valvuloplasty, 11
Perfusion techniques, 39, 40, 41
Pericardial closure, 51–52
Pericardial effusions, 189–191
Pericardial tamponade
 in children, 207–208
 delayed, 189–191
Pericarditis, 189–191
Peripheral nerve injury, 174–175
Peripheral vascular disease
 cardiac catheterization with, 6
 preoperative management of, 17
Peripheral vascular examination, 3, 6
PGE$_1$. See Prostaglandin E$_1$
pH
 and pulmonary circulation, 214, 215
 during reperfusion, 222
Phenobarbital
 pediatric dosage of, 271
 in renal failure, 279
 for seizures, 174
  in infants, 222
 serum concentration of, 271
Phentolamine, for low cardiac output, 117
Phenylephrine hydrochloride (Neo-Synephrine)
 adult dosage of, 267
 for hypotension, 71

 for low cardiac output, 111, 117–118
 pediatric dosage of, 270
Phenytoin sodium (Dilantin)
 adult dosage of, 267
 for arrhythmias, 127
 pediatric dosage of, 271
 in renal failure, 276
 for seizures, 174
  in infants, 222
 serum concentration of, 273
Phlebotomy, preoperative, with cyanotic congenital heart disease, 14
Phototherapy, for rejection of transplant, 249
Phrenic nerve injury, 143
Physical examination
 for low cardiac output, 107
 postoperative, 65–66
  of children, 204–206
 preoperative, 3–6
Phytonadione (AquaMEPHYTON), adult dosage of, 268
Plasmapheresis, preoperative, 13
Platelet abnormalities, postoperative bleeding due to, 157–158, 162
Platelet transfusion, 162
Pleural effusions, postoperative, 147–148
Pneumocystis prophylaxis, for transplantation, 250–251
Pneumonia, postoperative, 166
Pneumothorax, postoperative, 146–147
Polyclonal antibodies, for transplantation, 243
Polycythemia, in congenital heart disease, preoperative management of, 14
Positioning, 37
Positive end-expiratory pressure (PEEP), 79
 for ARDS, 146
 for bleeding, 160
 in children, 211
 pulmonary blood flow and, 215
Postoperative complications
 arrhythmias, 124–137
 late, 191–192
 with automatic implantable cardioverter defibrillator, 137–138

bleeding, 157–163
cardiac arrest, 121–124
coronary artery spasm, 140, 141
deep venous thrombosis, 176–177
endocarditis, 185–186
gastrointestinal, 169–171
graft failure, 184–185
infections, 166–169
of internal mammary artery mobilization, 175–176
low cardiac output, 105–121
myocardial ischemia and infarction, 138–140
neurologic, 171–175
pericarditis and delayed pericardial tamponade, 189–191
pulmonary, 140–148
pulmonary embolism, 176–177
with prosthetic valves, 187–189, 190–191
renal failure, 164–165
of saphenous vein harvesting, 175
of transplantation, 245–252, 253–254
Postoperative management
of acid-base balance, 88–91
of arrhythmias and cardioversion, 191–192
arterial blood gas determination in, 80
of blood pressure, 71–76
blood products used in, 91–94
of cardiac output, 70–71
cardiac rehabilitation in, 183–184
of cardiovascular function, 65–70
of children, 204–216
of coronary bypass grafts, 184–185
of diabetes, 95–97
diuretic therapy in, 95
of endocarditis, 185–186
of fluids and electrolytes, 83–88
of the hemodynamic state, 65–71
of hypertension, 71–76
of hypotension, 71
immediate, 62–65
intensive care flow sheet in, 62, 63
mechanical ventilators in, 77–79
nutritional support in, 97–100
pain control in, 94–95
of pericarditis and delayed pericardial tamponade, 189–191
postoperative orders in, 63, 64
pulmonary care in, 76–83
respiratory, 80–83
transfer orders in, 63, 65
of transfusion-acquired disease, 192–193
of valve surgery, 187–189, 190
Postoperative orders, 63, 64
Potassium, for renal failure, 165
Potassium levels
and alkalosis, 91
in children, 218–219
postoperative, 85–86
Prednisone
for rejection of transplant, 247
in renal failure, 279
for transplantation, 241, 243, 244
Pregnancy, preoperative management of, 17
Preload, 67
Premature ventricular contractions, 125, 136
Preoperative evaluation and management
blood conservation in, 23–24
of children, 201–202
database for, 2–3, 4–6
diagnostic studies in, 6–9. *See also specific study*
general considerations with, 1–2
history and physical examination in, 3–6
medications in, 19–21, 22
of special problems, 9–18
following transplantation, 229–231
Prinivil. *See* Lisinopril
Procainamide (Procan SR, Pronestyl)
adult dosage of, 268
for arrhythmias, 127
for atrial fibrillation and flutter, 135
in renal failure, 276

Procainamide — *Continued*
  serum concentration of, 273
  for ventricular tachycardia, 136, 137
  for wide QRS trachycardia, 130
Procardia. *See* Nifedipine
Prochlorperazine (Compazine), adult dosage of, 268
Profound hypothermia, 239–241
  in infants, 220–222
Propafenone, for atrial arrhythmias, 135
Prophylaxis. *See* Antibiotic prophylaxis
Propoxyphene napsylate and acetaminophen (Darvocet-N 100), adult dosage of, 263
Propranolol
  for arrhythmias, 127
  pediatric dosage of, 271
  preoperative use of, 19
  for prophylaxis of atrial arrhythmias, 132
  for prophylaxis of paradoxical hypertension, 219–220
  in renal failure, 276
Prostaglandin E_1 (PGE_1)
  for bronchospasm, 142
  for congenital anomalies, 202
  for cyanotic congenital heart disease, 18
  for low cardiac output, 117, 120
    in children, 207
  pediatric dosage of, 270
  for pulmonary hypertension, 213
  for transplantation, 234, 238
Prosthetic valve(s)
  in children, 223
  late postoperative complications of, 187–189
  malfunctioning, preoperative management of, 11–12
Prosthetic valve endocarditis, 185–186
Prostigmin, pediatric dosage of, 270
Protamine
  allergic response to, 49–51
  for postoperative bleeding, 162
  for reversal of heparin, 49–51, 158
Prothrombin time (PT), 158, 188–189, 190

Pulmonary artery catheters
  complications of, 29–30, 68
  in infants and children, 203–204
  insertion of
    intraoperative, 47, 50
    preoperative, 29–33, 34–35
  intraoperative, 29–33
  with oximetric capability, 203–204
  postoperative, 66–68
Pulmonary artery wedge pressure, with low cardiac output, 107–108
Pulmonary atresia, 199
Pulmonary blood flow, 214–215
Pulmonary capillary wedge pressure, 67
Pulmonary care, postoperative, 76–83
  of infants and children, 209–216
Pulmonary complications, postoperative, 140–148
Pulmonary embolism, 176–177
Pulmonary function testing, preoperative, 8–9
Pulmonary hypertension, in children, 210, 211, 212–213
Pulmonary vascular resistance (PVR), 68
  in transplantation, 230–231, 238
Pulmonary venous connection, total anomalous, 201
Pulseless electrical activity, 123–124
PVCs (premature ventricular contractions), 125, 136
Pyrimethamine, for toxoplasmosis prophylaxis following transplantation, 251

Quantitative coronary angiography, following transplantation, 253, 254
Quinidine
  adult dosage of, 268
  for arrhythmias, 127
  for atrial fibrillation and flutter, 135
  in renal failure, 277
  serum concentration of, 273

Q waves, in myocardial infarction, 139

Ranitidine (Zantac)
  adult dosage of, 268
  in renal failure, 279
  for ulcer disease, 170
Rapid atrial pacing, for atrial flutter, 44, 133
Recipient, transplant, preparation and operative management of, 235–239
Recombinant erythropoietin, and need for blood products, 93
Regitine. *See* Phentolamine
Regurgitation, valve, 11
Rehabilitation
  cardiac, 183–184
  after transplantation, 252–253
Rejection, of heart transplant, 245–249
Renal failure
  drug dosages with, 275–279
  hyperkalemia with, 86
  postoperative, 164–165
    in children, 222
  preoperative management of, 14
Renal function studies, after transplantation, 254
Reoperation, patient preparation for, 37–38
Replete with Fiber, 98
Reserpine, preoperative use of, 23
Residual lesions, in children, 208–209
Respirator. *See* Mechanical ventilation
Respiratory acidosis, 88–89
  in infants, 202
Respiratory alkalosis, 90
Respiratory insufficiency, prolonged, 143–145
Respiratory management, postoperative, 80–83
Resuscitation, 121–122
  of donor heart, 232
  of infants and children, 272
Retransplantation, 249
Rhythmol. *See* Propafenone
Right ventricular failure, low cardiac output due to, 119–121

Sandimmune. *See* Cyclosporine
Saphenous vein harvesting
  complications of, 175
  evaluation for, 3
  sites of, 37
Secobarbital, in renal failure, 279
Sedation, postoperative, 94
Seizures, 173–174
  in infants, 222
Sepsis. *See* Infection
Septal defects, in children, 197
Serum concentrations, of drugs, 273
Shock, cardiogenic. *See* Cardiogenic shock
Sickle cell trait, preoperative management of, 13–14
Sinus bradycardia
  intraoperative, 33–36
  postoperative, 124, 125
Sinus tachycardia, 125, 130–131
Skin
  preoperative evaluation of, 3
  preparation of, 37
Skin temperature, of infants, 204
Smoking, 77, 141
Sodium bicarbonate
  for cardiac arrest, 123
  for hyperkalemia, 86
  for metabolic acidosis, 89–90
  pediatric use of, 272
Sodium level, 86–87
Sodium nitroprusside. *See* Nitroprusside
Sodium polystyrene sulfonate (Kayexalate)
  for hyperkalemia, 86
  pediatric dosage of, 272
Solu-Medrol. *See* Methylprednisolone
Sotalol, for atrial arrhythmias, 135
Spherocytosis, hereditary, preoperative management of, 13
Spirometer, incentive, 77, 82
Spironolactone (Aldactone)
  adult dosage of, 268
  pediatric dosage of, 271
  in renal failure, 278
Spironolactone and hydrochlorothiazide (Aldactazide), adult dosage of, 263
Starling relationship, 110
Sternal stripe sign, 167

Sternal weave technique, 52
Sternotomy, 37–38
Steroids
  for allergic response to protamine, 51
  for bronchospasm, 142
  preoperative management of chronic use of, 15
  for rejection following transplantation, 247–248
Streptomycin, in renal failure, 275
Stroke, 171–173
  with prosthetic valve endocarditis, 186
Subclavian vein, for catheter insertion, 32
Succinylcholine, pediatric dosage of, 270
Sucralfate (Carafate)
  adult dosage of, 268
  for ulcer disease, 170
Suctioning, endotracheal, of children, 211
Sufentanil
  anesthesia with, 36
  in renal failure, 279
Sulfadiazine, for toxoplasmosis prophylaxis, 251
Sulfisoxazole, in renal failure, 276
Suplena, 99
Supreventricular tachycardia, 130–135
  paroxysmal, 125
Swan-Ganz catheter
  insertion of, 29–33, 34–35
  postoperative, 66
Sympathetic amines, for low cardiac output, 112–114
Synchronized intermittent mandatory ventilation (SIMV), 78–79
Synthroid (thyroxine), for transplant donor, 234
Systemic oxygen saturation, 213–214
Systemic vascular resistance, 68

Tachyarrhythmias
  postoperative, 128–137
  ventricular, 136–137
Tachycardia
  junctional ectopic, 135–136
  paroxysmal supraventricular, 125
  sinus, 125, 130–131
  supraventricular, 130–135
  ventricular, 125, 136–137
  wide QRS, 129–130
Tagamet. See Cimetidine
Tambocor. See Flecainide
Tamponade, 162–163
  in children, 207–208
  delayed, 189–191
Technetium-99m scan, to detect myocardial infarction, 139–140
Teeth, preoperative evaluation of, 3, 6
Temperature
  intraoperative monitoring of, 33
  skin, of infants, 204
Temperature regulation, in infants, 202, 220, 221
Temporary cardiac pacing, for bradyarrhythmia, 124, 128–129
Tenormin. See Atenolol
Tetracycline, in renal failure, 276
Tetralogy of Fallot, 18, 198–199
Thalidomide, for rejection following transplantation, 249
Thallium scintigraphy, preoperative, 8
Theophylline
  adult dosage of, 268
  for bronchospasm, 142
  serum concentration of, 273
Thermodilution cardiac output, 62, 67–70
Thermoregulation, in infants, 202, 220, 221
Thiazides, in renal failure, 278
Thiopental
  anesthesia with, 36
  pediatric dosage of, 271
Thorazine. See Chlorpromazine
Thrombin time (TT), 159
Thrombocytopenia, postoperative, 157
Thromboembolic complications, of prosthetic valves, 188–189
Thrush prophylaxis, following transplantation, 250

Thyroxine (Synthroid), for transplant donor, 234
Ticarcillin, pediatric dosage of, 271
Tidal volume, pulmonary blood flow and, 215
Tigan (trimethobenzamide), adult dosage of, 268
Tissue typing, for transplantation, 229–230
Tobramycin
  pediatric dosage of, 272
  in renal failure, 276
Tolerex, 98
Topical hypothermia, 42
Toradol (ketorolac), adult dosage of, 266
Total lymphoid irradiation, for refractory rejection following transplantation, 249
Toxoplasmosis, from transplantation, 233
  prophylaxis for, 251
Tracheostomy, 145
  in infants and children, 216
  infection with, 166–167
Trandate. See Labetalol
Transbronchial biopsy, of transplant patient, 245–246
Transcutaneous oxygen saturation monitor, 33
Transesophageal echocardiography
  of cardiac tamponade, 163
  postoperative, 108
  preoperative, 6
Transfer orders, 63, 65
Transfusion, 92–93
  of children, 219
Transfusion-acquired disease, 192–193
Transplantation
  antibiotic prophylaxis for, 250–252
  donor management for, 231–235
  early postoperative considerations with, 239–240
  immunosuppression for, 240–245
  infection and, 229, 250
  long-term follow-up of, 252–254

lung
  donor management for, 233–234
  donor operation for, 234, 235
  early postoperative considerations with, 239–240
  long-term complications after, 254
  operative management for, 236, 237
  rejection of, 245–246, 247, 248
  size matching for, 230, 231
  transbronchial biopsy of, 245–246
preoperative considerations with, 229–231
preoperative medication with, 20
recipient preparation and operative management of, 235–239
rejection of
  diagnosis and grading of, 246–247, 248
  surveillance for, 245–246
  treatment of, 247–249
retransplantation after, 249
size matching considerations for, 230–231
tissue typing and crossmatching for, 229–230
Transport, of patient, 53–54
Transposition of the great arteries, 199
Transthoracic monitoring lines, 45–47, 49, 50
Triamterene, postoperative use of, 95
Triamterene and hydrochlorothiazide (Dyazide), adult dosage of, 263
Tricuspid atresia, 200–201
Tricuspid valve insufficiency, cardiac output with, 68
Tricuspid valve vegetation, of donor heart, 232
Triiodothyronine, for low cardiac output, 116
Trimethobenzamide (Tigan), adult dosage of, 268
Trimethoprim-sulfamethoxazole, for pneumocystis prophylaxis, 250–251
Tromethamine, for metabolic acidosis, 90

Truncus arteriosus, 201
Tube feeding, 97–98
Tubocurarine, pediatric dosage of, 270

Ulcer disease, 169–170
Umbilical artery catheters, 204, 205
Umbilical venous lines, 204, 205
Univentricular heart, 200–201
Upper respiratory tract procedures, endocarditis prophylaxis for, 261–262
Urinary catheters, 33
Urine output, postoperative, 66

Valium. *See* Diazepam
Valve surgery, late postoperative issues, 187–189, 190
Vancomycin (Vancocin)
 adult dosage of, 268
 for endocarditis prophylaxis, 167, 262
 pediatric dosage of, 272
 in renal failure, 276
 serum concentration of, 273
Varicella-zoster virus (VZV), following transplantation, 252
Vasoactive drugs, for low cardiac output, 116–118
Vasoconstrictors, for low cardiac output, 117–118
Vasodilators
 for hypertension, 71–74
 for low cardiac output, 116–117
Vasotec. *See* Enalapril
Vecuronium bromide (Norcuron)
 adult dosage of, 269
 with anesthesia, 36
 pediatric dosage of, 270
 in renal failure, 279
Venous cannulation, 39
Ventilation, resumption of, 44
Ventilators. *See* Mechanical ventilation
Ventricular arrhythmias, preoperative electrophysiologic testing for, 9
Ventricular assist devices, for low cardiac output, 119
Ventricular decompression, in myocardial protection, 41

Ventricular fibrillation, 121–122
Ventricular septal defect
 in children, 197
  pulmonary atresia with, 199
 postinfarction, preoperative management of, 12
Ventricular tachyarrhythmias, 136–137
Ventricular tachycardia, 125, 136–137
Verapamil
 for arrhythmias, 127
 for atrial fibrillation and flutter, 134
 for coronary artery spasm, 140
 for hypertension, 75
 in renal failure, 277
Versed. *See* Midazolam
Vibratory therapy, 82
Vital High Nitrogen, 99
Vitamin K
 for transplantation, 235
 and warfarin, 20, 189
Vivonex T.E.N., 99
Volume replacement, 84–85, 93, 109
von Willebrand's disease, preoperative management of, 13

Warfarin (Coumadin)
 adult dosage of, 269
 in children, 223
 for deep venous thrombosis, 176
 factors that interfere with, 189, 190
 preoperative use of, 20
 prothrombin time and, 190
 with prosthetic valves, 188–189
 in renal failure, 278
 and transplantation, 235
Weaning parameters, 80, 82
Wide QRS tachycardia, 129–130
Worksheet, for preoperative patient information, 4–5
Wound infection, 166–168

Xylocaine. *See* Lidocaine

Zantac. *See* Ranitidine
Zaroxolyn. *See* Metalazone
Zestril. *See* Lisinopril